Morbidity, Performance and Quality in Primary Care

Dutch general practice on stage

Edited by

Gert P Westert
Lea Jabaaij

and

François G Schellevis

Foreword by

Els Borst-Eilers

Radcliffe Publishing
Oxford • Seattle

Radcliffe Publishing Ltd
18 Marcham Road
Abingdon
Oxon OX14 1AA
United Kingdom

www.radcliffe-oxford.com
Electronic catalogue and worldwide online ordering facility.

_____

British Library Cataloguing in Publication Data

A catalogue record for this book is available from the British Library

ISBN-10 1 84619 053 3
ISBN-13 978 184619 053 7

Typeset by Action Publishing Technology Ltd, Gloucester
Printed and bound by TJ International Ltd, Padstow, Cornwall

Contents

Foreword

The first national survey of general practice in the Netherlands was published in 1990. It described the position and role of the general practitioner (GP) in the late eighties. The second national survey covers the years 2000–2002. Data have been collected about roughly 200 GPs in 100 practices. The survey involved 400 000 patients, 1.5 million recorded GP–patient contacts and 2.1 million drug prescriptions. A team of 30 researchers and staff members was involved in the collection, analysis and reporting of the data. The general aim of this nation-wide study was to describe the GP's performance as gatekeeper of the Dutch healthcare system. What happens before people enter the 'gate', what happens when they are in and which patients pass through the gate?

This second survey was undertaken and analysed along six themes: the health of the population, inequalities in health, utilisation of care, quality of care, communication, organisation and workload. The results were presented and discussed at an international conference 'Dutch general practice on stage', which preceded the European World Organization of Family Doctors (WONCA) conference in Amsterdam in early June 2004. The chapters of this book give an overview of the results presented at that conference.

From this second national survey it can be concluded that GPs are still the gate-keepers of the Dutch healthcare system. The study also shows that, since the last survey, primary care has become more patient centred and that GPs have improved the efficiency and quality of their work. In comparison with other sectors of the healthcare system, general practice is still very cost-effective.

For two reasons, this survey appears at a timely moment. In the first place, it coincides with the recent interest in primary care in the Anglo-Saxon world.[1] This interest arises not only from the growing importance of cost containment in healthcare, but also from the now firmly established association between the life expectancy of a population and the existence of a strong primary care sector. The international interest in the Dutch situation is reflected in several chapters, where experts from all over the world put Dutch general practice into an international perspective.

In the second place, the Dutch healthcare system is about to undergo some fundamental changes. In 2006, a mandatory national healthcare insurance will replace the existing two-tier system. Furthermore, healthcare insurers will all be budgeted, which will drive them into the role of critical purchasers of care and will stimulate competition between providers. Although GPs will retain their role as gatekeepers, the changes might well influence general practice in some way. By comparing the results of the recent survey with those of a future, third national survey, this influence can be closely monitored.

Els Borst-Eilers MD PhD
Former Minister of Health, Welfare and Sports
Chair of the Board of Governors of the
Netherlands Institute for Health Services Research (NIVEL)
January 2006

Reference

1 Macinko J, Starfield B and Shi L (2003) The contribution of primary care systems to health outcomes within Organisation for Economic Cooperation and Development (OECD) countries, 1970–1998. *Health Serv Res.* **38**: 831–65.

About the editors

Gert P Westert is a scholar in medical sociology and trained in research methodology and statistics. Westert's thesis, titled *Variation in Use of Hospital Care*, was published in 1991 (Groningen University). As a health services researcher his research is focused on quality of healthcare and disparities in health and healthcare utilisation. In 1997 he was appointed as senior researcher at the National Institute for Public Health and the Environment (RIVM) and for a period of five years attached to the Netherlands Institute for Health Services Research (NIVEL) as project leader of the 2nd Dutch National Survey of General Practice. Gert Westert is professor of health services research at Tilburg University (2005).
Email: gert.westert@rivm.nl

Lea Jabaaij is a senior researcher at the NIVEL institute (Utrecht, the Netherlands). Since 2000 she has been involved with the Netherlands Information Network of General Practice (LINH), the base for the 2nd Dutch National Survey of General Practice (DNSGP-2). She has extensive experience in healthcare research, including GP care, midwifery care and mental healthcare in general hospitals. She has a degree in physiological psychology and wrote a thesis on stress-related immunomodulation in humans.
Email: l.jabaaij@nivel.nl

François G Schellevis was educated and worked as a GP in the Netherlands between 1982 and 1996. He changed gradually towards a research career and worked as researcher at the university departments of General Practice of the Nijmegen University and the Vrije Universiteit in Amsterdam. François finished his PhD titled *Chronic Diseases in General Practice; Comorbidity and Quality of Care* in 1993. In 1997 he was appointed as co-ordinator of the research programme of General Practice Care of the NIVEL institute and as project leader of the 2nd Dutch National Survey of General Practice. He is professor of General Practice, Vrije Universiteit Medical Centre, Amsterdam (2006).
Email: f.schellevis@nivel.nl

List of corresponding authors

MJ van den Berg MA, researcher, NIVEL, Netherlands Institute for Health Services Research, Utrecht, The Netherlands. m.vandenberg@nivel.nl

AH de Boer PHD, senior researcher, Social and Cultural Planning Office of the Netherlands (SCP), The Hague, The Netherlands. a.de.boer@scp.nl

JCC Braspenning PHD, senior researcher, Centre for Quality of Care Research (WOK), Radboud University Nijmegen Medical Centre, The Netherlands. j.braspenning@kwazo.umcn.nl

A van den Brink-Muinen PHD, senior researcher, NIVEL, Netherlands Institute for Health Services Research, Utrecht, The Netherlands. a.vandenbrink@nivel.nl

MW Calnan, Professor of Medical Sociology, Department of Social Medicine, MRC Health Services Research Collaboration, University of Bristol, UK. m.w.calnan@bristol.ac.uk

M Cardol PHD, senior researcher, NIVEL, Netherlands Institute for Health Services Research, Utrecht, The Netherlands. m.cardol@nivel.nl

V van Casteren MD, senior researcher, Unit of Epidemiology, Scientific Institute of Public Health (IPH), Brussels, Belgium. viviane.vancasteren@iph.fgov.be

PB Davis PHD, Professor of Sociology, Department of Sociology, University of Auckland, New Zealand. pb.davis@auckland.ac.nz

W Devillé PHD, MD, research co-ordinator, international and migrant health, NIVEL, Netherlands Institute for Health Services Research, Utrecht, The Netherlands. w.deville@nivel.nl

L van Dijk PHD, research co-ordinator pharmaceutical care, NIVEL, Netherlands Institute for Health Services Research, Utrecht, The Netherlands. L.vandijk@nivel.nl

M Droomers PHD, epidemiologist, National Institute for Public Health and the Environment (RIVM), Bilthoven, The Netherlands. mariel.droomers@rivm.nl

S van Dulmen PHD, research co-ordinator, NIVEL, Netherlands Institute for Health Services Research, Utrecht. s.vandulmen@nivel.nl

DM Fleming PHD, F MED SCI, Director of the Birmingham Research Unit, Royal College of General Practitioners, Birmingham, UK. dfleming@rcgpbhamresunit.nhs.uk

F Groenhof MA, researcher, Department of General Practice, University Medical Centre, Groningen, The Netherlands. f.groenhof@med.umcg.nl

E Hak PHD, clinical epidemiologist, Julius Center for Health Sciences and Primary Care, University Medical Center Utrecht, The Netherlands. e.hak@umcutrecht.nl

N Hoeymans PHD, senior research associate, Department for Public Health Forecasting, National Institute for Public Health and the Environment (RIVM), Bilthoven, The Netherlands. nancy.hoeymans@rivm.nl

P van den Hombergh PHD MD, senior researcher, Centre for Quality of Care Research, Radboud University Nijmegen Medical Centre, Nijmegen, The Netherlands. p.vd.hombergh@lhv.nl

RH Jones, Professor of General Practice, Kings College London School of Medicine and Health Schools Dean for Education, King's College London, UK. roger.jones@kcl.ac.uk

JD de Jong MSC, researcher, NIVEL, Netherlands Institute for Health Services Research, Utrecht, The Netherlands. j.dejong@nivel.nl

I Kawachi PHD, MD, Professor of Social Epidemiology, Harvard School of Public Health, Boston, USA. ichiro.kawachi@channing.harvard.edu

MW van der Linden PHD, MD, researcher, NIVEL, Netherlands Institute for Health Services Research, Utrecht, The Netherlands. mvanderlinden@med.uu.nl

H Otters PHD, MD, general practitioner, Department of General Practice, Erasmus MC-University Medical Center Rotterdam, The Netherlands. j.otters@erasmusmc.nl

JJ Polder PHD, project coordinator health services research, Centre for Public Health Forecasting, National Institute for Public Health and the Environment (RIVM), Bilthoven, The Netherlands. johan.polder@rivm.nl

HJ Sixma PHD, senior researcher, NIVEL, Netherlands Institute for Health Services Research, Utrecht, The Netherlands. h.sixma@nivel.nl

LFJ van der Velden PHD, senior researcher, NIVEL, Netherlands Institute for Health Services Research, Utrecht, The Netherlands. l.vandervelden@nivel.nl

PFM Verhaak PHD, research co-ordinator, NIVEL, Netherlands Institute for Health Services Research, Utrecht, The Netherlands. p.verhaak@nivel.nl

RA Verheij PHD, project leader of the Netherlands Information Network of General Practice (LINH), NIVEL, Netherlands Institute for Health Services Research, Utrecht, The Netherlands. r.verheij@nivel.nl

Abbreviations

ACE	angiotensin-converting enzyme
A&M	accident and medical
ARI	acute respiratory infections
ATC	Anatomical Therapeutic Chemical (classification)
AWBZ	Exceptional Medical Expenses Act
BP	blood pressure
CAGE	acronym for the four questions (Cut down drinking, Annoyed by criticising drinking, Guilty about drinking, Early drinking)
CEP	Clients Evaluate Practice
CHAPS	Consumer Assessment of Health Plans Study
CHD	coronary heart disease
CI	confidence interval
CIDI	Composite International Diagnostic Interview
CME	continuous medical education
COPD	chronic obstructive pulmonary disease
DDD	defined daily dose
df	degrees of freedom
DNSGP-1	first Dutch National Survey of General Practice
DNSGP-2	second Dutch National Survey of General Practice
DOSD	diseases of the oesophagus, stomach and duodenum
DSM	Diagnostic and Statistical Manual
ECG	electrocardiogram
ED	emergency department
EMR	electronic medical record
ENT	ear, nose and throat
EPR	electronic patient record
EVS	electronic prescribing system
fte	full-time equivalent
GDP	gross domestic product
GHQ	General Health Questionnaire
GLOBE	Gezondheid en LevensOmstandigheden Bevolking en omstreken [Population's Health and Living Conditions and Surroundings]
GMR	Global Medical Record
GP	general practitioner
GPAS	General Practice Assessment Survey
GPIS	general practitioner information system
HbA_{1c}	haemoglobin A_{1c}
HIS	Health Interview Survey
ICC	intra-class correlation
ICD	International Classification of Disease
ICPC	International Classification of Primary Care
IHD	ischaemic heart disease
IMA	Intermutualistic Agency

IPH	Scientific Institute of Public Health
LHV	Landelijke Huisartsen Vereniging [National Association of General Practitioners]
LINH	Dutch National Information Network of General Practice
LRTI	lower respiratory tract infection
LTMI	long-term mental illness
MOS	Medical Outcomes Study
MRI	magnetic resonance imaging
NEC	not elsewhere classified
NHG	Nederlands Huisartsen Genootschap [Dutch College of General Practitioners]
NICE	National Institute for Clinical Excellence
NIVEL	Nederlands Instituut Voor Onderzoek Van De Gezondheidszorg [Netherlands Institute for Health Services Research]
NSAID	non-steroidal anti-inflammatory drug
OECD	Organization for Economic Cooperation and Development
OPCS	Office of Population Censuses and Surveys
OR	odds ratio
PAP	Papanicolau
PDA	personal digital assistant
PHS	periarthrytis humero-scapularis
PHSF	Public Health Status and Forecasts
PSA	prostate-specific antigen
QA	quality assurance
QI	quality improvement
QoC	quality of care
QOF	Quality and Outcomes Framework
QUOTE	QUality Of care Through the Patient's Eyes
RIAS	Roters' Interaction Analysis System
RIVM	National Institute for Public Health and the Environment
RTI	respiratory tract infection
SCP	Social and Cultural Planning Office
SD	standard deviation
SPR	standardised prevalence rates
SSRI	selective serotonin reuptake inhibitor
TB	tuberculosis
TCA	tricyclic antidepressants
TIA	transient ischaemic attack
UCL	Université Catholique de Louvain
URTI	upper respiratory tract infection
UTI	urinary tract infection
VIP	practice visiting instrument
WGBO	Medical Treatment Act
WHO	World Health Organization
WOK	Centre for Quality of Care Research
WRS	Weekly Returns Service of the Royal College of General Practitioners
ZFW	Health Insurance Act

Part I

Introduction

General practice in the Netherlands: major findings from the second Dutch National Survey of General Practice

Gert Westert, François Schellevis and Jouke van der Zee

What is this chapter about?

This chapter presents the major findings of the second Dutch National Survey of General Practice (DNSGP-2). Empirical results show that general practitioners (GPs) in the early 2000s are still gatekeepers in the Dutch health system. Furthermore, it is observed that general practice in the Netherlands is accessible and community oriented. GPs take quality serious. The total quality score, which indicates the extent to which the actual performance in general practice is in accordance with the guidelines, is high. General practice has been shown also to be efficient: the approximately 8000 GPs in the Netherlands consume less than 5% of the Dutch healthcare budget.

Background

The Public Health Status and Forecasts report (1997) (PHSF) strongly advised the Dutch Ministry of Health to install a nationwide information and monitoring system, containing representative information on morbidity in the population, the use of health services at patient level, and its determinants.[1] In 2000, such a plan was put into action: the second Dutch National Survey of General Practice (DNSGP-2). In the Netherlands, like in the UK, the general practice setting is an optimal one for providing information on the population's health, because it is accessible to all and close to the community.[2,3] The study's starting point is general practice, and, therefore, the focus is on the entry of the Dutch healthcare system, which is almost universally general practice. Furthermore, general practice provides information about lifelong disease occurrence registered by medical professionals. The important epidemiological criterion of covering the whole population at risk is met, since almost all non-institutionalised Dutch citizens are registered with a GP.

Besides the need for valid and reliable information on the health of the Dutch population, the Ministry of Health – and other parties involved – wanted an update of existing information on the functioning and performance of general practice in the Netherlands. This update was particularly urgent since the last time that nationwide information was made available for this purpose was in 1987: the first Dutch National Survey of General Practice (DNSGP-1).

From this perspective, the objective of DNSGP-2 was to provide an up-to-date and nationally representative insight into the role, task and the position of general practice in healthcare in the Netherlands. The major topics covered are:

- frequency and type of health problems in general practice
- type of care provided in general practice, including its quality
- factors determining the presentation of health problems in general practice, the care and its quality
- changes in these topics compared to 1987.

DNSGP-2 data collection took place between April 2000 and April 2002, with approximately 85% of the data in the calendar year 2001. The design of the study is presented in Chapter 2.

DNSGP-2 was carried out in 104 general practices in the Netherlands in 2001, comprising 195 GPs (in total 165 GP full-time equivalents) and including 385 461 patients.

Performance has become a popular term in policy and in academic circles. Terms such as *health systems performance, performance management, performance measurement, indicators, measures, league tables*, and *value for money* dominate in policy documents and the scientific literature. Governments, and also the Dutch government, strive to monitor, measure, and improve the performance of their healthcare systems.[4] DNSGP-2 provided a huge empirically based information source that gives the opportunity to assess the performance of the GP, gate-keeper in the Dutch healthcare system. In the following paragraphs we present the major findings of DNSGP-2 for six separate themes (*see* Box 1.1). Finally, we draw conclusions about how general practice in the Netherlands performs on the target domains of quality of care, efficiency and accessibility.

Box 1.1

The results of DNSGP-2 are reported in six separate reports:

1   Health of the Dutch
2   Utilisation of care
3   Inequalities
4   Quality of GP care
5   Communication in general practice
6   Organisation and workload

Health of the Dutch

(Further reading Chapters 5, 6, 8, 9 and 11)

In 2001 over 80% rated their health as '(very) good'; this percentage is lower than in 1987

In 2001, 82% of the 270 000 people surveyed reported their own health to be 'good' or 'very good'. This means that the number of people who rate their health this highly has dropped by over 2% since 1987 after adjustments for demographic age-profile changes. More men than women reported good or very good health, i.e. 84% versus 80%.

More symptoms and conditions were reported in 2001, but GPs do not report a greater number of diseases

Compared with 1987, the difference in the rate of self-reported complaints and conditions and those presented to a GP appears to have increased somewhat. On the one hand, the number of self-reported complaints has increased; on the other hand the incidence of symptoms and conditions in general practice has remained more or less the same. People do consult their doctor more often (a higher average number of contacts with the GP or surgery), but this does not result in a higher number of diagnoses made by the GP compared with the 1987 figures. The increased number of self-reported symptoms and conditions is apparently not based on a higher incidence of diseases. People may show a greater tendency to report physical and mental symptoms and problems, with the frequency of illnesses presented to and diagnosed by the GP remaining more or less constant.

Mental health problems increased compared to 1987

Of those surveyed and aged over 18 years, over 20% have an increased risk of a mental health disorder. These results have been derived from the scores on a questionnaire. In 1987 the corresponding figure was 17%. The percentage is higher for women, single people and those from lower socio-economic groups.

Utilisation of care

(Further reading Chapters 12–15)

Demand for general practice care has risen compared to 1987. In 2001, over three-quarters of the population contacted the GP at least once

While this latter fraction has remained unchanged since 1987, the consultation rate per patient has increased by 10%. The increase is particularly marked among older patients.

In 2001, patients had an average of six contacts on annual basis with their GP's surgery (GPs and/or practice assistants). Patients aged over 75 years had an average of 16 contacts with their GP's surgery. Women show higher consultation rates than men. Patients with mental health problems and/or chronic conditions have the highest number of contacts with their GP's surgery.

Most contacts take place in the GP's office and prescription of medication is the most common intervention

Seventy-four per cent of contacts with the GP take place in the surgery; 8.5% are house calls. The remaining 18% of GP contacts are telephone calls or other (e.g. administrative) contacts. By comparison with 1987, the percentage of house calls has dropped from 17% to almost 9% of all contacts with GPs. The number of telephone contacts has increased from 4% to 11%. Of the interventions reviewed, the most common is prescribing medication: in 57% of all contacts GPs issue one or more prescriptions. The number of prescriptions per patient has increased since 1987, particularly for patients aged over 75 years.

GPs deal with 96% of all contacts themselves

In 4% of the contacts, referrals are made within primary care, or a new referral is made to secondary care. In this respect, the GP (still) acts as a gatekeeper for the Dutch healthcare system. By comparison with 1987, GPs in 2001 were conducting fewer interventions themselves. Practice assistants have assumed part of these tasks.

Inequalities

(Further reading Chapters 7 and 10)

People with lower socio-economic status report comparatively poorer health and unhealthier behaviour

Diabetes mellitus is much more prevalent among those of lower socio-economic status than in higher socio-economic groups. The gap in mental health between the socio-economic groups has widened significantly since 1987.

People with a lower socio-economic status are more likely to smoke, have generally unhealthier eating habits, are more prone to hard drug use and excessive alcohol consumption than those of a higher socio-economic status. There is little difference between the two groups in terms of the national standard for adequate physical exercise. However, people from a lower socio-economic background are more likely to be overweight or obese than others.

Older people report better health in 2001 than in 1987, whereas younger people report poorer health in 2001

Nowadays, older people report better health than they did in 1987. This is particularly true in the 45–64 years age group. Younger people, on the other hand, report somewhat poorer health than in 1987. Compared to 1987, the differences in mental health between older and younger age groups have, however, increased.

Immigrants report poorer health, but have comparable healthcare use

Besides this general point – immigrants reporting poorer health – there are significant differences between the immigrant subgroups. In general, people from a Turkish background report poorer health than those with a Moroccan, Antillean or Surinamese background.

Quality of GP care

(Further reading Chapters 21–25)

In three-quarters of the cases GPs adhere to national guidelines

There was an overall 74% rate of convergence between GP performance and the guidelines for more than 100 indicators (including diagnostics, prescribing and referrals). The rate varied from 10% to almost 100%, showing a considerable degree of divergence between practices. The information shows where there is room for improvement.

Nine out of ten patients say they receive the care they actually expect

Patients attach considerable importance to certain elements of the actual care given by the GP in the surgery. They want to be taken seriously, to receive an understandable explanation of their symptoms, and also to be properly informed about the nature and purpose of the proposed treatment. Rating their contacts with the GP, an average of nine out of ten patients say that they receive the actual care that they expect. Some 10% of the patients indicate that the content of the care given by their GP was of 'inadequate quality'.

Contact frequencies vary substantially from one general practice to another

There is considerable variation between GPs and practices in the contact frequencies of older patients and those who rate their health as 'not good'. The differences remain apparent even when differences in the registered practice populations are taken into account.

Communication in general practice

(Further reading Chapters 19 and 20)

GPs involve their patients more often in the decision-making process than in the 1980s

Communication in the GP's surgery and the communication styles of GPs and patients have changed over time. Nowadays, GPs give more information – especially on medical matters. On the other hand, however, they are less affective:

they show less concern and less empathy than previously. Patients are generally more involved in the decision-making process, but are less involved in other aspects of the consultation.

Consultations with highly educated patients take longer

Consultations with highly educated patients take longer than with those who are less well educated, and the GP and patient both talk more. GPs are more patient centred in these consultations. This difference is particularly marked during the decision-making phase of the consultation. Patients' assertiveness increases with their level of education. GPs are more likely to involve highly educated patients in decisions about their treatment.

GPs are more instrumental with immigrant patients

With persons from immigrant groups there is less talk between patient and doctor in consultations. GPs are more patient centred in consultations with patients of Dutch origin. Dutch and western immigrants talk more to the GPs. In comparison, GPs talk more about medical topics in consultations with non-westerners and less about psychosocial problems.

Organisation and workload

(Further reading Chapters 16–18)

GPs do more in less time

A clear shift has taken place towards less labour-intensive and time-consuming contacts. In 1987, over 16% of all contacts consisted of house calls; in 2001 this percentage had dropped to 8.5%. At the same time, telephone contacts increased from 4.4% to 10.8%. This enabled GPs to gain a lot of time. However, the average consultation duration remained the same at almost 10 minutes. Furthermore, access to the GP has become more regulated. Walk-in consultation hours are being increasingly replaced by consultations-by-appointment; some 50% of the GPs operate a policy of telephone consultations by return phone call, and over half of the practice assistants independently give advice by phone for a selected number of problems.

GPs now delegate more medical tasks

Task delegation continues to be seen as an important means to contain the workload of GPs and to possibly address the consequences of a future shortage of GPs. The deployment of practice assistants has increased in a qualitative sense during the period under review. Quantitatively, there has been a slight increase, but the qualitative changes have been more significant. The job of practice assistant has professionalised.

Job satisfaction decreased from 88% to 74%

Approximately three-quarters of the GPs were satisfied or very satisfied with their work in 2001. Compared to 14 years ago, this represents a distinct decline. Despite a considerable increase in the demand for care in absolute terms, GPs are working fewer hours per week. This puts extra pressure on the time spent at work. The decline in satisfaction is not so much related to work as to material aspects of the job, such as income. On the other hand, GPs showed fewer symptoms of burnout than a decade ago.

How is general practice performing?

This chapter has presented the core findings of the study in a nutshell. From these findings we can draw a few general conclusions with respect to the quality of care, efficiency and accessibility of general practice in the Netherlands.

Quality of care

Dutch GPs deliver high quality of care: on average they adhere in 74% of cases to national guidelines and 90% of the patients are satisfied with the care they receive.

Efficiency of care

Dutch GPs have organised their work in a more efficient way since 1987: they see more patients in less time. GPs are still the gatekeepers in the Dutch healthcare system: they deal with 96% of all contacts themselves without referring the patient, and they do that for less than 5% of the Dutch healthcare budget.

Accessibility

General practice is accessible for the entire population. Despite existing differences in health between different sociodemographic subgroups, they all visit the GP according to their needs.

Therefore we conclude that general practice is a high-quality, efficient and accessible element in the Dutch healthcare system.

References

1 Ruwaard D and Kramers PGN (1998) *Public Health Status and Forecasts 1997. Health prevention and health care in the Netherlands until 2015*. Elsevier/de Tijdstroom, Maarsen.
2 van der Velden J (1999) *General Practice at Work*. PhD Thesis. NIVEL, Utrecht.
3 Fleming DM (1991) The design and management of national morbidity surveys. *Methods Inf Med.* **30**: 284–8.
4 Arah OA (2005) *Performance Re-examined*. PhD Thesis. UvA/AMC, Amsterdam.

Chapter 2

The design of the second Dutch National Survey of General Practice

François Schellevis and Gert Westert

What is this chapter about?

In this chapter the design of the second Dutch National Survey of General Practice (DNSGP-2) and its methods of data collection and data analyses are described. The first section provides a short introduction into the research questions that have guided the design and measurements. In the next sections the recruitment of the participating practices, the patient population, the data collection modules and measurements are described. The last sections deal with issues such as the representativeness, the statistical power of the study, and the comparability of the second and the first Dutch National Surveys of General Practice.

For a quick overview the sections 'Design' and 'Data collection modules' provide the essentials.

Aim and research themes

The aim of the study was 'to provide an actual and nationally representative insight into the role and function of general practice in Dutch healthcare'.

Based on this aim the research questions of the DNSGP-2 were categorised into six research themes:

- health and health problems in the population and in general practice
- the use of healthcare services
- inequalities in health and healthcare utilisation between social groups
- quality of general practice care
- doctor–patient communication
- organisation and workload in general practice.

The underlying research questions were to be answered in studies carried out by NIVEL (Netherlands Institute for Health Services Research) in co-operation with the Dutch National Institute of Public Health and the Environment (RIVM) and the Centre for Quality of Care Research (WOK) of the Radboud University in Nijmegen. Also, many additional research projects and secondary analyses were planned in co-operation with research groups in the Netherlands and abroad. Different chapters in this book are based on these additional studies.

Design

The collection of the data, necessary to answer the research questions, took place in 104 general practices throughout the Netherlands with 195 general practitioners (GPs) and a practice population of approximately $n = 400\ 000$. In these practices a number of data collections took place within different (sub)populations:

- census of the total practice population to collect sociodemographic data
- health interview survey among a random sample of 5% of the total practice population (all ages) and a second health interview survey among a random sample of Turkish, Moroccan, Surinamese and Antillean migrants aged 18 years and older
- data regarding all contacts between patients and the practices via the electronic medical record during one calendar year; these data include contact diagnoses, prescriptions, and referrals
- videotaping of GP–patient consultations during consultation hours of GPs
- audit visits of the practices with additional written questionnaires for GPs and assisting personnel.

An important feature of the DNSGP-2 was the use of unique identifiers in the collection of data which enables the interlinkage of all data on all measurement levels.

The DNSGP-2 took place in 104 general practices throughout the Netherlands with 195 GPs and a practice population of approximately n = 400 000.

Practices and GPs

At first, practices already participating in the Dutch National Information Network of General Practice (LINH) were invited to participate in the DNSGP-2. This network was chosen as basis for the DNSGP-2 because many of these GPs were experienced in the use of electronic medical records. Data from electronic medical records have been used by LINH since 1992 to analyse healthcare utilisation in general practice (consultation frequency, prescription of medication and referrals). Sixty-one LINH practices were prepared to participate in the DNSGP-2. To recruit more practices, a mailing was sent out to a sample of practices (drawn from the national NIVEL register of GPs) selected on the basis of region, urbanisation level and status of 'deprived area', in order to increase the representativeness of the participating practices. The invitation was accompanied by a letter from the Dutch College of General Practitioners and the Dutch Association of General Practitioners recommending participation. This led to another 43 practices being willing to participate. The 104 participating practices included 195 GPs equivalent to 165 full-time working GPs.

Patient population

In the Netherlands, individuals with public health insurance (approximately 65% of the population) are obliged to be registered in a general practice. Individuals with private health insurance usually comply with this rule voluntarily. Therefore, the patient lists of all participating practices were used as the population denominator for the DNSGP-2. The patient lists were derived from the practice computers at the beginning and at the end of the study. For some parts of the data collection, the population at the start of the study ($n = 399\ 068$) were used as the denominator; for other parts, the mid-time population (the mathematical mean of the population at the start and at the end of the study; $n = 400\ 912$) was used.

Data collection modules

Census

A written questionnaire with 14 items in 4 languages (Dutch, English, Turkish and Arabic) was sent to all patients registered in the participating practices at the start of the study ($n = 385\ 461$). Questionnaires were sent in one envelope per address with an introduction letter signed by the GP and an information leaflet about the study and the aim of this part of the data collection. Questionnaires could be sent back free of charge, and the questions could also be answered via the internet on a secure website. One reminder was sent and a personal approach in certain practices with low response rates was applied in order to optimise the response rate. Data from 294 999 persons were available for analysis, representing a response rate of 76.5%.

The data include civil status, household composition, living arrangement, health insurance, ethnic origin (based on country of birth of the respondent and both parents), number of years living in the Netherlands, education level, occupation, work status, and the '1–item scale' on perceived health.[1]

The census resulted in data from 294 999 persons, representing a response rate of 76.5%.

Health interview survey

A 5% all-age random sample of the practice population was invited to participate in an extensive health interview survey. A letter from the GP accompanied the invitations. The computer-assisted personal interview was carried out at the person's home by a trained interviewer. The average interview duration was 90 minutes. The interviews were randomly distributed over the calendar year 2001. Of the 19 685 invited persons, data from 12 699 valid interviews could be used for the analyses (response = 64.5%).

The core part of the interview included validated instruments to measure health status and healthcare utilisation, and determinants of health status and healthcare utilisation including coping, social support, opinions and attitudes.

For children aged under 12 years, a restricted proxy-interview was held with one of the parents; during interviews with children aged between 12 and 18 years, a parent was nearby.

Health interview survey among migrants

For a comparable health interview survey, a random sample of the respondents on the census questionnaire (*see* above) was drawn from the 7355 persons of 18 years and older reporting to be of Turkish, Moroccan, Surinamese or Netherlands Antillean origin. The oral interview took place at the person's home with the help of a paper questionnaire. In total 2682 persons were invited to participate in this survey, of whom 1339 responded (49.9%).

The interview included more or less the same instruments as mentioned above. In addition, an instrument measuring the degree of acculturation in Dutch society was administered.

Data from the electronic medical record

Data about contacts of patients with the practice were derived from the routine registration in the electronic medical records ($n = 1.5$ million contacts). For some data, additional software was installed to remind GPs and practice personnel to complete the data or to provide additional information. In every practice, the data were collected over a period of 12 months; 87% of the data were collected in 2001. Data extraction software was applied every 3 months and the data were subsequently stored in a database. An overview of the data derived from the electronic medical record is provided in Table 2.1.

Data relating to 1.5 million contacts of patients with the practice were derived from the routine registration in the electronic medical records.

Videotaping of consultations

On a voluntary basis, 142 GPs (72.8% of the participating GPs) agreed to have GP–patient consultations videotaped. A total of 2784 consultations were recorded during regular consultation hours of the GPs; 11.9% of the eligible patients refused participation. Patients filled in written questionnaires before, immediately after and 2 weeks after the consultation. The videotaped consultations were observed by trained observers using standardised observation schemes (Roter Interaction Process Analysis System[2]) and additional checklists. Observation was carried out on verbal and non-verbal communication style, patient participation, and content of the consultation (information, advice). Patient questionnaires included measuring instruments regarding health status, reason to consult the GP, preferences to see a specific GP, and the patient's opinion about the consultation.

A total of 2784 consultations were recorded on video during regular consultation hours of the GPs.

Table 2.1 Data derived from the electronic medical record

Data	Measurement	Remarks
Morbidity		
reason for encounter	Free text	Recorded during 12 months
disease episode	Contact diagnosis (ICPC-coded); episode type (new/ongoing)	Recorded during 12 months; disease episodes were constructed on the basis of contact diagnosis and episode type
somatic/psychosocial background of the contact diagnosis	5-point Likert-scale	Recorded during 6 weeks
diagnosis-specific data	Additional data for a selection of ICPC-codes, related to guidelines of the Dutch College of GPs	Recorded during 3 months
Contact details		
type of contact	Categories: consultation, home visit, telephone, request for repeat prescription, etc.	Recorded during 6 weeks
contact duration	Categories: 1–5, 6–10, 11–15 minutes etc	Recorded during 6 weeks
Interventions		
drug prescriptions	Product name	The product name maps to different drug characteristics (e.g. ATC-code, defined daily dose); recorded during 12 months
diagnostic interventions	Categories: blood pressure measurement, weight measurement, blood testing, urine testing, ECG, diagnostic imaging, function test, etc.	Recorded during 6 weeks
therapeutic interventions	Categories: ear wax removal, wound care, minor surgery, intra-uterine device, etc	Recorded during 6 weeks
information/advice	Categories: sick leave, return to work, self-care medication	Recorded during 6 weeks
referral	New referral to: • physical therapy • exercise therapy • logopedist • mental care • medical specialist (incl. type of specialist)	Recorded during 12 months

ATC: Anatomical Therapeutic Chemical classification; ECG: electrocardiogram; ICPC: International Classification of Primary Care

Practice visits and questionnaires for GPs and practice assistants

A systematic practice visiting instrument (VIP) has been used for audit visits to the participating practices.[3] This was realised for 98 out of the 104 practices (94%), including 181 GPs and their assisting personnel. The practice visits took place in the years 2000–2002. With the help of the VIP, six dimensions of the practice organisation could be assessed: (1) practice equipment; (2) task delegation; (3) service and organisation; (4) registration; (5) quality system; (6) workload. The practice visits were carried out by trained auditors. Data collection includes questionnaires to be filled in by GPs, practice assistants and patients visiting the practice.

In addition to the data collected with the VIP, questionnaires were sent to GPs and practice assistants, to collect data about topics not covered by the VIP (e.g. opinions and attitudes). Response rates for the different questionnaires varied between 78% and 96%.

Representativeness of GPs and practice population

The GPs participating in the survey were, in most relevant aspects, representative of the Dutch GP population, e.g. sex, age, part-time/full-time working, urbanisation level of the practice location and geographical distribution (*see* Figure 2.1). However, with regard to practice type, GPs working solo were relatively under-represented in the study population (31% versus 43%).

The total practice population of the participating practices was comparable to the population of the Netherlands with respect to sex, age and type of healthcare insurance (*see* Table 2.2).

Table 2.2 The total practice population of the participating practices compared with the total population of the Netherlands on 1 January 2001 (source: Statistics Netherlands) by age and type of healthcare insurance

Age (years)/type of healthcare insurance	Total practice population (n = 399 068) (%)	Population of the Netherlands (n = 15 987 075) (%)
0–4	5.1	6.3
5–14	12.4	12.4
15–24	12.3	11.8
25–44	32.7	31.3
45–64	24.5	24.6
65–74	7.1	7.5
≥75	5.9	6.1
Public health insurance	64.6	66.5
Private health insurance	35.4	33.5

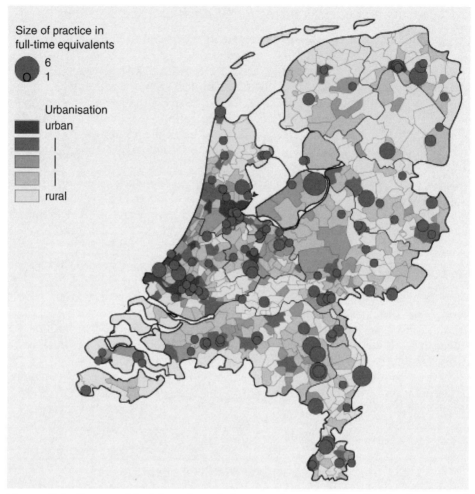

Figure 2.1 Geographical location of the practices participating in the second Dutch National Survey of General Practice (DNSGP-2): urbanisation level and number of GPs per practice.

Statistical power

In determining the required number of participating GPs, the comparability of the results with the first Dutch National Survey of General Practice of 1987 was of primary concern. The number of 161 participating GPs in the 1987 survey was established on the basis of:

- the national nature of the study
- sampling among established GPs
- enabling reliable analyses of differences between regions in the Netherlands, urbanisation levels, and distance between the practice and the nearest hospital
- the feasibility of the study.

An important difference between the 1987 and 2001 survey was the recruitment method: in 1987 a non-proportionally stratified random sample of GPs was invited to participate; in 2001 the starting point was an existing registration network of GPs.

Post hoc power analyses were carried out to establish the level of precision and statistical power for different research questions. These analyses revealed the following results for the different study populations:

- diseases with an incidence rate of 3 per 1000 patients per year or higher are considered to be relevant to measure in a general practice population in terms of reliability.[4] In a total population of n = 400 000, this incidence rate can be measured with a 95% confidence interval of ±0.2 per 1000 patients per year
- the size of the population participating in the health interview survey allows the representation of at least 10 persons with a rare disease, e.g. the prevalence of multiple sclerosis is 0.8 per 1000; in an all-age population sample of n = 12 699 the expected number of multiple sclerosis patients is 10 (95% confidence interval: 3–12)
- quality indicators, representing the degree of compliance with guidelines for optimal care, are calculated on GP level. In previous research an average level of 61% compliance was found.[5] With 195 participating GPs a 20% difference between groups of equal size can be established with α = 0.05 and β = 0.20.

Table 2.3 Comparability of different aspects of the surveys in 1987 and 2001

	Methods	Data
Recruitment of practices	1987: random sample; 2001: existing registration network (LINH)	
Census	1987: in the practices and by mail; 2001: by mail	1987 and 2001 identical
Health interview survey	Identical	In 2001 more validated instruments than in 1987
Health interview survey among migrants	Not performed in 1987	
Data about contacts of patients with the practice	1987: paper forms during 3 months; 2001: electronic medical records during 12 months	1987: central coding by clerks; reason for encounter coded; 2001: coding by GP; reason for encounter not coded
Videotaping of consultations	1987: performed among selected GPs; 2001: performed among volunteering GPs	
Practice visits	Not performed in 1987	
Questionnaires for GPs and practice assistants	Identical	In 2001 more validated instruments than in 1987

Comparability of the first (1987) and second (2001) Dutch National Surveys

An important aim of the second Dutch National Survey was to compare the results of 2001 with those from the first survey of 1987. This required as much comparability as possible in the design of both surveys. In general, the comparability is strong. However, developments over time made it inevitable that some aspects of the survey had to change in 2001. Most changes represent an improvement. Table 2.3 summarises the main differences of the two surveys. The main differences relate to the data about contacts of patients with the practice. Comparisons between the two surveys should be carried out with caution due to differences in the data collection method (paper forms versus electronic medical records), the classification of health problems (by clerks versus by GPs), and the data collection period (3 months versus 12 months).

References

1 Mossey JM and Shapiro E (1982) Self-rated health: a predictor of mortality among the elderly. *Am J Pub Health*. **72**: 800–8.
2 Roter DL (1991) *The Roter Method of Interaction Process Analysis. RIAS Manual*. Johns Hopkins University, Baltimore.
3 van den Hombergh P, Grol R, van den Hoogen HJM and van den Bosch WJHM (1998) Assessment of management in general practice: validation of a practice visit method. *Br J Gen Pract*. **48**: 1743–50.
4 Marinus AMF (1993) *Interdoktervariatie in de Huisartspraktijk* [Inter-doctor variation in general practice] (PhD thesis). University of Amsterdam, Amsterdam.
5 Grol R, Dalhuijsen J, Thomas S, In't Veld C, Rutten G and Mokkink H (1998) Attributes of clinical guidelines that influence use of guidelines in general practice: observational study. *BMJ*. **317**: 858–61.

Chapter 3

The Dutch healthcare system: how are we organised?

Lea Jabaaij

What is this chapter about?

The Netherlands has a unique and complex healthcare organisation and financing system. Insight into the peculiarities of the Dutch system helps one to understand the position of general practice. This chapter opens with a short outline of Dutch demographics: who are we and how many are we? Subsequently, the funding of healthcare is discussed, and the way it is organised. The chapter ends with some future developments.

Who are we: demographics

In 2001, 16 000 000 people were living in the Netherlands, 49.5% being male (*see* Figure 3.1).[1] The number of people in the age cohorts 30–34 to 50–54 years are comparable. The same is true of the number of people in the younger age cohorts, but because their size is lower, the Netherlands will face an ageing population in the near future.

In 2001, 9.3% of the population was of non-western origin (first and second generation). With 320 000 people, the Turkish form the largest part, followed by 309 000 Surinamese people (a former Dutch colony), 270 000 Moroccans, and 117 000 people coming from the Dutch Antilles and Aruba. More than 460 000 people originate from a range of other non-western countries.[2] Another 9% of the population consists of foreigners originating from other western countries.

In 2001, 200 000 children were born and 140 000 people died.

How do we finance it?

Changes are on their way, but in 2001, the year in which data were collected for the second Dutch National Survey of General Practice (DNSGP-2), the financing of Dutch healthcare system was composed of a mix of public and private insurance. The system was divided into three compartments:[3]

- the first compartment is the Exceptional Medical Expenses Act (AWBZ)
- the second compartment is the statutory public health insurance based on the Health Insurance Act (ZFW), and private insurance
- the third compartment is supplementary (private) insurance.

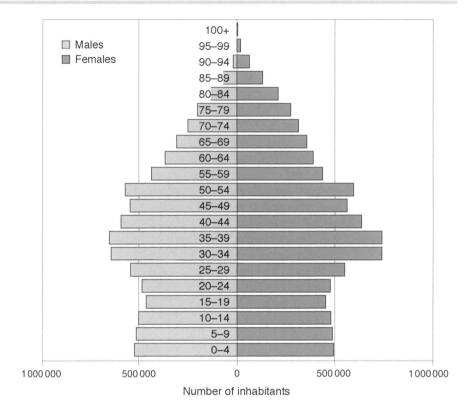

Figure 3.1 Age distribution of the population in 2001.

The first compartment

The AWBZ was created in order to ensure that all inhabitants of the Netherlands have insurance coverage for long-term care and uninsurable risks. It refers to areas such as nursing homes, care for the disabled, home care, and care for the mentally ill. All inhabitants of the Netherlands participate compulsorily in the AWBZ. In this compartment there is no competition or operation of market forces. The government is responsible for cost control. The budget comes from compulsory payment of taxes.

The second compartment

The second compartment concerns curative care. Insurers are free to contract care providers. People with a relatively low income are publicly insured; people with a higher income are privately insured. Approximately 63% of the Dutch population is publicly insured via the Health Insurance Act. A limited market operation applies to this compartment.

Health Insurance Act: income-related public health insurance

The government determines the care package. In 2001, the insurance covered basic medical care, such as general practitioners (GPs) and medical specialists, hospital care, drugs, physiotherapy and dental treatment for children. The size of the premium is to a large degree income related; the care insurer sets only a small portion of the premium (the nominal premium).

The following groups are compulsorily insured according to the Health Insurance Act (public insurance): employees with an income below the cut-off level (for 2001 this has been set at €29 864), their (non-earning) partners and their children, people over 65 years (with an income up to €19 000), recipients of social insurance benefits, and the self-employed and their (non-earning) partners and children, with an income up to €19 091.[4]

Private medical expenses insurance

People who do not qualify for public insurance can contract private medical expenses insurance. The coverage is by and large comparable with the public insurance, but more variation is allowed. For example, in 2001 one could choose not to insure care provided by the GP. Premiums are not income related, but depend on age and the package insured. Taking a high 'own risk' reduces the premium. In addition to a nominal premium, the privately insured also pay a statutory solidarity supplement. Since the number of older people covered by public insurance is far greater than that covered by private insurance, the state tries to compensate for this by this supplement.

The third compartment

The third compartment concerns all care that is not covered by the first two, as for example dental healthcare for adults, (more) physiotherapy sessions, psychotherapy, glasses or exercise therapy. Care insurers offer this care in policies that are supplementary to the statutory health insurance fund or the standard package policy. The content of these packages varies substantially as does the premium and any own-risk cover.

With the introduction of a new healthcare insurance system in January 2006, the distinction between public and private insurance has disappeared.

How do we organise it?

Because this book is about care by GPs, we focus on their role in the system. Other healthcare deliverers will be discussed only briefly.

The Dutch GP

Gatekeeper

The GP has a central position in Dutch healthcare. Somebody with health complaints first contacts the GP for advice, if he or she thinks self-care is insufficient. All non-institutionalised inhabitants are registered with their own GPs. GPs treat most complaints themselves. Only patients with complex problems or complaints needing specialised treatment are referred to other healthcare workers in primary or secondary care. In general, these are only accessible through referral. The GP functions as a 'gatekeeper' or navigator in the health-care system.

Male/female differences

In 2001, three-quarters of the GPs were male. But a feminisation of the profession is on its way: 60% of all young GPs (under age 35 years) are female (*see* Tables 3.1 and 3.2).[5] Three-quarters of all male GPs work full-time, but only one of every five female GPs work full-time (*see* Table 3.3).[5] The mean number of full-time equivalents (ftes) worked a week is 0.87, but differs for men and women: 0.93 and 0.69 respectively.

Table 3.1 Number of GPs in 2001

	Absolute number	% of all GPs
Independent GPs	7270	94
male	5631	
female	1639	
HIDHA[a]	493	6
male	87	
female	406	
All		
male	5718	74
female	2045	26
Total	7763	100

Source: NIVEL.[5]
[a]A qualified GP working for an independent GP.

Table 3.2 Age distribution of independent GPs on 1 January 2001

Age (years)	Male (%)	Female (%)	All
<35	2.2	10.7	4.1
35–39	9.8	25.9	13.4
40–49	45.0	48.6	45.9
50–54	26.8	11.9	23.5
55–59	12.9	2.5	10.5
>60	3.3	0.4	2.6
	100	100	100

Source: NIVEL.[5]

Practice organisation

A typical Dutch GP is independent, the owner of the premises and assisted by a receptionist or practice assistant. Because almost half of the GPs work single-handed, two-thirds of the practices are single-handed (*see* Table 3.4).[5] The number of qualified GPs employed by a colleague GP is low (*see* Table 3.1). Most of them are part-time working women. In 2001, the normative list size –

the number of patients registered per GP to earn the normative income – was 2350 patients.

Table 3.3 Number of hours worked per GP in 2001

Hours worked (fte)	Male	Female	All
<0.40	0.2	2.2	0.7
0.40–0.60	4.6	28.3	10.4
0.60–0.80	8	33.5	14.2
0.80 – 1	11.8	14.4	12.5
1 (full-time)	75.2	21.6	62.2

Source: NIVEL.[5]

Table 3.4 Number of GPs working in a practice in 2001

	GPs		GP practices	
	Absolute number	%	Absolute number	%
Single-handed practice[a]	3059	42	3059	64
Partnership (duo)[b]	2400	33	1210	26
Group practice[c]	1811	25	481	10
Total	7270	100	4750	100

Source: NIVEL.[5]
[a]Practice with one independent GP who might or might not have employed a qualified GP working in the practice.
[b]Practice with two independent GPs working in one building.
[c]Practice with at least three independent GPs working in one building.

Care

For most diagnostic procedures, GPs rely on external facilities. A diminishing proportion of GPs (9% in 2001) owns a practice pharmacy. Traditionally, GPs delivered obstetric care, but in 2001 only 11% of all GPs were still active in obstetric care (personal communication, Trees Wiegers, Netherlands Institute for Health Services Research (NIVEL)). Home visits belong to the normal tasks, but the number of home visits has decreased during the last 30 years (*see also* Chapter 12 of this book).

Out-of-office care

GPs are responsible for 7 × 24 h services. This was usually achieved on a rota basis in small local or regional tenancy groups. To make out-of-office-hours healthcare more efficient and lower the workload for GPs, so-called central GP posts have been initiated. These posts are physically located on a fixed spot and GPs are on duty by turn. Their service area is not local but regional with up to

150 000 people per central GP post.[6] GPs on duty in these posts have assistants and a car, with a driver at their disposal.

Payment

Payment of GP care differs for publicly and privately insured patients. For publicly insured patients the GP receives a capitation fee. GPs are compensated for groups of patients who need more care, such as senior citizens or inhabitants of deprived areas. Privately insured patients pay a 'fee for service'. Practice costs are included in the fees.

Other primary care services

Midwives, physiotherapists, dentists, pharmacists, speech therapists, exercise therapists, podotherapists and community nurses all deliver primary care health services. Some of them are freely accessible, others only through referral. They are paid on a fee-for-service basis (excluding community nurses). Because each has his or her own expertise, co-operation and co-ordination are often complex. Since the 1970s, the government has been stimulating teamwork in healthcare centres, where several primary care workers co-operate, including GPs. In 1998, there were 148 healthcare centres employing 3210 healthcare workers and serving more than a million people. A typical healthcare centre accommodates GPs, community nurses, social workers, physiotherapists, dieticians, speech therapists, and a pharmacy. Most healthcare centres are located in urban areas.

Medical specialists' care: outpatient and hospital care

In 2001, there were 140 hospital locations in the Netherlands and 38 outpatient hospitals, organised in 94 organisations and 8 university hospitals.[2,7] In general, all hospitals offer a wide range of care, with university hospitals offering the most specialised care. However, hospital organisations tend to choose more differentiated care for each hospital and concentrate specific functions in one location. Virtually all outpatient specialist care is provided in hospitals.

The total number of beds is 53 247 with a mean of about 400 per hospital, ranging from 138 for the smallest and 1 368 beds for the largest hospital. The number of beds was 3.7 per 1000 inhabitants in 1999.

In 2001, the number of admissions was 1 479 000 with a total of 12 778 000 inpatient nursing days and 938 000 daycare treatments.[2] The number of admissions is decreasing, as well as the number of days hospitalised (an average of 8.2 days in 2001).[8] Daycare and outpatient treatment is increasing. In 2001 5.4% of the population was hospitalised in a year, and 38% was treated by medical specialists. In 2001, 11 515 medical specialists were working in the Netherlands.[9] In general, they are associated with a hospital.

Hospital care is by far the most expensive service in healthcare. In 1999, 30% of the budget for healthcare was consumed by hospital-delivered care. In comparison, GP care consumed only 3% of the total budget for healthcare.[10]

The future

Dutch GPs are looking for creative solutions to decrease their workload. Tasks are delegated to physician assistants, practice nurses or nurse practitioners. Care delivered during out-of-office hours is to an increasing degree organised in GP co-operatives. This reduces the number of shifts enormously and also the workload experienced (*see* Chapters 16 and 18).

Fundamental changes in financing healthcare were introduced in January 2006. The distinction between public and private insurance has disappeared. By and large the new system has the following features.[3]

All Dutch inhabitants now have a compulsory insurance for all basic healthcare. The government determines which medical care is covered in this standard package. This is financed in two ways: a nominal fee for individual insured people and an income-related contribution to the scheme. Insurers are obligated to accept all applicants for the standard package. It is expected that competition between insurers will be stimulated by giving citizens choices in insurance packages, nominal premiums, payback arrangements (in natura or restitution) and own risk covers. Above this, a 'no-claim' system rewards those insured who claim nothing or less than 255 euro (2006). They recover (part of) this amount on their insurance fee the next year. Care delivered by general practitioners is not included in this 'no claim' system, so the free and low threshold access to the general practitioner is not at stake. Besides the compulsory standard insurance, the citizen can voluntarily take out an additional insurance, for which no compulsory acceptance applies.

At the time of writing this chapter, the system has just been introduced. What effect it will have on cost-control, quality of care, efficiency and accessibility is still unclear.

References

1 www.cbs.nl/en-GB/menu/themas/mens-maatschappij/bevolking/cijfers/default.htm (accessed 6 October 2005).
2 http://statline.cbs.nl
3 Website of Dutch Health Care insurers [Zorgverzekeraars Nederland (ZN)] www.zn.nl (accessed 8 October 2005).
4 www.salarisinfostartpagina.nl/tarieven_en_premies_2001.htm#boven (accessed 12 September 2005).
5 NIVEL (1980–2004) *NIVEL Registratie van Huisartsen* [NIVEL GP registration]. NIVEL, Utrecht. *See also* www.nivel.nl
6 Inspectie voor de Gezondheidszorg. Huisartsenposten in Nederland. Nieuwe structuren met veel kinderziekten. [Health Care Inspectorate. Central points for general practitioners in the Netherlands. New structures with many initial problems.] IGZ, Den Haag, 2004. For a map see www.rivm.nl/vtv/data/atlas/cure_huis_haps.htm (accessed 12 September 2005).
7 www.rivm.nl (accessed 12 September 2005).
8 www.prismant.nl (accessed 12 September 2005).
9 www.brancherapporten.minvws.nl/object_document/o317n680.html (accessed 12 September 2005).
10 www.rivm.nl/kostenvanziekten/site_nl/index1.htm (accessed 12 September 2005).

Chapter 4

Primary healthcare as a determinant of population health: a social epidemiologist's view

Ichiro Kawachi

What is this chapter about?

Social epidemiologists state that medical care makes only a relatively modest contribution to population health. Others say they are too harsh. Since the 1950s medical care has contributed substantially to the decline in mortality. Does that mean that the more you spend, the healthier your population? Surprisingly, it is not only how much you spend on medical care, but also how spending is allocated across sectors that matters. Primary healthcare seems to be a key determinant of the health of the nations.

Medical care makes a modest contribution to population health

Among social epidemiologists, medical care has often been relegated to a secondary role as a determinant of population health.[1,2] This view originated from influential works such as René Dubos' *Mirage of Health*,[3] Ivan Illich's *Medical Nemesis*,[4] and Thomas McKeown's *The Role of Medicine*.[5] Together, these classic works contributed to the formulation of received wisdom among social epidemiologists that medical care has made a relatively modest contribution to population health. For example, McKeown[5] argued from the historical analysis of mortality trends in Britain that most of the decline in mortality between 1860 and 1960 from specific causes, such as respiratory tuberculosis and whooping cough, had occurred well before the introduction of effective medical cures.[5] In turn, Illich coined the term 'iatrogenic disease' to describe the contribution of medicine in *creating* illness and disease.[4] Although the extent of iatrogenic disease is sometimes exaggerated, even credible sources, such as the report from the Institute of Medicine of the US National Academy of Sciences, have estimated that medical errors are responsible for between 44 000 and 98 000 deaths annually in that country.[6] If one adds to that figure the number of deaths due to 'adverse events' (for example, side-effects of medication), John Bunker has estimated that upwards of 150 000 iatrogenic deaths occur in the United States annually, equivalent to the loss of between 6 to 12 months of life expectancy.[7] If Bunker's estimates are correct, that would make iatrogenic deaths the fourth leading cause of mortality in the US, after coronary heart disease (725 000 deaths), malignant neoplasms (549 800 deaths), and cerebrovascular disease (167 300 deaths).

Iatrogenic deaths: the fourth leading cause of mortality in the US.

A separate line of reasoning that questions the contribution of medicine to population health focuses on the empirical relationship between national expenditures on medical care and life expectancies in different countries, which reveals very little association between the two.[8] For example, the United States spends over half of every medical dollar expended on the planet, yet achieves a level of health that is lower than that of most other industrialised countries that spend considerably less.[9]

Medical care as 'the ambulance waiting at the bottom of the cliff'

Does all this mean that medical care is unimportant in determining a population's level of health? Social epidemiologists have not disputed the relevance of medical care as a determinant of population health, but at the same time, they have also tended to downgrade its significance relative to other *social* determinants, such as the distribution of income, schooling, employment and working conditions, social exclusion, and housing.[10,11] The social epidemiologist's traditional stance is summarised by Daniels *et al.* (p.4):[2]

> *Health is produced not merely by having access to medical prevention and treatment, but also, to a measurably greater extent, by the cumulative experience of social conditions over the course of one's life. By the time a sixty-year old heart attack victim arrives at the emergency room, bodily insults have accumulated over a lifetime. For such a person, medical care is, figuratively speaking, 'the ambulance waiting at the bottom of the cliff'.*

Have critics been too harsh on the role of medical care?

A reconsideration of the social epidemiologist's traditional position suggests that perhaps the profession has been too harsh, especially in the light of careful quantitative assessments of the contribution of medical care to population health improvements.[12,13] McKeown was probably right concluding that the major part of the decline in cause-specific mortality in Britain between the mid-19th and 20th centuries occurred prior to the discovery of medical cures.[5] But his examples were mostly confined to infectious diseases, such as tuberculosis (TB), whooping cough, measles, and his time series ended around 1960. What has happened since 1960?

Decline in mortality occurred prior to the discovery of medical cures, but . . .

Bunker and colleagues attempted to answer this question by developing a comprehensive inventory of medical benefits.[14] Based on clinical trial evidence and the timing of the introduction of different medical innovations, they attempted to quantify the population health impacts of a range of preventive and curative medical services. According to Bunker *et al.*, about 5 years of the 30 year gain in life expectancy which occurred in the United States during the last century (1900 to 1995) could be attributed to medical care.[14] This may seem like a modest benefit. However, their analysis also suggested that the contribution of medicine to population health had been growing in the most recent decades, i.e. the period after McKeown's analysis ends. Thus, of the 7.6 year gain in life expectancy among Americans between 1950 and 1995, fully 50% could be attributed to medical care.[14] Other studies agree with the conclusions of Bunker and his colleagues. For example, Hunink and colleagues attempted to estimate the contribution of medical care to the observed decline of coronary heart disease deaths in the United States between 1980 and 1990.[15] Based on a sophisticated forecasting model incorporating demographic structure, risk factor trends, and evidence-based estimates of the benefits of medical and surgical treatment for heart attacks, Hunink *et al.* concluded that medical care accounted for fully 70% of the observed decline in heart disease mortality during that decade, with the remainder attributable primarily to secular declines in smoking.[15] Medicine, therefore, 'matters after all'.[12] This inescapable conclusion is echoed by David Cutler's recent book, *Your Money or Your Life*, in which he has argued that:[16]

> *Since 1950 the modern medical system has been more important in extending life. A reduction in the number of cases of cardiovascular disease and infant death are the most significant in contributing to longer life. Physical disability has decreased as well. In the post-1950 era, health improvements have more directly followed medical advances. (p. 9).*

Who is right: the social epidemiologists or the defenders of medical care?

The answer is that both groups are telling some part of the truth. Medical care has undoubtedly made a major contribution to population health gains in the last five decades, but, at the same time, the level of spending on medical care cannot explain cross-national variations in health achievement – for example, the fact that the United States (US) spends nearly 14% of gross domestic product (GDP) on medical care, yet remains near the bottom of the international 'league table' of life expectancies.[17] In other words, Bunker, Cutler and others are asking a different question ('What explains the historical trends in improved life expectancy during the past half century?') from the question that social epidemiologists usually pose ('Why are some societies healthy and others not?'). The contribution of medicine varies according to the question being asked.

Although 14% of GDP is spent on medical care, the US is near the bottom of the international 'league table' of life expectancies.

Primary healthcare is a key determinant of population health

How large a role does medicine play, then, in explaining the cross-national variations in health status? As already alluded to, sceptics point out that aggregate national spending on medical care correlates very little with average health status. On the other hand, aggregate medical spending is a crude basis for evaluating the contribution that healthcare could *potentially* make to national health performance. It matters not just how much is spent on medical care, but also *how* spending is allocated across sectors, as well as questions relating to the efficiency and equity of spending, institutional structures and practices, and the strength of healthcare delivery systems. Growing evidence has highlighted the importance of primary healthcare systems as a key determinant of the health of nations.

In a series of articles, Barbara Starfield, Leiyu Shi and colleagues have demonstrated the role of primary healthcare as a key ingredient of population health.[18-20] In a pooled, cross-sectional time series analysis of 18 wealthy Organization for Economic Cooperation and Development (OECD) countries from 1970 to 1998, Shi and coworkers found that the strength of a country's primary healthcare system was inversely associated with (1) all-cause mortality; (b) all-cause premature mortality; and (c) cause-specific premature mortality from preventable causes including asthmas and bronchitis, pneumonia, and cardiovascular disease ($P < 0.05$ in fixed effects, multivariable adjusted regression analyses).[19] These associations were robust after control for other country-level variables, including GDP per capita, total physicians per 1000 of population, and percentage of elderly people in the population.

It matters not just how much is spent on medical care, but also *how* spending is allocated across sectors.

The authors evaluated the strength of each country's primary healthcare system by adopting a multidimensional index which incorporated institutional and policy characteristics such as geographic regulation (do specific national policies exist to regulate the distribution of primary care providers and facilities?), financing (what is the method of financing healthcare for the majority of the population?), access (what is the level of cost sharing for primary care visits?), longitudinality (are individual patient lists required for all primary care visits?), co-ordination (are guidelines for the transfer of information between primary care and other levels available and required?), and community-orientation (is there a policy that requires the use of community-based data and/or the presence of community members in primary care management or priority setting?).

The ranking of individual countries revealed some striking variations in the strength of primary care systems. For example, those countries with predominantly tax-based health financing also tended to score higher on the index of primary healthcare system performance – e.g. the UK (ranked at the top of 18 countries), Denmark (2nd), as well as neighbouring Nordic countries (Finland, 6th; Norway 7th, Sweden 10th). The authors noted that the Netherlands (ranked 4th) was the exception to the generalisation:

Although it does not have a purely tax-based health financing system, the Netherlands does share other features of primary care (such as few barriers to access, geographic regulation of primary care, use of family practitioners as gatekeepers, and a family-orientation) with its Scandinavian neighbours, all of which have high primary care scores (pp. 845–6).[20]

In countries with a strong primary healthcare system, the population is healthier and mortality is lower.

Based on the predominantly private financing of healthcare, absence of geographic regulation, high levels of primary care visit copayments, lack of co-ordination and community orientation, and the paucity of general practitioners (GPs), it comes as no surprise that the United States ranked near the bottom of the countries studied (tied for 16th out of 18 OECD countries). In a separate analysis conducted by the same group of researchers, primary care was inversely associated with population health *within* the US from 1980 to 1995.[21] Both contemporaneous and time-lagged analyses showed that the primary care physician-to-population ratios in each of the 50 US states were significantly associated with lower all-cause mortality rates ($P < 0.05$ across all time periods). By contrast, higher specialty care indicators were associated with higher mortality rates. These studies suggest the potential contribution that strong primary care systems could make to population health, even in a country like the United States.

The challenge of health disparities

One of the chief challenges for population health remains the existence and persistence of health disparities, whether by socio-economic status, sex, race/ethnicity, or immigrant status.[11] The second Dutch National Survey of General Practice (DNSGP-2) has revealed the existence of these health disparities in the Netherlands (*see* Chapter 7). What is the role of primary healthcare in reducing such disparities?

Healthcare, by itself, is insufficient to eliminate health disparities. This is perhaps the most basic tenet of social epidemiology and of the field of the social determinants of health in general.[2] In a country like the US where upwards of 43 million citizens lack health insurance, universal healthcare remains one of the top priorities for reducing health disparities. However, even if universal healthcare could be achieved in the US, it is unlikely to *eliminate* health disparities, because many other factors besides access to medical care determine the observed social inequalities in health and disease prognosis.[22] The introduction of the National Health Service in Britain following the Second World War did not eliminate health disparities in that nation. Socio-economic inequalities in health have been observed in all societies, not just the United States where one in six citizens goes without health insurance.[23]

Healthcare, by itself, is insufficient to eliminate health disparities.

Here again, it is important to avoid falling into the trap of polarised discussions about the comparative contributions of medical care and the so-called social determinants of health disparities. Strengthening healthcare systems (especially primary care) and social conditions are not competing objectives. For example, both primary care and income inequality (a *social* determinant of population health and health disparities) have been shown to be associated with levels of health within US communities.

A strong primary care has been shown to mitigate the adverse association of income inequality with population health.

Good primary care experience, in particular enhanced accessibility and conti-nuity, are associated with better self-reported physical and mental health.[18] Conversely, higher levels of income inequality have been associated with worse population health and wider socio-economic disparities in health.[17] Importantly, strong primary care has been shown to mitigate the adverse asso-ciation of income inequality with population health; it is especially beneficial in communities with the highest levels of income inequality.[18,21] In essence, primary care and social determinants are complementary inputs to the goal of reducing health disparities.

Medicine matters after all, especially primary care!

The key message of social epidemiology is that there are many determinants of population health and health disparities besides what takes place within the healthcare sector. But the critics of the social determinants perspective make a valid point: that in the general enthusiasm to get their message out, social epidemiologists have undervalued the potential contribution of medical care. As argued by Bunker:[12]

> *The provision of medical care, the development of healthier personal habits, and the creation of a more just social environment each harbour the potential to improve health ... Each strategy can potentially lessen inequalities in health. All deserve government consideration, and it is a question of how much to invest in each. The government, if it hopes to 'improve the health of everyone, and the health of the worst off in particular', must not place its hopes too heavily on lifestyle changes, nor should it expect that social reform, however desirable in the name of social justice, will resolve the problem of inequalities in health (pp. 90–1).*

Strong healthcare systems, especially those emphasising primary care, are an essential ingredient for advancing population health and tackling health dispar-ities. Any strategy to improve the health of the nation that ignores the contribution of general practice does so at its peril.

References

1 Wilkinson R (1996) *Unhealthy Societies. The afflictions of inequality.* Routledge, London.

2 Daniels N, Kennedy B and Kawachi I (2000) *Is Inequality Bad for Our Health?* Beacon Press, Boston.

3 Dubos R (1959) *Mirage of Health: utopias, progress and biological change.* George Allen & Unwin, London.

4 Illich I (1975) *Medical Nemesis.* Calder and Boyars, London.

5 McKeown T (1976) *The Role of Medicine: dream, mirage, or nemesis?* Nuffield Provincial Hospitals Trust, London.

6 Kohn LT, Corrigan JM, Donaldson MS (2000) *To Err is Human: building a safer health system.* National Academy Press, Washington DC.

7 Bunker J (2001) The role of medical care in population health. *Int J Epidemiol.* **30**: 1260–3.

8 House JS and Williams DR (2000) Understanding and reducing socioeconomic and racial/ethnic disparities in health. In: Smedley BD and Syme SL (eds) *Promoting Health. Intervention strategies from social and behavioral research.* National Academy Press, Washington DC, pp. 81–124.

9 Starfield B (2000) Is US health really the best in the world? *JAMA.* **284**: 483–5.

10 Marmot M and Wilkinson RG (eds) (1999) *Social Determinants of Health.* Oxford University Press, Oxford.

11 Berkman LF and Kawachi I (eds) (2000) *Social Epidemiology.* Oxford University Press, New York.

12 Bunker J (2001) *Medicine Matters After All. Measuring the benefits of medical care, a healthy lifestyle, and a just social environment.* Nuffield Trust Series, No. 15. The Stationery Office, London.

13 Cutler DM (2004) *Your Money or Your Life.* Oxford University Press, New York.

14 Bunker J, Frazier HP and Mosteller F (1995). The role of medical care in determining health: Creating an inventory of benefits. In: Amick III BC, Levine S, Tarlov AR, Chapman Walsh D (eds) *Society and Health.* Oxford University Press, New York, pp. 305–41.

15 Hunink MGM, Goldman L, Tosteson ANA and Weinstein MC (1997) The recent decline in mortality from coronary heart disease, 1980–1990: The effect of secular trends in risk factors and treatment. *JAMA.* **277**: 535–42.

16 Cutler D (2004) *Your Money or Your Life.* Oxford University Press, Oxford.

17 Kawachi I and Kennedy BP (2002) *The Health of Nations. Why inequality is harmful to your health.* The New Press, New York.

18 Shi L, Starfield B, Politzer R and Regan J (2002) Primary care, self-rated health, and reductions in social disparities in health. *Health Serv Res.* **37**: 529–50.

19 Shi L, Macinko J, Starfield B, Xu J and Politzer R (2003) Primary care, income inequality, and stroke mortality in the United States: a longitudinal analysis, 1985–1995. *Stroke.* **34**: 1957–64.

20 Macinko J, Starfield B and Shi L (2003) The contribution of primary care systems to health outcomes within Organization for Economic Cooperation and Development (OECD) countries, 1970–1998. *Health Serv Res.* **38**: 831–65.

21 Shi L, Macinko J, Starfield B *et al.* (2003) The relationship between primary care, income inequality, and mortality in US states, 1980–1995. *J Am Board Fam Pract.* **16**: 412–22.

22 Adler NE, Boyce T, Chesney MA, Folkman S and Syme SL (1993) Socioeconomic inequalities in health: No easy solution. *JAMA.* **269**: 3140–5.

23 Marmot M, Bobak M, Davey Smith G (1995) Explanations for social inequalities in health. In: Amick III BC , Levine S, Tarlov AR, Chapman Walsh D (eds) *Society and Health.* Oxford University Press, New York, pp. 172–210.

Part 2

Health and disparities

Chapter 5

Morbidity in the population and in general practice

Michiel van der Linden, François Schellevis and Gert Westert

What is this chapter about?

This chapter uses data from the second Dutch National Survey of General Practice (DNSGP-2) to describe the health status of the population and health problems presented to general practice in 2001. The results will be compared with data from the first Dutch National Survey of General Practice (DNSGP-1), 1987. We conclude that the health status of the Dutch people has undeniably changed during the last 15 years. More people than in 1987 reported having health problems, especially locomotory symptoms, fatigue and sleeping problems. The demand for general practice care has increased, but this has not resulted in an increase in the number of diagnoses. There is a relative increase in the number of conditions of the skin and the locomotory tract presented to the general practitioner (GP), but not of psychosocial problems.

Introduction

Reference data with regard to the frequency of complaints and conditions are important for policy makers and researchers in the field of general practice. Such data, derived from a nationwide, representative network of simultaneously recording GPs, allow uniform analyses and are a valuable source for research and healthcare planning. The desirability of such an information infrastructure has been expressed in the Dutch Public Health Forecast Report of 1997.[1] The first and second Dutch National Surveys have been designed to allow the collection of comprehensive data on the health status of the Dutch, their use of care and the performance of Dutch GPs. The information goes beyond the domain of general practice and includes self-care and informal care, and the care provided by other primary and secondary care professionals.

This chapter gives an overview of symptoms, conditions and other aspects of the population's health as recorded by the DNSGP-2. Both the health status as reported by the population and the health status as recorded by the GPs are included. Comparison with the results from the DNSGP-1 of 1987 makes it possible to show differences in the population's health status over 15 years.

How was it done?

For a description of the methods of the first and second Dutch National Surveys of General Practice, DNSGP-1 of 1987 and DNSGP-2 of 2001, *see* Chapter 2. The following is specific for the study described in this chapter.

Self-reported health

Data about self-reported health were derived from a written questionnaire and a health interview. For the written questionnaire, all patients listed in the participating practices were approached. As in 1987, the questionnaire included questions about sociodemographic characteristics and the one-item question on perceived health:[2] the participants could rate their health in five categories ranging from 'very bad' to 'very good'. The questionnaire was sent to 385 461 persons and 294 999 responded (76.5%). The health interview was administered to a random sample of approximately 4% of the listed population ($n =$ 19 685, response $n =$ 12 699, i.e. 65%). The interview included questions directed at various aspects of health, including recent complaints, short-term conditions and long-term conditions. For this, validated instruments were used: the 'list of acute symptoms', and the 'list of long-term conditions'.[3] Functional status was investigated using the medical outcomes study (MOS) short-form-36, a 36–item questionnaire containing eight health dimensions.[4] Dimension scores were calculated according to the standard instructions on a 0–100 scale, with high scores indicating good functional status. To assess mental wellbeing, the 12–item version of the General Health Questionnaire (GHQ) was included in the health interview.[5] A score of 2 or higher indicates a higher risk for psychological problems.

Morbidity in general practice

Morbidity presented to the GP was derived from diagnoses made in contacts between patients and the GP recorded in the electronic medical records of the practice information system. Contact diagnoses were coded using the International Classification of Primary Care (ICPC).[6] Contacts for the same medical problem were clustered into episodes of care. Episodes were used to calculate annual incidence and prevalence rates. Incidence refers to the number of newly presented episodes of disease; period prevalence refers to the number of people with at least one disease episode. For each ICPC code, annual rates were calculated across sex and age groups. Detailed tables with incidence and prevalence rates by ICPC code can be found on www.NIVEL.nl/nationalestudie.

What was found?

Self-reported health

Table 5.1 shows the self-reported health as derived from the one-item questionnaire.

Table 5.1 Perceived health (scores on the 'one-item' questionnaire) by sex (all ages)

	Males (n = 130 684) (%)	Females (n = 140 640) (%)	Total (n = 271 324) (%)
Very good	26.0	22.1	24.0
Good	58.1	58.3	58.2
Neither good nor bad	13.6	16.9	15.3
Bad	2.0	2.3	2.2
Very bad	0.4	0.4	0.4

Compared to 1987, the percentage of people reporting (very) good health in 2001 was 2.3% lower after adjustment for age.

From the list of 31 acute symptoms, 88.6% of the respondents reported having suffered from one or more symptoms in the previous fortnight. The average number of reported symptoms was 4.0 (standard deviation (SD) 3.7). Table 5.2 shows the 10 most frequently reported symptoms.

Long-term conditions were reported by almost 57% of the respondents. Migraine, osteoarthritis and hypertension were among the most frequently reported conditions (see Table 5.3).

Compared to 1987, 8% more people reported suffering from a chronic condition.

Functional health status can be considered as good with dimension scores ranging from 65.4 to 89.6 on a 0–100 scale (see Table 5.4). A comparison with

Table 5.2 Frequency of 10 most frequently reported symptoms during 2 weeks preceding the health interview by sex (all ages)

	Males (n = 5845) (%)	Females (n = 6827) (%)	Total (n = 12 672) (%)
Fatigue	28.4	42.5	36.0
Headache	25.5	40.7	33.7
Sleeplessness, bad sleeping	18.1	28.4	23.6
Pain in neck, shoulder, upper back	15.3	26.1	21.1
Stuffed-up nose	20.6	21.0	20.8
Low back pain	16.6	22.2	19.6
Coughing	17.3	18.3	17.8
Being nervous, anxious, stressed, tensed	13.1	20.6	17.2
Pain in hip or knee	10.0	15.1	12.8
Feeling aggressive, easily angry or irritated	11.6	12.6	12.2

Table 5.3 Frequency of 10 most frequently reported chronic conditions during 12 months preceding the health interview by sex (all ages)

	Males (n = 5860) (%)	Females (n = 6839) (%)	Total (n = 12 699) (%)
Migraine or regularly serious headache	9.5	20.9	15.7
Osteoarthritis of hip or knee	9.9	14.9	12.6
Hypertension	10.3	13.8	12.2
Serious or persistent disorder of the neck or shoulder	7.6	12.7	10.4
Serious or persistent disorder of the back, including herniation of the intervertebral disc	9.4	11.2	10.4
Serious or persistent disorder of the elbow, wrist or hand	5.0	9.0	7.1
Asthma, chronic bronchitis, or emphysema	8.2	8.4	8.3
Unintentional loss of urine (incontinence)	1.8	10.3	6.5
Chronic eczema	6.7	6.6	6.7
Cancer	3.6	4.7	4.2

Table 5.4 Functional health status (SF-36 scores on eight dimensions) of respondents 16 years and older in the DNSGP-2 (2001) compared with Dutch reference data (1996)

	2001 (n = 9969) mean (SD)	1996 (n = 1742) mean (SD)	Difference 2001–1996
Physical functioning	86.1 (21.7)	83.0 (22.8)	+3.1
Social functioning	86.4 (20.1)	84.0 (22.4)	+2.4
Role limitations: physical	79.6 (35.6)	76.4 (36.3)	+3.2
Role limitations: emotional	89.6 (26.5)	82.3 (32.9)	+7.3
Mental health	80.1 (15.8)	76.8 (17.4)	+3.3
Vitality	69.6 (18.9)	68.6 (19.3)	+1.0
Bodily pain	65.4 (21.6)	74.9 (23.4)	−9.5
General medical health	69.1 (20.1)	70.7 (20.7)	−1.6

SD: standard deviation.

1987 is not possible because this instrument was not available at the time. Comparison with other Dutch reference data showed no statistically significant differences.[7]

The scores on the GHQ-12 indicate that 22.8% of the adult respondents (18 years and older) are at risk for psychopathology (*see* Table 5.5). This proportion is 6.0% higher than in 1987.

In summary, the vast majority of people consider their health as good or very good, although they frequently experience common symptoms; half of the population reports suffering from a chronic condition and one-fifth is at risk for psychopathology. Moreover, this picture has worsened since 1987.

Table 5.5 Mental wellbeing (scores on GHQ-12) in respondents of 18 years and older by sex

GHQ score	Males (n = 4328) (%)	Females (n = 5357) (%)	Total (n = 9685) (%)	Total cumulative %
0	68.6	59.9	63.8	63.8
1	12.1	14.5	13.4	77.2
2	6.0	7.2	6.7	83.9
3	3.5	4.3	4.0	87.9
4	2.1	3.3	2.8	90.6
5–8	5.8	7.6	6.8	97.4
9–12	1.8	3.1	2.6	100.0

Morbidity in general practice

The annual proportion of listed patients who consulted their GP at least once was 77% and this has not changed since 1987. However, the frequency of consultations of those patients that do visit their GP has increased (*see* Chapter 12). This increase has not led to an increase in the number of diagnoses made.

Table 5.6 shows the incidence and prevalence rates of diseases presented to GPs in 2001, clustered according to organ systems (ICPC chapters). Compared to 1987, cardiovascular and psychological problems have proportionally decreased the most, and skin and musculoskeletal problems have increased the most.

Publicly insured people showed generally higher incidence and prevalence rates than privately insured people. This was most apparent for neurological problems, psychological problems, female genital system problems and problems related to pregnancy, childbearing and family planning. People of non-western origin showed higher incidence and prevalence rates than native Dutch people, especially for problems of the digestive tract, the respiratory tract, the skin and musculoskeletal problems.

Table 5.7 shows the rates of the 10 most frequent newly presented diseases (incidences) for males and females.

Table 5.8 shows the 10 most frequently encountered diseases in general practice.

Self-reported health and morbidity in general practice compared

Not all health problems experienced by people will be presented to the GP; this is usually referred to as the 'iceberg phenomenon'.[8] Table 5.9 shows the frequency of chronic conditions as reported by respondents on the health interview, and the frequency of the same chronic conditions presented in general practice.

This table shows that in general more people report suffering from a chronic condition than the frequency of this condition in general practice would suggest. The difference is smaller for conditions with a clear diagnosis such as diabetes mellitus and hypertension.

Table 5.6 Frequency of symptoms and diseases presented to general practice by ICPC chapter; annual incidence rates and prevalence rates per 1000 registered patients (all ages) per year (n = 375 899)

ICPC chapter		Incidence rate (per 1000 per year)	Period prevalence rate (per 1000 in 1 year)
A	General and unspecified	79	119
B	Blood, blood-forming organs and immune mechanism	12	22
D	Digestive	103	178
F	Eye	53	79
H	Ear	86	114
K	Circulatory	52	171
L	Musculoskeletal	267	397
N	Neurological	40	74
P	Psychological	52	125
R	Respiratory	214	318
S	Skin	240	361
T	Endocrine, metabolic and nutritional	19	74
U	Urinary system	49	65
W	Pregnancy, childbearing, family planning	74[a]	196[a]
X	Female genital system (including breast)	106[a]	178[a]
Y	Male genital system	33[b]	53[b]
Z	Social problems	17	26

[a]Per 1000 females.
[b]Per 1000 males.

Table 5.7 Frequency of the 10 most frequently newly presented diseases to general practice; incidence rates per 1000 registered patients (all ages) per year

ICPC code		Incidence rate (per 1000 per year)		
		Males (n = 186 727)	Females (n = 189 172)	Total (n = 375 899)
R74	Acute upper respiratory infection	45.6	57.0	51.3
R05	Cough	29.5	38.7	34.1
U71	Cystitis/other urinary infection	7.7	58.5	33.3
S74	Dermatophytosis	30.4	31.4	30.9
L03	Low back symptom/complaint	27.0	26.2	26.6
S88	Contact dermatitis/other eczema	21.0	31.8	26.4
H81	Excessive ear wax	26.5	23.9	25.2
R75	Acute/chronic sinusitis	15.2	28.8	22.1
R78	Acute bronchitis/bronchiolitis	19.9	23.0	21.5
A04	General weakness/tiredness	12.5	24.3	18.5

Table 5.8 Frequency of 10 most frequently presented diseases to general practice; period prevalence rates per 1000 registered patients (all ages) in one year

ICPC code		Period prevalence rate (per 1000 in one year)		
		Males (n = 186 727)	Females (n = 189 172)	Total (n = 375 899)
K86	Uncomplicated hypertension	43.8	70.8	57.1
R74	Acute upper respiratory infection	49.9	63.4	56.4
S74	Dermatophytosis	46.5	47.7	46.9
R05	Cough	39.4	54.1	46.6
S88	Contact dermatitis/other eczema	36.5	53.9	45.1
L03	Low back symptom/complaint	39.2	40.6	39.7
U71	Cystitis/other urinary infection	9.5	67.6	38.5
H81	Excessive ear wax	34.1	30.9	32.3
R97	Hay fever/allergic rhinitis	25.1	30.8	27.8
R75	Acute/chronic sinusitis	19.3	35.8	27.4

Table 5.9 Number of self-reported chronic conditions during 12 months preceding the health interview and frequency of these conditions presented to general practice in one year in persons of 25 years and older

	Self-reported ($n = 8940$) (%)	Presented in general practice per 100 in one year ($n = 260\ 899$)
Migraine or regularly serious headache	18.3	3.8
Osteoarthritis of hip or knee	14.9	2.5
Hypertension	14.3	11.5
Serious or persistent disorder of the neck or shoulder	14.0	8.8
Serious or persistent disorder of the back, including herniation of the intervertebral disc	13.9	9.6
Serious or persistent disorder of the elbow, wrist or hand	9.6	2.4
Asthma, chronic bronchitis, or emphysema	7.8	3.8
Unintentional loss of urine (incontinence)	7.5	0.9
Chronic eczema	6.1	6.8
Cancer	5.9	1.7
Chronic arthritis	5.1	1.7
Diabetes mellitus	4.5	4.0
Vertigo with falling	4.2	1.8
Myocardial infarction	3.8	1.4
Serious or persistent bowel disorders of more than three months' duration	3.7	1.8
Narrowing of blood vessels in abdomen or legs	3.4	0.5
Stroke	2.8	1.0
Other serious heart disease (e.g. angina pectoris, heart failure)	2.6	4.3
Psoriasis	2.6	0.7

What to think about it

The number of self-reported conditions increased compared with 1987, and also the number of people rating their health in general as (very) good decreased. Among self-reported recent complaints, sleep problems and fatigue are high on the list. The number of participants that indicated having 'no chronic condition' has also decreased. Reported frequencies of individual chronic conditions in subgroups have increased as much as 10–fold (osteoarthritis among women). Assessment of mental wellbeing showed an increase in the number of participants with a score over the threshold value, indicating that more people are at risk for psychological problems than in 1987.

With regard to the nature of the morbidity presented to the general practice, there have been shifts in the conditions presented since 1987. Differences in incidence and prevalence rates between the sexes, and between ethnic groups (after standardisation for age) are largely in accordance with literature.

Important findings are a relative increase in problems of the skin and the locomotory system, and a relative decrease in mental and social problems.

Demand on general practice has increased during the last 15 years, but the number of diagnoses made did not change.

The worsening of self-reported health is not reflected in higher morbidity rates in general practice. One explanation could be that the threshold for reporting health problems in a health interview has lowered, in the sense that people more easily perceive their health as impaired. The differences between the frequency of self-reported chronic conditions and those in general practice are not only explained by the fact that these chronic conditions occur mainly among patients who do not consult the GP very often. There are many explanations for this lack of agreement between patient and doctor. Explanations may differ by population subgroup and by condition. Conditions with strict diagnostic criteria, such as diabetes mellitus and hypertension, are characterised by a larger degree of agreement. For these diagnoses it is essential that the patient pays a visit to the practice and undergoes ongoing treatment or follow-up.

Conclusion

The health status of the Dutch has undeniably changed during the last 15 years. In summary, we observed the following:

Self-reported health

- 18% of the population report their health as less than 'good', an increase of approximately 2% since 1987.
- The proportion of persons who report recent symptoms has increased from 78% to 89%.
- With regard to chronic conditions, locomotory complaints have increased strongly (e.g. osteoarthritis in women, from 1.4% to 14.9%).
- Functional health status has not clearly changed. The proportion of people scoring above the threshold score of 2 on the GHQ-12 – indicating a higher risk for psychological problems – has increased from 17% in 1987 to 23% in 2001.

Health problems presented to general practice

- From the listed population, 77% presented at least one condition to general practice in the course of one year. This did not change since 1987. Age and sex, and socio-economic disparities of the presented morbidity were in accordance with the literature.
- Of all conditions, essential hypertension comes out as the most frequent, and of newly diagnosed conditions, upper respiratory tract infections as the most frequent.

- Since 1987, there has been a relative increase in conditions of the skin and locomotory tract.
- The frequency of chronic conditions by self-report and diagnosed in general practice differed most for severe headache/migraine (difference of 15%) and least for diabetes mellitus (difference 0.5%).

Many people indicated they have more health problems, especially locomotory complaints, fatigue and sleeping problems. The demand made on general practice has increased, but this is not translated into an increase in the number of diagnoses made. There is a relative increase in general practice in the number of conditions of the skin and locomotory tract, but not of psychosocial problems.

References

1 Ruwaard D and Kramers PGN (eds) (1998) *Public Health Status and Forecasts 1997. Health prevention and health care in the Netherlands until 2015.* Elsevier/de Tijdstroom, Maarsen.
2 Mossey JM and Shapiro E (1982) Self-rated health: a predictor of mortality among the elderly. *Am J Pub Health.* **72**: 800–8.
3 CBS (NL Statistics Netherlands) (2003) *POLS/Gezondheidmonitor Bevolking.* [Health Monitor.] Statistics Netherlands, Voorburg/Heerlen.
4 Ware JE and Sherbourne CD (1992) The MOS 36–item short-form health survey (SF-36). I Conceptual framework and item selection. *Med Care.* **30**: 473–83.
5 Goldberg DP (1972) *The Detection of Psychiatric Illness by Questionnaire.* Oxford University Press, London.
6 Lamberts H and Wood M (eds) (1987) *The International Classification of Primary Care.* Oxford University Press, Oxford.
7 Aaronson NK, Muller M, Cohen PD *et al.* (1998) Translation, validation, and norming of the Dutch language version of the SF-36 Health Survey in community and chronic disease populations. *J Clin Epidemiol.* **51**: 1055–68.
8 Last JM (1963) The iceberg: 'completing the clinical picture' in general practice. *Lancet.* **ii**: 28–31.

Chapter 6

A comparison of disease prevalence in general practice in the Netherlands and in England and Wales

Douglas Fleming, François Schellevis, Michiel van der Linden and Gert Westert

What is this chapter about?

General practice-based morbidity surveys have been conducted in the Netherlands and in England and Wales primarily to estimate disease prevalence and examine health inequalities. We have compared disease prevalence in general practice reported in the second Dutch National Survey of General Practice (DNSGP-2) with prevalence data collected in the same year (2001) in the Weekly Returns Service (WRS) in England and Wales. Diseases were selected according to interest and compatibility of classification (International Classification of Primary Care (ICPC-1), DNSGP-2; Read-International Classification of Disease (ICD)-9, WRS). Age- and sex-specific prevalence rates were standardised to the national census population of England and Wales (2001). Differences between the surveys were determined from non-overlapping 99% confidence intervals. Although many small differences were identified, the similarities were more striking. Important differences included higher prevalence of lung cancer, diabetes mellitus, mental disorders and musculoskeletal conditions in the Netherlands, and lower prevalence of prostate cancer (but not of benign prostatic hypertrophy), hypothyroidism and respiratory infections. Some of the differences identified may have been influenced by the use of different classification systems, others may relate to differing consulting behaviour, and some reflect true national differences.

Introduction

National morbidity surveys in general practice serve many purposes, chief of which is to describe the incidence and prevalence of disease in general practice indicating the morbidity profile in the community. For the majority of conditions, persons presenting to healthcare provide particularly useful information since they reflect the demand on healthcare facilities, and the knowledge and opinion of the community on the ability of the health service to respond to their needs and provide a basis for resource allocation. With few exceptions, conditions excluded from healthcare do not require essential treatment. Practice-based morbidity surveys also permit comparisons between groups and over time. Surveys in differing countries provide a basis for international comparison of health problems, and opportunities to refine recording methods in the interests of harmonisation and of creating a truly comparative international framework for disease monitoring, as has been envisaged at a European level.[1]

In England and Wales, the history of national morbidity surveys started with the Survey of Sickness 1943–52 which was based on patient-reported symptoms/diseases and was very difficult to interpret.[2] The first major survey in general practice was conducted in 1956 and was based on the general practitioners' (GPs') interpretation and diagnosis for presented problems which were recorded on summary cards and analysed according to the rubrics of the International Classification of Disease (ICD) version 7.[3] Other national surveys followed in 1970/1971, 1980/1981, and 1991/1992.[4–6] The first two involved recording diagnoses in diagnostic indexes and the last of these collected data on patient-specific electronic medical records (EMR). All these data included patient-specific data on socio-economic and demographic characteristics. Data on referrals and – to a limited extent – on patient investigation were also collected. All diagnoses were analysed according to the ICD, most recently based on version 9 though data entry in the most recent survey was facilitated using the Read Code Thesaurus.[7] The recording methods established for that survey have been continued in the Weekly Returns Service of the Royal College of General Practitioners (WRS) and annual reports on disease prevalence are now available from this network.[8,9]

In the Netherlands, the first major general practice-based morbidity survey was conducted in 1987 and the second in 2001. The first survey was limited to a morbidity registration during a 3-months period per practice; the second survey included data from a full 12-months period.[10,11] Both surveys collected diagnostic data which were coded to the rubrics of the International Classification of Primary Care version 1 (ICPC-1).[12] In the 1987 survey, coding was carried out by trained clerks; in the 2001 survey the participating GPs coded the diagnostic information themselves. In both surveys, the GPs were specifically encouraged to report their interpretation of the consultation rather than merely record the symptoms prompting the reason for encounter. Both studies included patient-specific, sociodemographic data, and both examined other elements of practice activity including referrals to secondary care and prescriptions issued.

Similar research designs made comparison of morbidity patterns between UK and the Netherlands possible.

This study compares the findings on the prevalence of selected diseases as reported in the national morbidity study in the Netherlands in 2001 (second Dutch National Survey of General Practice – DNSGP-2),[11] with those reported in the WRS estimation of annual prevalence in the same year.[9] The selection of diseases was made on the basis of potential interest, compatibility of classifications and relative frequency.

How was it done?

Design

For a description of the methods of the DNSGP-2, *see* Chapter 2 of this book. For the study prescribed in this chapter the data of 8 of the 104 practices were excluded from the analyses; from three because of problems with data transfer, and from five because recording standards were not met. In total, data from 96 practices (185 GPs) were used in this study.

The WRS 2001 survey included data from 38 practices (163 GPs) out of the total 78 (378 GPs) who provided weekly returns in that year. Recruited practices were restricted to those with computer software capable of delivering an analysis over a full 12–month period. The standard software was originally designed to provide weekly and not annual data returns. Apart from the population monitored (considered below) the representativeness of these GPs and their practices has not been studied.

Population denominator

In the DNSGP-2, the total practice population was determined on the basis of the administrative registration of the patient in the practice computer; personalised data about age and sex were extracted. Population data were extracted at the beginning and at the end of the registration period, and the mathematical average (mid-time) was used as the epidemiological denominator (*n* all ages = 375 899) in all age groups, except children aged less than 12 months, where for the purpose of comparison with the national population, we estimated the population at risk from the number of person days included in the 12–month study period.

The WRS population was defined from a count of all persons registered at the midpoint of the survey (*n* all ages = 325 850).

Disease prevalence

The one-year period prevalence of disease was examined in the respective 12–month survey periods (DNSGP-2 12 months per participating practice between May 2000 and April 2002, 87% in calendar year 2001; WRS 1 January to 31 December 2001) on the basis of a consultation with the recording GP on at least one occasion in this period for the specified condition or group of conditions. Conditions were grouped into clusters to match as well as possible the ICD-9 three-digit and major subgroup categories. Conditions creating substantial difficulty for matching were either excluded from this study or considered at a lower level of precision – e.g. by ICD chapter. Diseases and groups of diseases examined are detailed by the codes in the two classification systems in Appendix 6.1.

Prevalence rates per 10 000 were generated separately by gender and in age groups (<1, 1–4, 5–14, 15–24, 25–44, 45–64, 65–74, 75 years and over). Gender-specific age-standardised prevalence rates (SPR) were calculated by applying the age-specific incidence rates from both surveys to the national population estimate for England and Wales established in the national census for 2001.[13] Confidence intervals (99%) were calculated, based on the proportion of the population consulting, and study differences were defined as non-overlapping confidence intervals.

What was found?

The populations surveyed, and the percentage of the respective national populations are given in Table 6.1: differences between the survey populations and the national populations with regard to the age and sex distribution are small.

Data on selected diseases are reported as gender-specific SPRs in ICD chapter order in Table 6.2.

SPRs for infectious diseases show differences between the Netherlands and England and Wales with respect to chickenpox (approximately 50% lower in the Netherlands), herpes simplex in females (lower in the Netherlands), infectious mononucleosis (approximately 50% higher in the Netherlands) and candidiasis in females (lower in the Netherlands).

The SPRs for breast and bladder cancer were similar; for lung and bronchial cancer SPRs in the Netherlands exceeded the rates of England and Wales for males; and for prostate cancer the rate in the Netherlands was lower. SPRs for all benign neoplasms were similar, but SPRs were lower in the Netherlands for those involving the skin.

SPRs for diabetes mellitus reported in the Netherlands were approximately 30% higher than in England and Wales. Also, in the Netherlands, the SPR for females exceeded the male equivalent, whereas the opposite was observed in England and Wales. For hypothyroidism, rates among females were lower in the Netherlands than in England and Wales. Male SPRs for gout were identical, but in females the SPR was higher in England and Wales. Differences between the countries in the prevalence of hypothyroidism and diabetes were explored further in persons aged over 25 years (*see* Figure 6.1, p. 50). For hypothyroidism, the prevalence in the Netherlands fell after the age of 65 years, whereas for diabetes mellitus it increased: the opposite was reported for England and Wales.

Table 6.1 Size of the survey populations and percentages of national populations by age and sex

| Age (years) | The Netherlands | | | | England and Wales | | | |
| | Male | | Female | | Male | | Female | |
	n	%	n	%	n	%	n	%
<1	2 258	2.13	2 123	2.10	1 937	0.65	1 861	0.65
1–4	9 516	2.34	8 777	2.27	8 083	0.62	7 577	0.62
5–14	24 002	2.38	22 792	2.36	21 664	0.63	20 652	0.63
15–24	22 984	2.39	23 552	2.53	20 117	0.63	20 010	0.64
25–44	61 538	2.42	59 676	2.43	50 671	0.68	49 419	0.64
45–64	46 811	2.35	44 968	2.31	39 583	0.65	39 131	0.63
65–74	12 498	2.25	14 407	2.22	11 665	0.57	12 969	0.56
75+	7 638	2.25	13 364	2.11	7 491	0.52	13 020	0.52
Total	186 727	2.36	189 172	2.37	161 211	0.64	164 639	0.62

Table 6.2 Standardised prevalence rates for selected diseases and disease groups in the Netherlands (NL) and England and Wales (E&W) by sex, by ICD chapters and ICD codes (per 10000)

	Males		Females	
	NL	E&W	NL	E&W
Chapter I: infectious diseases				
infectious intestinal disease	214	200	238	222
chickenpox	25[a]	46	22[a]	39
herpes simplex	16	20	35[a]	50
infectious mononucleosis	10[a]	6	14[a]	7
candidiasis	56	62	239[a]	271
Chapter II: neoplasms				
carcinoma lung/bronchus	16[a]	9	7	5
carcinoma prostate (males) breast (females)	25[a]	36	43	40
carcinoma bladder	5	6	2	2
all benign neoplasms	137	129	231	213
benign neoplasms skin	76[a]	95	127[a]	162
Chapter III: metabolic disorders				
hypothyroidism	18	24	104[a]	135
diabetes mellitus	271[a]	214	317[a]	173
gout	72	73	25[a]	17
Chapter IV: blood and blood-forming organs				
iron deficiency anaemia	32[a]	21	121[a]	68
other deficiency anaemias	18	14	33[a]	21
Chapter V: mental disorders				
mental disorders	828[a]	625	1325[a]	964
anxiety neuroses	151	177	328[a]	427
depression	166[a]	78	362[a]	177
Chapter VI: diseases of the nervous system and sense organs				
Parkinson's disease	13	15	15	12
epilepsy	32	37	31	30
multiple sclerosis	3	5	7[a]	12
glaucoma	16	23	25	27
cataract	27	33	44[a]	58
acute otitis media	239[a]	267	233[a]	282
otitis externa	169	172	172	182
Chapter VII: diseases of the cardiovascular system				
hypertensive disease	599[a]	528	755[a]	712
ischaemic heart disease	226	233	156	149
heart failure	85[a]	58	102[a]	59
cerebrovascular disease	91[a]	68	103[a]	67
varicose veins	31[a]	50	105	92
haemorrhoids	67	70	103[a]	86
Chapter VIII: diseases of the respiratory system				
acute respiratory infection	1015[a]	1569	1335[a]	2149
acute sinusitis	265[a]	550	488[a]	1260
chronic obstructive pulmonary disease	372[a]	457	400[a]	488

	Males		Females	
	NL	E&W	NL	E&W
Chapter IX: diseases of the digestive system				
diseases of the oesophagus and stomach	213[a]	250	241[a]	280
inguinal hernia	48	57	6	6
Chapter X: diseases of the genito-urinary system				
urinary tract infection	107[a]	143	696[a]	590
benign prostatic hypertrophy	66[a]	62	–	–
Chapter XII : diseases of the skin and subcutaneous tissue				
skin infections	297[a]	392	293[a]	463
eczema/dermatitis	516[a]	588	664[a]	763
psoriasis	56	60	50[a]	70
Chapter XIII: diseases of the musculoskeletal system				
rheumatoid arthritis	32[a]	20	71[a]	48
dorsopathies	721[a]	492	846[a]	688

[a]Non-overlapping 99% confidence intervals between NL and E&W within sex.

SPRs for iron deficiency anaemia and for other deficiency anaemias were higher in the Netherlands, the latter only in women.

The SPRs for mental illness were higher in the Netherlands. More detailed analysis disclosed lower levels of anxiety among females but higher levels of depression both in males and females.

Among nervous system disorders, SPRs for Parkinson's disease, epilepsy, glaucoma, and external otitis were similar, but for multiple sclerosis the rates in the Netherlands were lower although the twofold male excess over female was

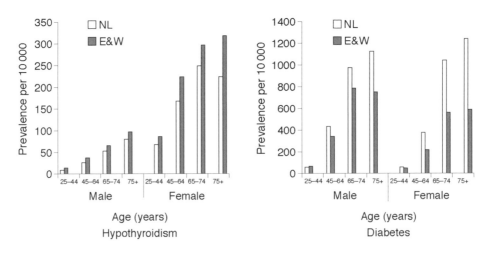

Figure 6.1 Hypothyroidism and diabetes. Prevalence per 10 000 by age and sex. NL: Netherlands; E&W: England & Wales.

similar in both countries. SPRs for cataract in females and for acute otitis media were lower in the Netherlands.

SPRs for hypertensive disease were higher in the Netherlands. SPRs for heart failure and cerebrovascular disease were substantially higher in the Netherlands. For ischaemic heart disease no differences between the two countries could be found. The male SPR for varicose veins was lower and the female SPR for haemorrhoids higher in the Netherlands.

SPRs for all three diseases of the respiratory system under study were considerably lower in the Netherlands.

The SPRs for diseases of the oesophagus, stomach and duodenum (DOSD) were lower in the Netherlands, but SPRs for inguinal hernia did not differ.

Rates in the Netherlands for urinary tract infections were lower in males but higher in females than their equivalents for England and Wales. SPRs for benign prostatic hypertrophy were similar in both countries.

SPRs for skin conditions were lower in the Netherlands than in England and Wales. Age-specific data for psoriasis (*see* Figure 6.2) suggest that GPs in the Netherlands reported fewer young people with psoriasis than GPs in England and Wales. SPRs for dorsopathies and rheumatoid arthritis were higher in the Netherlands.

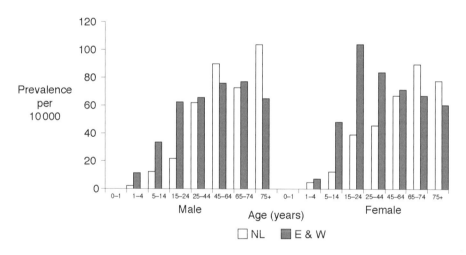

Figure 6.2 Psoriasis. Prevalence per 10 000 by age and sex.
NL: Netherlands; E&W: England and Wales.

What to think about it

These results are discussed from two perspectives: the practical issues surrounding international comparative studies, and the clinical significance of the differences identified.

Comparative studies

We experienced serious limitations in trying to compare data collected in ICPC-1 codes (DNSGP-2) with data collected as Read codes mapped to ICD-9 (WRS).

The Read code is a hierarchical thesaurus with many more terms than are found in ICD and thus grouping to three-digit ICD-coded categories was straightforward. There are fewer ICPC-1 codes than ICD codes and, therefore, we were only able to map several ICPC-1 codes to ICD in broader groups. Even then problems occurred related to the inherent structures of the respective coding systems. For example, herpes simplex and herpes zoster are classified as part of the infectious disease chapter in ICD, but are part of the skin chapter in ICPC; malignancies are grouped together in ICD but are included in the appropriate anatomical chapter in ICPC. The ICD presents problems where conditions can be coded in more than one place – e.g. several infections can be coded by causative organism or clinical manifestation, or coded in both places. The ICPC classification does not allow for dual classification in this way though where possible it integrates symptoms within particular chapters of the classification. It involves the collection of symptoms that may be entered as an alternative to a diagnosis. When considering the prevalence of intestinal infectious diseases, it is necessary to search a wide range of symptomatic and diagnostic codes. In the ICD, non-specific symptom codes are included in Chapter 16 'Symptoms, signs and ill-defined conditions', and are used where there is no reasonable diagnostic alternative. The net result of these constraints was the considerable restriction in the number of conditions compared, and the limitation to those diagnostic groups where an acceptable level of coding comparability was achieved.

Comparison between ICPC and ICD-9 classified illnesses is possible, but only for a restricted set of conditions.

This comparison of national data concerned disease prevalence and was possible because person-specific data were examined. Comparisons of episodes of illness would be more difficult. The WRS protocol requires doctors to define the episode type at each consultation, whereas the DNSGP-2 definition of episode is based on a retrospective clustering of the data on the basis of the episode typing. This distinction relates partly to the fact that the WRS is rooted in the provision of weekly surveillance data. WRS data were extracted from the practices as tabular summaries, and individual patient-specific data were not collected. DNSGP-2 data were collected as an anonymised person-specific linked data set. Linked person-specific data permit more detailed study of morbidity and socio-economic variables and of linked morbidities. However, collection of linked data increases the costs and complexity of morbidity surveys, not the least because of the ethical issues surrounding the capture of sociodemographic data.

Clinical significance of the findings

The two national datasets were obtained in countries operating within broadly similar healthcare systems in which patient registration and the gatekeeper role for GPs with restricted access to secondary care is usual. Though there are certainly differences, and these are statistically significant because of the large population samples, and because we have used person- rather than practice-based data to calculate the confidence intervals, the similarities are more striking than the differences. These are seen in a wide variety of conditions. In contrast, for some conditions the differences could be very important and they require further research. Some of these are considered here.

Diabetes mellitus and hypothyroidism

The opposing differences in the two countries could be real, but our findings suggest that the GPs in the Netherlands may be missing cases of hypothyroidism, and GPs in England and Wales may be missing cases of diabetes mellitus, both in the older population. The natural history of conditions which are essentially degenerative diseases prompts an expectation of increasing prevalence with age.

Prostatic cancer

The differing SPRs for prostatic cancer contrast with similar results for breast and bladder cancer, and are particularly interesting when set against the similar SPRs for benign prostatic hypertrophy. No structured screening programmes based on estimation of prostate-specific antigen (PSA) levels in blood exist in either country, though the routine investigation of men with symptoms suggestive of urinary obstruction would normally involve investigation of the level of PSA. Differing intensity of investigation by biopsy might also partly explain the differences in national rates.

Respiratory infections

SPRs for respiratory disorders were approximately 25% higher in England and Wales, though sex distribution was similar in both surveys. In both countries the incidence of respiratory infections has reduced considerably over the last 10 years. These reductions are evident in both upper and lower respiratory infections. Interestingly, the SPRs for otitis media were reduced in the Netherlands, compared with those in England and Wales, by a similar amount as other respiratory infections. The SPRs for otitis externa was similar in both countries. The twofold female excess over males for acute sinusitis reported in both surveys, and the much more frequent use of this diagnosis in the Netherlands, call for further investigation.

Musculoskeletal conditions

Back problems are a major cause of illness and carry high economic costs. Prevalence rates were higher in the Netherlands than in England and Wales, but it seems unlikely that the total community prevalence for back conditions is greater in the Netherlands. Accordingly, this difference may reflect a different attitude to healthcare interventions for back problems. Physiotherapy and related services are available by referral from GPs and privately by open access in both countries and the arrangements in both are similar. In the Netherlands, GPs do not undertake sickness certification, whereas in England and Wales sickness certification is required for persons absent from work for more than a week.

Conclusions

Though there were differences in disease prevalence between these national surveys measuring healthcare utilisation in primary care, the similarities were more striking. The high consistency of the gender relativity for many conditions was particularly interesting, and attention is drawn to diabetes where this was not the case. Many conditions showed large and, even if previously known, unexplained sex differences, calling for further investigation – for example multiple sclerosis, acute sinusitis and rheumatoid arthritis. The respective national systems for primary healthcare provision are similar, but differences in patients' expectations may influence the results of this type of comparison, as illustrated here for musculoskeletal problems. There may also be systematic differences in the diagnostic preferences of doctors, as illustrated in the contrasting results for anxiety and depression, the high prevalence of acute sinusitis but otherwise lower prevalence of respiratory infections in DNSGP-2. The comparison has also highlighted differences which may reflect the alertness of doctors; for example the opposing differences in the prevalence of hypothyroidism and of diabetes, and the differing prevalence of prostatic cancer. The age-specific data presented in the figures suggest that doctors in the two countries are weighting diagnostic decisions differently according to the person's age. Not all differences can be readily explained, and these probably reflect true differences between the countries concerned including infectious mononucleosis, carcinoma of the lung and bronchus, respiratory infections and possibly diabetes and rheumatoid arthritis.

References

1 Kramers P (2001) *Design for a set of European Community Health Indicators. Report of the ECHI Project.* National Institute of Public Health and the Environment (RIVM), Bilthoven.

2 Logan WPD and Brooke EM (1957) *The Survey of Sickness 1943–1952, Studies on General Medical and Population Subject.* No 12. HMSO, London.

3 Logan WPD and Cushion AA (1958) *Morbidity Statistics from General Practice Volume I (general), Studies on Medical Population Subjects.* No 14. HMSO, London.

4 Royal College of General Practitioners (RCGP), Office of Population Consuses and Surveys (OPCS) and Department of Health (DH) (1979) *Morbidity Statistics from General Practice 1971–72: second national study (MSGP2).* SMPS No 36. HMSO, London.

5 RCGP, OPCS and DH (1990) *Morbidity Statistics from General Practice 1981–82: third national study (MSGP3): socio-economic analyses* [including microfiche]. Series MB5 No 2. HMSO, London.

6 RCGP, OPCS and DH (1995) *Morbidity Statistics from General Practice: fourth national study, 1991–1992.* Series MB5 No 3. HMSO, London.

7 Read JD and Benson TJR (1986) Comprehensive coding. *Br J Health Care Computing.* 3: 22–5.

8 Fleming DM (1999) Weekly Returns Service of the Royal College of General Practitioners. *Commun Dis Public Health.* 2: 96–100.

9 Fleming DM, Cross KW and Barley MA (2005) Recent changes in the prevalence of diseases presenting for health care. *Br J Gen Pract.* 55: 589–95.

10 van der Velden J, de Bakker DH, Claessens AAMC and Schellevis FG (1992) *Dutch National Survey of General Practice. Morbidity in general practice.* Netherlands Insititue of Primary Health Care (NIVEL), Utrecht.

11 Westert GP, Schellevis FG, de Bakker DH *et al.* (2005) Monitoring health inequalities through general practice: the Second Dutch National Survey of General Practice. *Eur J Public Health.* **15**: 59–65.

12 Wood M and Lamberts H (eds) (1987) *International Classification of Primary Care (ICPC).* Oxford University Press, Oxford.

13 www.statistics.gov.uk (accessed 12 September 2005).

Appendix 6.1 Mapping of selected clusters and separate diseases of comparable ICD-9 and ICPC-1 codes

Disease (cluster)	ICD-9 code	ICPC-1 code
Infectious intestinal diseases	001–009	D11, D70, D73
Chickenpox	052	A72
Herpes simplex	054	S71, X90, Y72
Infectious mononucleosis	075	A75
Candidiasis	112	S75, X72, Y75
Carcinoma lung, bronchus	162	R84
Carcinoma prostate (male)	185	Y77
Carcinoma breast (female)	174	X76
Carcinoma bladder	188	U76
All benign neoplasms	210–229	B75, D78, F74, H75, K72, L71, N75, R86, S78, S79, T72, T73, U78, W73, X78,X79, X80, Y79
Benign neoplasm of the skin	216	S79
Hypothyroidism	244	T86
Diabetes mellitus	250	T90
Gout	274	T92
Iron deficiency anaemia	280	B80
Other deficiency anaemias	281	B81
Mental disorders	290–319	P01–P29, P70–P99
Anxiety neuroses	300	P01, P74
Depression	300.4,311	P03, P76
Parkinson's disease	332	N87
Epilepsy	345	N88
Multiple sclerosis	340	N86
Glaucoma	365	F93
Cataract	366	F92
Acute otitis media	381,382	H71
Otitis externa	380	H70
Hypertensive disease	401–405	K86
Ischaemic heart disease	410–414	K74, K75, K76
Heart failure	428	K77
Cerebrovascular disease	430–438	K89, K90
Varicose veins	454	K95
Haemorrhoids	455	K96
Acute respiratory infection	460–466	R74, R75, R76, R77, R78
Acute sinusitis	461	R75
Chronic obstructive pulmonary disease	490–496	R91, R95, R96
Diseases of the oesophagus, stomach and duodenum	530–537	D84, D85, D86, D87
Inguinal hernia	550	D89
Urinary tract infection	595 599	U71
Benign prostatic hypertrophy	600	Y85
Skin and subcutaneous tissue infections	680–686	S09, S10, S11
Eczema/dermatitis	691, 692	S87, S88
Psoriasis	696	S91
Rheumatoid arthritis and allied conditions	714, 720	L88
Dorsopathies	720–724	L02, L03, L83, L84, L86

Chapter 7

A matter of disparities: risk groups for unhealthy lifestyle and poor health

Mariël Droomers, Hanneke van Lindert and Gert Westert

What it this chapter about?

This chapter addresses the results of the second Dutch National Survey of General Practice (DNSGP-2) with regard to differences in health and lifestyle according to age, socio-economic status, and working status in recent years. First, disparities in health and lifestyle will be presented, and secondly disparities according to age, socio-economic status and working status will be further elaborated upon. Sex, ethnic origin, and urbanisation level will be included in the description of the results where relevant. Also, comparisons with 1987 (based on the results of the DNSGP-1) are made, where possible. Besides presenting recent results on health and lifestyle disparities in the Netherlands, we explore how these results relate to previous Dutch studies.

How was it done?

The results described below are based on self-reported information, collected during interviews at the respondents' homes. From all 12 699 Dutch speaking patients who completed the health interview (*see* Chapter 2), a subsample of approximately 9000 respondents aged 25 years or older answered questions about health and lifestyle issues. Apart from age, the distribution of the respondents according to sex and place of residence is comparable with the original sample population. Additional interviews were held to collect information on lifestyle and health of 1151 migrants, i.e. people from Surinamese, Antillean, Moroccan and Turkish origin, aged 25 years and older. The statistics described here are based on univariate analyses; however, all described relations show statistical significance in the multivariate models when adjusted for the other variables.

What was found?

Disparities in health

Logically, elderly people are worse off healthwise than younger people. The health differences between the young and the old have, however, declined since 1987, due to the fact that elderly people now rate their health better than in 1987 (67% versus 69.5% in good health), while the evaluation of their own health by youngsters has deteriorated slightly between 1987 and 2001. Other Dutch studies conclude that younger people live less healthy lives, but at the same time enjoy better health and use less healthcare than older people.[1]

Results from DNSGP-2 show also that people from a lower educational background rated their health lower (58.9% versus 86.8% in good health) and reported more acute conditions, chronic conditions and poorer mental health. Moreover, socio-economic differences in perceived health and mental health have increased between 1987 and 2001. In 1987, people with a lower educational attainment reported in 17.4% of cases a relatively high score on the General Health Questionnaire (GHQ) (2 or higher); this was 25.6% in 2001. People with a high educational background scored 19.4% in 1987 and 23.9% in 2001. The GLOBE study on the extent of and reasons for socio-economic health differences in the Netherlands concluded that people from a lower socio-economic background have more health problems and a higher mortality rate.[2] Another study confirms the increasing socio-economic health differences in the Netherlands in recent decades.[3]

Poor health is reported most often by occupationally disabled people, as well as Turks, lower educated persons and the unemployed.

Occupationally disabled people score the lowest on all health indicators included in the DNSGP-2, e.g. perceived health, acute complaints and diseases, chronic conditions, limitations and mental health. The poorer health of the occupationally disabled is confirmed in a number of other studies.[4,5]

Migrants report poorer health than the Dutch native population. People from ethnic minorities rate their health as poorer and report on average more health problems. Persons with an ethnic (non-western) background report in 37.3% of cases less than good health. Compared to the native Dutch population (21.9%), this is a large difference. Chronic conditions do not follow this rule. Some chronic conditions are more prevalent among migrant groups, whereas other are more prevalent among the indigenous population. The reporting of chronic conditions, and their order of prevalence rates vary among the different ethnic groups. Other studies confirm that migrants are generally less healthy than nationals.[6,7] Similar to the DNSGP-2 results, two studies report that migrants have a higher rate of diabetes mellitus.[8,9]

We found significant differences among the migrant groups themselves (*see* Table 7.1). In general, people of Turkish origin report a poorer health than those of Moroccan, Antillean or Surinamese origin. Turks report the poorest health; they are the least positive about their health and report more health complaints and chronic conditions than any of the other three migrant groups. Only mental health is not worse in Turkish people than in the other three groups.

In general, the health of women is poorer than that of men. Compared to 1987, health differences between men and women have increased slightly. Women rate their health lower than men (21.2% versus 17.6% report less than good health): they report more acute symptoms, more chronic conditions, more physical limitations and poorer mental health. These results corroborate the ruling view that women report more physical and mental problems than men

Table 7.1 Poor health by ethnic origin

	Dutch native	Moroccan	Antillean	Turkish	Surinamese
Perceived health less than good (%)	17.9	40.2	33.4	46.7	33.1
Number of chronic conditions (mean)	1.53	1.18	1.27	1.87	1.74
Anxious or worried (%)	33.2	25.5	39.7	25.2	33.9
Depressed or down (%)	27.5	24.7	37.0	31.9	34.9

and that the health situation of women has deteriorated in recent decades, whereas that of men has remained unchanged.[10,11]

Residents of highly urbanised areas report poorer health than those living in non-urban areas (22.1% versus 15% reported 'less than good health' in cities versus rural areas). This is true both for their own health evaluation and for the reported acute health problems, chronic illnesses, physical limitations and mental health. These differences between town and countryside have not increased between 1987 and 2001. The results show strong similarities with earlier research in the Netherlands concerning the differences between urban and rural areas.[12,13]

Disparities in lifestyle

Dutch people with lower socio-economic status smoke more often (29.4% smokers), are overweight more frequently, and take physical activity less frequently than people from higher socio-economic groups. This is in accordance with the results of the GLOBE study.[2,14,15]

Those who are unemployed or have been certified unfit to work report a comparatively less healthy lifestyle. They smoke more often (48.9% smokers), consume alcohol more often (19.3% heavy drinkers), are less physically active, and have poorer eating habits than people who are employed (36.3% smokers and 16% heavy drinkers). Additionally, the occupationally disabled are obese more often than the population on average (17.4% versus 10.8%). Other Dutch studies report that the occupationally disabled have a less healthy lifestyle than the working population, but that there is little or no difference between the employed and the unemployed in this respect.[4] However, results from the DNSGP-2 point out that it is often jobless people who report the least healthy lifestyles, certainly in terms of smoking, excessive alcohol consumption and drugs use.

Women generally report a healthier lifestyle than men. They smoke (25.7% versus 34.1%) and drink less (4% versus 19.5%), and have better eating habits than men. An exception to the healthier lifestyle of women is physical activity and weight. Women are less physically active and more overweight than men. Contrary to our finding of stable differences between men and women, Swinkels and Neve (1998) assert that the behaviour of women nowadays resembles more and more the lifestyle of men. They point out that in recent decades, fewer women than men have stopped smoking and that greater numbers of women now drink alcohol, whereas the percentage among men has remained stable.[11]

DNSGP-2 shows that, although migrants generally report a less healthy lifestyle, there are also differences between the different migrant groups. Male migrants, especially Turks (46.9% smoking), smoke more often than Dutch males (28.4% smoking). With regard to women, only the Turkish women smoke more often than Dutch women, while almost no Moroccan women smoke. People from migrant communities take physical activity less frequently than their Dutch counterparts, in particular Turkish and Moroccan people. Almost all ethnic minorities are more often overweight or obese than the Dutch native population. However, they are less prone to excessive alcohol consumption. Exceptions are Surinamese men and Antillean men and women, who are more often heavy drinkers.

Other Dutch studies reported that people from ethnic minority communities smoke less frequently than those from the native population.[7,8] Other studies on alcohol consumption, physical activity patterns and body weight of migrants report findings in keeping with ours. People from migrant communities are less often heavy drinkers, but are physically active less frequently, and are more likely to be overweight than their Dutch counterparts.[1,6,7]

People living in cities generally report a less healthy lifestyle than residents of moderately urban or non-urban areas. City dwellers are more likely to smoke (32% versus 25.1%), use soft or hard drugs (3.6% versus 0.7%) and take insufficient physical activity (54% versus 48.9%) than people living in non-urban areas. Women living in cities are more prone to excessive alcohol consumption. On the other hand, those living in rural areas are more likely to be overweight (48.4% versus 44%).

Although healthy behaviour in terms of smoking and alcohol consumption has improved since 1987, the increasing prevalence of overweight and obesity is alarming (*see* Figure 7.1). The DNSGP-2 results indicate that an unhealthy lifestyle is reported mostly by men, youngsters, lower educated persons, immigrants, the unemployed or occupationally disabled, and urban dwellers.

Age disparities

Younger people live less healthily, but at the same time enjoy better health than older people. As mentioned above, older people generally live in a healthier way than younger people. After the age of 50 years, many smokers have apparently quit the habit (*see* Figure 7.2).

Excessive alcohol consumption is also less frequent after this age. Older people are more physically active and generally report a healthier diet than younger people. A stain on the healthy lifestyle of elderly is overweight and obesity that increase with age.

Although older people generally live in a healthier way than younger people, they suffer from more health problems than younger people due to ageing. An exception to this rule is, however, mental health. People aged under 45 years report poorer mental health than those over 45 years of age.

The five most-often reported symptoms vary according to the different age groups. Children most often complain of a blocked nose and cough, followed by tiredness, headache and 'feeling aggressive'. The over 65 age group most

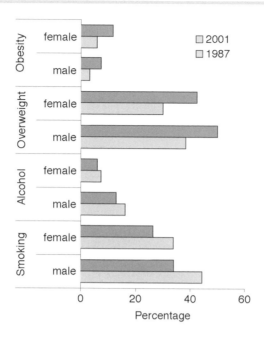

Figure 7.1 Changes in lifestyle between 1987 and 2001 (DNSGP); percentages of smokers, excessive alcohol consumers, people who are overweight (BMI > 25) and obese (BMI > 30) by sex.

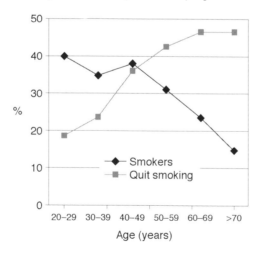

Figure 7.2 Percentage of respondents that report smoking and to have quit smoking by age group, 2001.

frequently report low back pain, tiredness, sleeplessness, neck or shoulder pain and impaired hearing. The majority of chronic conditions are also most prevalent among higher age groups. By contrast, the prevalence rates of migraine, serious headache and eczema seem to diminish with increasing age.

The good news is that since 1987 the differences in perceived health between younger and older people have decreased. Nowadays, older people report better health than they did in 1987 (*see* Figure 7.3). This is particularly true for the 45–64 years age group. Younger people, on the other hand, report a somewhat poorer health than in 1987. Compared to 1987, the differences in mental health between older and younger age groups have, however, increased.

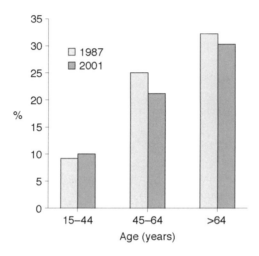

Figure 7.3 Poor self-rated health (% less than good) by age groups in 1987 and 2001.

Socio-economic differences

Lower socio-economic groups report comparatively poorer health and unhealthier behaviour than people from higher socio-economic backgrounds.

People with lower socio-economic status are more likely to smoke (29.4%) and have generally unhealthier eating habits than those with higher socio-economic status. People from a lower socio-economic background are more likely to be overweight or obese than others. There is, however, little difference between the two groups in terms of the national standard for adequate physical activity. The latter contradicts another Dutch study that reports that lower socio-economic groups take less physical activity.[14]

Finally, DNSGP-2 results show that between 1987 and 2001, socio-economic differences in smoking behaviour and excessive alcohol consumption have stabilised, while socio-economic differences in overweight and obesity have diminished since 1987.

We found that people from a lower socio-economic background rate their health lower and report more acute conditions, chronic conditions and poorer mental health. The GLOBE study reports similar socio-economic differences in health.[2] DNSGP-2 reports that socio-economic differences in perceived health and mental health have increased since 1987, as well as differences in the occurrence of diabetes mellitus. Socio-economic differences in the reported frequency of migraine or serious headache appear to have lessened. The increase of socio-economic health differences in recent decades in the Netherlands is corroborated by Dalstra *et al.* (2002).[3]

Differences related to working status

Those who are unemployed or have been certified unfit to work generally have a comparatively less healthy lifestyle. They smoke more frequently (48.9%, 43.3% and 36.3% respectively), consume alcohol more often, and take insufficient physical activity more often. They also skip breakfast or dinner more often. Additionally, the occupationally disabled are more often obese than the population average. The unhealthier lifestyle of the occupationally disabled compared with the employed is corroborated by van Deursen (1997),[4] but little or no difference between the employed and the unemployed was reported in this respect. By contrast, in our study population, it is often jobless people who report the least healthy lifestyles, certainly in terms of smoking, excessive alcohol consumption and drugs use.

The unemployed and occupationally disabled report poorer health than those in paid employment. They report more health complaints, chronic conditions and poorer mental health. The disabled also have more physical limitations. The poorer health of the occupationally disabled is confirmed in a number of studies.[4,5] Studies on the health of the unemployed report poorer physical health among the unemployed as compared to the employed,[5,16] as well as similar health for unemployed and employed people.[4] The DNSGP-2 results concur with the first.

Since 1987, this health gap between these groups and employed people has increased, due to the deterioration of the health situation of the occupationally disabled and unemployed. For instance, the percentage of unemployed people who rate their health as 'poor' or 'bad' has increased, whereas this is not true of those with a job (*see* Figure 7.4). Also acute health problems, migraine and poor mental health have increased more sharply among the unemployed than among other groups.

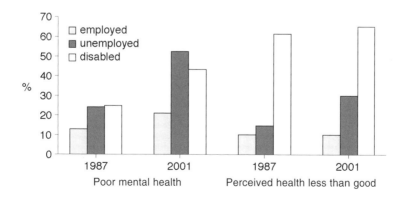

Figure 7.4 Poor perceived mental health and health by working status, 1987 and 2001.

What to think about it

This chapter presents an updated profile of the existing disparities in health and lifestyle in the population of the Netherlands. Where possible, comparisons are made over time. The results show that differences in health have not disappeared. The groups with poorer lifestyle and health tend to be the unemployed, the occupationally disabled, the less well educated, ethnic minorities and the elderly. Indeed, the health gap appears to have widened in some cases. Also striking is the deterioration of mental health among the unemployed, the occupationally disabled and the less well educated.

Need for caution

It is not always the less healthy groups who have a less healthy lifestyle. For instance, excessive alcohol consumption is higher among the Dutch native population than among migrant groups, while migrants report generally a poorer health status. Also, young people and men tend to behave more unhealthily, while older people and women are the ones who report poorer health.

Compared to 1987, the lifestyle of the Dutch population has deteriorated in a number of areas; at the same time it has improved in other areas. For instance, the number of overweight people has increased, but smoking has declined, as has excessive alcohol consumption.

Public health policy issues

In the government report *Langer Gezond Leven* (A longer healthy life) of the Health Ministry (2003), smoking, obesity and diabetes mellitus were appointed spearheads in the area of prevention.[17] According to the DNSGP-2 results highlighted in this chapter, this choice of topics simultaneously addresses the issue of disparities, since these problems show clear sociodemographic differences. For example, smoking, obesity and diabetes mellitus are more prevalent among lower socio-economic groups and ethnic minorities, with the exception of smoking among immigrant women.

The government report also prioritises a number of chronic diseases: cardiovascular diseases, cancer, asthma/chronic obstructive pulmonary disease (COPD), diabetes mellitus, mental conditions and mobility problems. Our results reported above show that chronic conditions are not evenly distributed among sociodemographic groups. In particular, the high prevalence of mobility problems, especially osteoarthritis, among those with a lower educational level is striking. Another notable result from DNSGP-2 in this respect is the poor mental health of the unemployed and occupationally disabled and lower-educated people.

Additionally to the above-mentioned prioritising of specific illnesses and prevention spearheads, public health should pay special attention to the situation of the unemployed and occupationally disabled. The results of DNSGP-2 show that these groups appear to be worse off on all fronts. Public health policy should especially focus on the deteriorating health of the unemployed and the occupationally disabled. These people are at a marked disadvantage and are increasingly becoming a vulnerable group in Dutch society.

References

1 van Oers JAM (ed) (2002) *Health on Course? The 2002 Dutch Public Health Status and Forecasts Report.* Report No: 270551002. RIVM, Bohn Stafleu van Loghum, Bilthoven, Houten.

2 van Lenthe FJ, Droomers M, Schrijvers CT and Mackenbach JP (2000) Socio-demographic variables and 6 year change in body mass index: longitudinal results from the GLOBE study. *Int J Obesity Rel Metab Disorders.* **24**: 1077–84.

3 Dalstra AA, Kunst AE, Geurts JJM, Frenken FJM and Mackenbach JP (2002) Trends in socioeconomic health inequalities in the Netherlands, 1981–1999. *J Epidemiol Community Health.* **56**: 927–34.

4 van Deursen CGL (1997) *De Gezondheidstoestand van Werklozen en Arbeidsongeschikten.* [The health situation of jobless people and the occupationally disabled.] In: Mackenbach JP and Verkleij H (eds) *Volksgezondheid Toekomst Verkenning 1997. Deel II. Gezondheidsverschillen.* RIVM, Bilthoven.

5 Hoff S and Jehoel-Gijsbers G (1998) *Een Bestaan zonder Baan. Een vergelijkende studie onder werklozen, arbeidsongeschikten en werkenden* (1974–1995). [A life without a job. A comparative study among jobless people, occupationally disabled people and working people (1974–1995).] SCP, Den Haag.

6 Brussaard JH, van Erp-Baart MA, Brants HA, Hulshof KF and Lowik M (2001) Nutrition and health among migrants in the Netherlands. *Public Health Nutr.* **4**: 659–64.

7 Reijneveld SA (1998) Reported health, lifestyles, and use of health care of first generation immigrants in the Netherlands: do socioeconomic factors explain their adverse position? *J Epidemiol Community Health.* **52**: 298–304.

8 Bindraban NR, Stronks K and Klazinga NS (2001) Cardiovasculaire risicofactoren bij Surinamers in Nederland: een literatuuroverzicht. [Cardiovascular risk factors in Surinamese people in the Netherlands.] *Ned Tijdschr Geneeskd.* **147**: 1591–4.

9 Dijkshoorn H, Uitenbroek DG and Middelkoop BJ (2003) Prevalentie van diabetes mellitus en hart-en vaatziekten onder immigranten uit Turkije of Marokko en de autochtone Nederlandse bevolking. [Prevalence of diabetes mellitus and cadiovascular diseases among immigrants from Turkey or Morocco and the native Dutch.] *Ned Tijdschr Geneeskd.* **147**: 1362–6.

10 Bensing J (1994) Vrouw in de gezondheidszorg: een factor van betekenis. [Women in health care: an important factor.] In: Noordenbos G and Winants Y (eds) *Feiten en Fricties: sekse-asymmetrieën in zorgsystemen.* [Facts and frictions: sex-asymmetries in care systems.] Vrouwenstudies, Congresverslag Maastricht, pp. 97–111.

11 Swinkels H and Neve R (1998) *Emancipatie en Gezondheid: ontwikkelingen in leefstijl, gezondheid en medische consumptie bij mannen en vrouwen in de periode 1981–1996.* [Emancipation and health; developments in lifestyle, health and medical consumption in men and women over the period 1981–1996.] *Maandbericht Gezondheidsstatistiek.* **17**: 12–25.

12 van der Lucht F and Verkleij H (2001) *Gezondheid in de Grote Steden. Achterstanden en kansen.* [NL Health in large cities. Backwardness and opportunities.] RIVM, Bilthoven.

13 Verkleij H and Verheij RA (2003) *Zorg in de Grote Steden.* [Care in large cities.] RIVM, Bilthoven.

14 Droomers M (2002) *Socioeconomic Differences in Health Related Behaviour* (PhD thesis). PPI, Enschede.

15 Stronks K, van de Mheen HD, Looman CW and Mackenbach JP (1997) Smoking 1998. Cultural, material, and psychosocial correlates of the socioeconomic gradient in smoking behavior among adults. *Prev Med.* **26**: 754–66.

16 Fengler M, Joung IMA and Mackenbach JP (1997) Sociaal-demografische kenmerken en gezondheid: hun relatief belang en onderlinge relaties. [Sociodemographic char-

acteristics and health: importance and interrelations.] In: Mackenbach JP and Verkleij H (eds). *Volksgezondheid Toekomst Verkenning 1997. Deel II Gezondheidsverschillen.* RIVM, Bilthoven.

17 Ministry of Health (2003) *Langer Gezond Leven* [A longer healthy life.] Ministry of Health, Den Haag.

Chapter 8

Child health and general practitioners' management, 1987–2001

Hanneke Otters and François Schellevis

What is this chapter about?

This contribution compares the presentation and management of childhood morbidity (0–17 years) in general practice in 2001 with that in 1987. In the Netherlands, childhood morbidity presented to the general practitioner (GP) has changed: (infectious) skin problems have become more important. In 2001, incidence rates of most respiratory infections and acute otitis media were much lower. Although efforts to improve antibiotic prescription have intensified (e.g. introduction of guidelines), children with respiratory infections and acute otitis media were prescribed antibiotics more often in 2001 than in 1987. This can probably partly be explained by a change in consultation threshold in 2001. Overall, GPs referred fewer children to specialists in 2001.

Introduction

Children consult their general practitioner (GP) frequently and Dutch GPs deal with childhood morbidity in their surgery daily. The first Dutch National Survey of General Practice (DNSGP-1) provided detailed information of childhood health problems and GPs' management.[1] Over the past decades, there have been several changes that may have affected children's health and GPs' management. For example, vaccination schemes have changed, allergy-related diseases are rising, and also childhood demographics have changed.[2–4]

Since the first national survey was performed, several evidence-based guidelines for childhood diseases have been developed and published by the Dutch College of General Practitioners.[5] These guidelines help decision making for referral to specialist care and rationalise drug prescriptions such as antibiotics. These guidelines are generally accepted and widely used by Dutch GPs.[6]

With an ageing population we run the risk that the childrens' health tends to become a neglected area in health (care) research.

These changes, among other things, will probably have affected both childhood morbidity presented to general practice and GPs' management.[7]

The objective was to gain insight into childhood morbidity (0–17 years) presented in general practice in 2001 and to compare this with childhood morbidity in 1987 (0–17 years). Incidence rates of the most frequently encountered health problems in 2001 are examined and compared with those in 1987. GPs' management of these health problems is compared with that in 1987 by comparing referral and antibiotic prescription rates.

How was it done?

For a description of the methods of the (first and) second Dutch National Survey of General Practice (DNSGP-1, 1987 and DNSGP-2, 2001), *see* Chapter 2. The following is specific for the study described in this chapter.

From the second survey, data were analysed from all 0–17 years olds, a total of 82 053 children (mid-time population). From the first survey, data from 86 577 children aged 0–17 years were analysed. Both surveys were episode orientated, meaning that different consultations concerning the same health problem were linked to one episode. The most recent diagnosis made by the GP was considered to be the diagnosis of the disease episode.

Incidence rates of health problems presented in general practice were calculated by dividing the number of new episodes by the number of children-years followed. Referrals and prescriptions are evaluated per 100 presented disease episodes.[8,9] New referrals to secondary care were evaluated with the referring diagnosis, which is the diagnosis at the time the referral was made. The referral rate was calculated as the number of referrals per 100 episodes. The antibiotic prescription rate was calculated as the number of antibiotic prescriptions per 100 disease episodes.

What was found?

Childhood morbidity

Figure 8.1 shows the distribution of all episodes of disease by organ systems for 2001 and 1987. The bars represent the proportion of disease episodes that was presented in each organ system. In both surveys, health problems concerning the respiratory tract were presented most often (23.3% in 2001 and 25.5% in 1987), followed by skin problems which increased from 17.8% in 1987 to 23.0% in 2001.

Skin problems increased between 1987 and 2001.

Top 10 diagnoses

The most frequently encountered health problems in children are illustrated in Figure 8.2. The top 10 incidence rates of 2001 were compared with those of 1987. Incidence rates for upper respiratory tract infection and acute bronchitis had decreased by 50% or more in 2001. The incidence rate of cough was higher in 2001 than in 1987. Rates for dermatomycosis and impetigo increased significantly in 2001. Acute otitis media is the second most important health problem in both surveys and in 2001 the incidence rate decreased by approximately 30%.

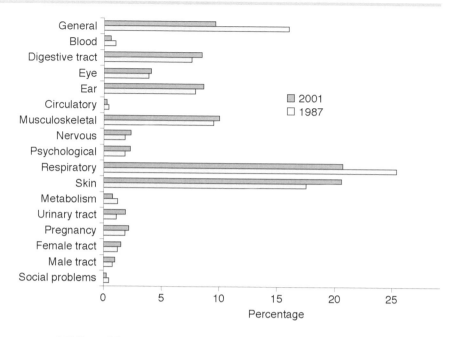

Figure 8.1 Childhood health problems presented in general practice, percentage of presented episodes per organ system, 2001 (DNSGP-2) and 1987 (DNSGP-1).

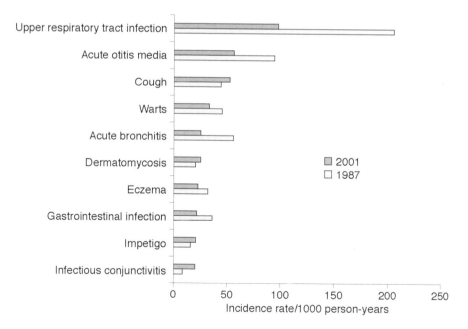

Figure 8.2 Incidence rates of top 10 diagnoses in 2001 (DNSGP-2), compared with 1987 (DNSGP-1).

Upper respiratory tract infections halved between 1987 and 2001, but are still the most frequent reason to visit a GP.

General practitioners' management

GPs' management for these frequently encountered childhood health problems is presented in Table 8.1. In 2001, antibiotic prescription rates for respiratory tract problems, such as acute respiratory tract infection, cough and acute bronchitis, had not decreased. Referral rates for these diagnoses are low in both surveys: one or two children were referred to medical specialists per 100 encountered episodes. Children with acute otitis media were prescribed antibiotics more often in 2001 than in 1987 (56/100 episodes in 2001 versus 34/100 episodes in 1987), but were referred to specialists less often (3.1/100 episodes in 2001 versus 7.5/100 episodes in 1987). Compared with 1987, referral rates for most skin problems have decreased significantly in 2001. In particular, children with warts were referred less often to secondary care in 2001 (2.2/100 episodes in 2001 versus 7.6/100 episodes in 1987).

For the top 10 diagnoses GPs refer fewer children to medical specialists.

Table 8.1 Antibiotic prescription rates[8] and referral rates[9] per 100 episodes, 1987 and 2001

Diagnosis	Prescription rates per 100 episodes		Referral rates per 100 episodes	
	1987	2001	1987	2001
Acute respiratory tract infection	16.4	17.0	1.5	1.1
Acute otitis media	33.5	55.8	7.5	3.1
Cough	7.0	8.8	0.3	1.5
Warts	0.3	0	7.6	2.2
Acute bronchitis	75.2	83.5	2.9	1.9
Dermatomycosis	0.5	0.2	4.4	1.5
Eczema NEC	1.8	0.7	5.2	3.7
Gastrointestinal infection	2.0	1.2	1.6	1.5
Impetigo	35.6	30.4	0.8	1.2
Infectious conjunctivitis	0.8	0.8	0.8	1.2

What to think about it

Childhood morbidity patterns presented in Dutch general practice have changed considerably during the past decades. Compared with 1987, fewer health problems concerning the respiratory tract were presented, but children presented significantly more skin problems. GPs' management has changed as well; they were less likely to refer children to specialists for the most common health problems; however, they do prescribe somewhat more antibiotics for respiratory health problems.

Respiratory tract diseases

We observed a significant decline in respiratory health problems in children, illustrated by the large (50%) decrease in incidence rates of specific respiratory tract infections. For example, the incidence rate of acute upper respiratory tract infection – the number-one health problem in both surveys – decreased from 209 per 1000 person-years in 1987 to 96 per 1000 person-years in 2001.

Parents are better informed about causes and treatment of respiratory tract infections and otitis media.

Decreasing incidence rates of respiratory tract problems, presented by children in general practice, have been reported by others as well,[10] and there are several possible explanations for this decline.

Particularly in the case of respiratory tract infections, parents nowadays may be better informed how to handle these infections themselves and know when they should consult a GP. Moreover, parents may have become increasingly aware of the viral origin of respiratory infections and the (non-)usefulness of antibiotics in these infections. As a consequence, parents may wait before contacting the GP and also will consult the GP with a child that is more severely ill. Therefore, the GPs of 2001 may see children with more severe symptoms, and that could also explain why the number of antibiotic prescriptions has not decreased for these infections. Unfortunately, there is no information on severity of disease in both surveys and therefore this explanation remains inconclusive. Another explanation for the decrease in the presentation of respiratory problems could be that, in 2001, cough medications are no longer reimbursed by health insurance. In 1987, many of the prescribed cough medications were reimbursed by insurance companies and could have been a reason to consult the GP in 1987.

But it is also possible that there may be a decrease of respiratory tract infections in the general population. Fleming *et al.* suggested that this is a possible and reasonable explanation.[10] However, interview data from the first and second survey, mirroring true morbidity trends in the population, do not support this theory. In both surveys, a subanalysis of young (0–4 years old) children showed that a similar proportion of children reported that they had coughed during the past 14 days.

Acute otitis media

Acute otitis media was presented less often in general practice in 2001, and the GPs managed this health problem increasingly themselves. However, parallel with the decrease in referral rates for acute otitis media, antibiotics were prescribed more often: the antibiotic prescription rate increased by 65%. This finding was rather unexpected and surprising because the acute otitis media guideline, rationalising judicious antibiotic prescription, was one of the first guidelines to be introduced by the Dutch College of General Practitioners.[11] Moreover, several studies performed in primary care settings have shown that antibiotics only have a modest effect in acute otitis media in young children, and these studies have also reported that 'watchful waiting' seems to be justified for this health problem.[12,13] One could assume that the children with acute otitis media that were not referred to an ear, nose and throat (ENT) specialist received antibiotics instead. However, the decrease in referral rate is not fully substituted by an increase in the antibiotic prescription rate for this diagnosis.

It is possible that particularly in children with earache, parents are nowadays better informed when to consult general practice. In that case, GPs are not more inclined to prescribe antibiotics but are contacted by children with more severe disease. Yet, on the other hand, it is a conflicting finding that in a disease for which a guideline has been implemented recommending judicious prescribing, antibiotics prescription rates increase.

Skin disease

Skin problems have become more important over time. We observed increasing incidence rates of impetigo and dermatomycosis in particular. One possible explanation for this finding could be that the increasing use of day care facilities and after-school activities is associated with the higher occurrence of these infectious skin problems.

Impetigo and dermatomycosis: what about daycare facilities?

Although the incidence rates for skin problems have increased markedly, this is not reflected in higher referral rates for skin diseases. On the contrary, GPs manage skin problems more themselves in 2001 than they did in 1987. In particular, the referral rates for warts have decreased since 1987.

Implications for general practice and policy

Childhood morbidity presented to general practice, and GPs' management have changed over the past decades. Skin problems have become more important and GPs manage childhood health problems increasingly themselves. It is possible that the children that were presented to general practice were more severely ill in 2001 compared to 1987 and this could explain the stable and higher antibiotic prescription rates for many respiratory infections.

References

1 Bruijnzeels MA, van Suijlekom-Smit LWA, van der Velden J and van der Wouden JC (1993) *The Child in General Practice, Dutch National Survey of Morbidity and Interventions in General Practice*. Erasmus University, Rotterdam.

2 Conyn-van Spaendonck MA, Veldhuijzen IK, Suijkerbuijk AW and Hirasing RA (2000) Sterke daling van het aantal invasieve infecties door Haemophilus influenzae in de eerste 4 jaar na de introductie van de vaccinatie van kinderen tegen H. influenzae type b. [Strong decline in the number of invasive infections by *Haemophilus influenzae* during the first 4 years after vaccination of children against *H. influenzae* type b has been introduced.] *Ned Tijdschr Geneeskd*. 144: 1069–73.

3 Strachan DP (2000) Family size, infection and atopy: the first decade of the 'hygiene hypothesis'. *Thorax*. 55 (Suppl 1): S2–10.

4 www.cbs.nl

5 *NHG Standaarden*. [NHG standards.] http://nhg.artsennet.nl/index (accessed 13 September 2005).

6 Grol R (2001) Successes and failures in the implementation of evidence-based guidelines for clinical practice. *Med Care*. **39** (Suppl 2): S46–54.

7 Ferris TG, Saglam D, Stafford RS *et al*. (1998) Changes in the daily practice of primary care for children. *Arch Pediatr Adolesc Med*. **152**: 227–33.

8 Otters HB, van der Wouden JC, Schellevis FG, van Suijlekom-Smit LW and Koes BW (2004) Trends in prescribing antibiotics for children in Dutch general practice. *J Antimicrob Chemother*. **53**: 361–6.

9 Otters H, van der Wouden JC, Schellevis FG, van Suijlekom-Smit LW and Koes BW (2004) Dutch general practitioners' referral of children to specialists: a comparison between 1987 and 2001. *Br J Gen Pract*. **54**: 848–52.

10 Fleming DM, Ross AM, Cross KW and Kendall H (2003) The reducing incidence of respiratory tract infection and its relation to antibiotic prescribing. *Br J Gen Pract*. **53**: 778–83.

11 Appelman CLM BP, Dunk JHM, Lisdonk EH, de Melker RA and van Weert HCPM (1990) NHG standard Otitis Media Acuta. *Huisarts Wet*. **33**: 242–5.

12 Damoiseaux RA, van Balen FA, Hoes AW, Verheij TJ and de Melker RA (2000) Primary care based randomised, double blind trial of amoxicillin versus placebo for acute otitis media in children aged under 2 years. *BMJ*. **320**: 350–4.

13 Glasziou PP, Del Mar CB, Sanders SL and Hayem M (2004) *Antibiotics for acute otitis media in children*. The Cochrane Database of Systematic Reviews, Issue 1.

Chapter 9

Patients with a psychiatric diagnosis in general practice: (co)morbidity and contacts

Peter Verhaak, Anita Volkers and Jasper Nuyen

What is this chapter about?

In this study we give a detailed account of the morbidity of patients with a psychiatric disorder, as diagnosed by general practitioners (GPs), during one year. We have found that about half of the patients with a psychiatric disorder according to a standardised psychiatric interview are diagnosed by the GP as such. Depending on their psychiatric disorder, 30–40% of these patients only present somatic problems that are not indicative for psychological or psychiatric problems.

Patients with a psychiatric disorder have relatively more psychological or psychiatric diagnoses recorded by their GPs than the practice population as a whole. However, the list of most common diagnoses is comparable with the list of most common diagnoses of the practice population. Patients with a psychiatric disorder stand out especially by a higher contact rate, for somatic illnesses as well as for psychological ones or psychiatric problems.

Introduction

Psychiatric disorders are much more prevalent in the community than statistics from primary care would suggest. A large World Health Organization (WHO)-consortium reported recently prevalences according to the Diagnostic and Statistical Manual for Mental Disorders (DSM-IV) diagnoses in 14 countries all over the world.[1] One-year prevalences of any psychiatric disorder, measured among more than 60 000 community adults between 2001 and 2003, varied between 5% and 26% with 15% for the Netherlands. Anxiety disorder was assessed for 2% to 18% of the respondents, with 9% for the Netherlands. Mood disorder ranged from 1% to 10%; in the Netherlands it was 7%. Substance abuse was diagnosed for 0.1% up to 4%, with 3% in the Netherlands. Earlier population studies in the 1990s, with a comparable design, using DSM-III-compatible diagnoses, reported comparable ranges and prevalences.[2]

Nevertheless, psychiatric morbidity as diagnosed by general practitioners (GPs) seems lower. Lamberts *et al.* used the International Classification of Primary Care (ICPC) and showed in 1991 a 2.9% prevalence of psychiatric diagnoses.[3] The second National Survey of General Practice presented a prevalence of 4.7% psychiatric diagnoses according to ICPC.[4] For more specific diagnoses in general practice in 1990 and 2001 respectively, the figures are: anxiety disorder: 0.5–0.7%, for depression 1.1–2.1% and for substance abuse 0.8–0.5%. For the record, symptoms registered by GPs, such as sleeping disorders or feeling agitated, are not included in these prevalence figures. But patients with only one or two psychological symptoms would not be considered as a DSM-IV case as well. The conclusion can be drawn that patients with a classified psychiatric disorder are only partly represented in the diagnostic statistics of general practice, especially when specific diagnoses are taken into account.

Patients with a classified psychiatric disorder are only partly represented in the diagnostic statistics of general practice.

This conclusion fits with another finding from these population surveys. Most patients with disorders, traced in these population surveys, did not receive any treatment, according to the respondents. In the two worldwide surveys mentioned above, any kind of healthcare treatment was reported by 1–15% of respondents with any DSM-disorder. In the Netherlands, this was 13% and 11% respectively.[1,2] However, there was a gradient: people with severe disorders had a 66% chance of professional treatment, while the chances for moderate and mild disorders were considerably lower. If Dutch patients with a DSM-III-compatible disorder received care, primary care was involved in 27% of the cases, mental healthcare in 15% of the cases and residential mental healthcare for 1%.[5] About two-thirds of patients with a DSM-III disorder did not receive any care for that disorder.

Nevertheless, although patients with psychiatric disorders are to some extent apparently not treated for these disorders, they make more use of healthcare facilities, in primary care as well as in secondary care.[6,7] This raises a number of questions, as far as primary care is concerned. Are there differences in the morbidity pattern of patients with a psychiatric disorder, compared to an average practice population? To what extent has the psychiatric status of a patient been recognised by the GP? Are there possible triggers for the GP, to distinguish between the morbidity pattern of a patient with a psychiatric disorder and that of patients without such a disorder?

Research questions

- What is the morbidity pattern in general practice of patients with a classified psychiatric diagnosis during one year?
- Are there differences between patients with a classified psychiatric diagnosis and the average practice population regarding morbidity pattern and contact frequencies?
- Are there differences between patients with severe and less severe psychiatric diagnosis regarding morbidity pattern and contact frequencies?

How was it done?

Design and patients

For a description of the methods of the second Dutch National Survey of General Practice (DNSGP-2, 2001), *see* Chapter 2 of this book. The following is specific to the study described in this chapter. Two screening instruments, the General Health Questionnaire (GHQ-12) for general psychopathology,[8] and CAGE for alcohol abuse,[9] were completed by respondents aged ≥18 years. Respondents with a GHQ score ≥4 (later lowered to ≥3, in order to include a sufficient number of patients with psychopathology) and/or a CAGE-score of 4 were invited for a standardised psychiatric interview, the Composite International Diagnostic Interview (CIDI).[10] The CIDI was successfully administered to 811 persons. A total of 1379 respondents met the cut-off point on one or both of the screeners. Of these, 1120 agreed to participate in the follow-up assessment, and 811 (58.8%) completed the CIDI. No significant differences were found between patients who completed the CIDI regarding age, sex and scores on the two screening instruments and those who did not (data not shown). However, the interviewed persons had a significantly higher educational level (*P* < 0.01) The present study includes patients who have completed the CIDI. In this study, we have used the computerised Dutch version of the 12–month CIDI (CIDI-Auto 2.1). The following five sections were assessed: demographics, phobic and anxiety disorders, depressive disorders and dysthymic disorder, manic and bipolar disorders, and disorders resulting from the use of alcohol.

CIDI-data were combined with data concerning morbidity presented to the GP by these patients during one year in the period of the interview. For 795 persons, CIDI data could successfully be combined with morbidity data concerning 6102 doctor–patient contacts during one year. About 90% of the morbidity was presented in contacts within a period of 9 months before or after the interview, 75% of the data within a period of half a year.

Psychiatric morbidity

CIDI diagnoses indicate psychiatric morbidity during the past 12 months. By means of diagnostic algorithms diagnoses according to criteria of the Diagnostic and Statistical Manual for Mental Disorders (DSM-IV) were provided.[11] A diagnosis was considered positive when all diagnostic criteria, inclusion as well as exclusion criteria, were fulfilled. In our analysis, we distinguished between patients with more and less severe psychiatric disorders. Those with moderate or severe major depressive disorder, bipolar disorder, any recurrent major depressive disorder, panic disorder, compulsive–obsessive disorder and each patient with more than one DSM-IV diagnosis were classified as more severe. Those with a single mild major depressive disorder, generalised anxiety disorder, phobia without panic and alcohol abuse were categorised as less severe.

Morbidity in general practice

Of all patients with a DSM-IV diagnosis, data about all contacts with their GPs during one year were recorded. During each contact with a patient, the GP registered the diagnosis in an electronic medical record coded according to the ICPC.[12] Separate attention has been paid to somatic symptoms that are considered indicative of depression or anxiety: cold chills, tired, abundant transpiration, nausea, palpitations, tightness of the chest and lack of appetite. Apart from morbidity, attention will be paid to the number of contacts during one year and to the number of episodes of illness during one year (one episode of illness may take more than one contact).

What was found?

Of the 795 persons with a successful CIDI and traceable morbidity data, 376 persons could be included with at least one DSM-IV diagnosis, within the realm of 'mood disorder', 'anxiety disorder' or 'alcohol abuse' (see Table 9.1). About two-thirds of the respondents with a psychiatric disorder had a mood disorder (major depression, dysthymia or bipolar disorder). About 60% had an anxiety disorder and about 10% had an alcohol disorder.

Comorbidity between several diagnoses is not uncommon (see Table 9.2). In fact, about half of the patients with alcohol abuse or anxiety disorder were

Table 9.1 Specific diagnoses of respondents with at least one DSM-IV diagnosis according to the CIDI ($n = 376$)

Disorder	Number of diagnoses
Alcohol disorder	41
Mood disorder[a]	252
bipolar disorder	8
dysthymia	41
Major depressive disorder	
single mild[a]	196
single moderate	67
single severe	52
recurrent mild	15
recurrent moderate	6
recurrent severe	3
Anxiety disorder[b]	232
panic disorder without agoraphobia	18
panic disorder with agoraphobia	20
agoraphobia without panic disorder	49
social phobia	52
generalised anxiety disorder	113
specific phobia	113

[a]Different depressive disorders are mutually exclusive, but bipolar disorder and dysthymia can be comorbid.
[b]Different anxiety disorders are not mutually exclusive.

Table 9.2 Psychiatric comorbidity among patients with a CIDI diagnosis

DSM-IV diagnosis	Any DSM-IV (n = 376) %	DSM-IV: alcohol (n = 41) %	DSM-IV: mood disorder (n = 252) %	DSM-IV: anxiety (n = 232) %
Alcohol	19	100	8	5
Mood disorder	67	46	100	3
Anxiety	62	29	49	100

diagnosed with a mood disorder as well. About half of the patients with a mood disorder and one-third of those with alcohol abuse were diagnosed with an anxiety disorder as well.

Morbidity depends on the DSM-IV diagnosis

During one year, 91% of patients with at least one DSM-IV diagnosis had at least one contact with their GP (*see* Table 9.3).

Patients with a DSM-IV diagnosis who did not visit their GP during one year were significantly younger than patients who had at least one contact. The two groups did not differ significantly in sex, education, psychiatric morbidity or severity of psychiatric morbidity.

Table 9.3 Contacts and GP diagnoses for patients with any DSM-IV disorder (in percentages)

	Any DSM-IV (n = 376)	DSM-IV: Alcohol (n = 252) %	DSM-IV: Mood disorder (n = 41) %	DSM-IV: anxiety (n = 232) %
Contacts with GP				
no contact during 1 year	9	15	7	9
at least one contact	91	85	93	91
At least one diagnosis in ICPC chapter P:[a]	52	57	60	53
alcohol (P15)	1	3	1	–
depression (P03; P76)	23	29	28	23
anxiety (P01; P74)	13	3	13	16
overworking (P78)	11	9	15	13
affective psychosis (P73)	1	3	1	1
At least one diagnosis in ICPC chapter Z	11	3	14	9
Somatic symptom of anxiety[b]	14	11	14	15
Somatic symptom of depression[c]	8	5	8	9
None of the GP diagnoses above	39	37	31	38

[a] Only a limited number of subcategories is mentioned.
[b] Cold chills, tired, abundant transpiration, nausea, palpitations, tightness of the chest.
[c] Tired, lack of appetite.

More than 50% of the patients who visit their GPs are diagnosed by their GPs at least once as having a psychological or psychiatric symptom or diagnosis. The most common diagnosis in general practice is depression followed by anxiety and stress/overworking. About 10% of visiting patients with a psychiatric disorder receive a diagnosis at least once within the ICPC chapter 'Social problems'. About 15% are diagnosed during that year with symptoms possibly indicating an anxiety disorder and about 10% with symptoms indicating a depressive disorder. About 39% of the patients with a DSM-IV diagnosis according to the CIDI did not receive any of these psychological or psychiatric or related diagnoses during one year. This proportion is slightly lower for patients with a DSM-IV diagnosis of mood disorder than for patients within other categories.

Considering the three main categories separately, it can be observed that about a quarter of patients with a DSM-IV diagnosis of a mood disorder are diagnosed during one year with a diagnosis of depression, while about 15% of patients with an anxiety disorder and less than 5% of those with alcohol abuse are diagnosed by their GPs as such. Nevertheless, about 60% of the patients with a DSM-IV diagnosis receive some GP diagnosis reflecting the psychological nature of their symptoms.

There is a difference in this respect between patients with a more severe and a less severe diagnosis. The proportion of GP diagnoses among patients with a severe DSM-IV diagnosis is larger (38%) than among patients with a mild diagnosis (16%). Of the former, 30% of those visiting their GPs are restricted to non-related somatic diagnoses, of the latter this is nearly 50% ($\chi^2 = 22.6$, df = 4, $P < 0.000$).

Patients with a DSM-IV diagnosis differ from the practice population

Table 9.4 gives a number of basic figures regarding the use of GP services and morbidity of patients with a DSM-IV diagnosis compared with the total practice population in the participating practices. Patients with a DSM-IV diagnosis (column 1) are divided into patients with a severe diagnosis (column 2) and patients with a less severe diagnosis (column 3). Patient characteristics are presented in the first rows. Patients with a DSM-IV diagnosis are comparable with the total practice population regarding age and education level. However, among patients with a psychiatric diagnosis, the proportion of women is considerably larger. Differences in contact rate and morbidity distribution have been tested for both sexes separately.

Patients with a DSM-IV diagnosis distinguish themselves from the 'average' patient by their frequency of use of GP-services (*see* Table 9.4). More than 90% of the patients with a DSM-IV diagnosis had at least one contact with the GP practice in 2001, while only 76% of the practice population did so. Especially when the psychiatric disorder is considered severe, the number of disease episodes is 1.7 times higher than the average. Those with a severe psychiatric disorder have almost twice as many contacts as the average population. For patients with a less severe DSM-IV diagnosis this difference is smaller. They have 1.4 times as many disease episodes and 1.5 as many contacts. Women account to a higher degree than men for the difference in contact frequency between the average population and the patients with a DSM-IV diagnosis. Women with a psychiatric diagnosis have 1.5 as many contacts as women from

Table 9.4 Contact data of patients with a DSM-diagnosis (more and less severe) compared with the practice population, adjusted for age and sex (2001)

	Patients with a DSM diagnosis (n = 376)	Patients with a severe DSM diagnosis (n = 201)	Patients with a less severe DSM diagnosis (n = 175)	Practice population DNSGP-2 (≥18 years) (n = 303 786)
Patient characteristics				
Age (mean)	44.3	44.1	44.7	45.8
% male	34	35	32	50
Education (%):				
low	16	19	12	17
middle	61	57	67	62
high	23	25	20	21
Contact data:				
no contact in 2001 (%)	9	9	8	24
at least one contact (%)	91	91	92	76
Episodes per visiting patient	5.8	6.3	5.1	3.9
Contacts per episode	1.58	1.62	1.52	1.46
Distribution of somatic, psychological and social diagnoses (contacts per visitor)				
Somatic (excluding vegetative)	7.06	7.74	6.29	5.15
Somatic/vegetative	0.23	0.26	0.20	0.16
Psychological	1.60	2.08	1.04	0.35
Social	0.19	0.21	0.18	0.06
Top 10 most common diagnoses				
1	Depression (3.8%)	Depression (5.5%)	Depression (4.8%)	Hypertension (3.3%)
2	Anxiety (2.1%)	Hypertension (3.9%)	Anxiety (3.2%)	Cough (1.8%)
3	Sleeping problems (1.8%)	Anxiety (2.6%)	Symptoms neck (2.3%)	Menopausal symptoms (1.7%)
4	Cough (1.6%)	Sleeping problems (1.6%)	Hypertension (2.2%)	Low back pain (1.5%)
5	Menopausal symptoms (1.6%)	Stress/ overworking (1.6%)	Sleeping problems (2.2%)	Urinary infection (1.2%)
6	Hypertension (1.6%)	Cough (1.4%)	Cough (1.8%)	Upper respiratory. infection (1.2%)
7	Dermatophytosis (1.4%)	Dermatophytosis (1.4%)	Diabetes (1.6%)	Depression (1.0%)
8	Stress/ overworking (1.3%)	Low back pain (1.4%)	Menopausal symptoms (1.6%)	Sleeping problems (1.0%)
9	Eczema (1.3%)	Personality disorder (1.2%)	Eczema (1.5%)	Bronchitis (1.0%)
10	Symptoms neck (1.2%)	Constipation (1.2%)	Warts (1.4%)	Excessive ear wax (1.0%)

the average population, while men only have 1.2 as many contacts (data not shown).

The more severe the psychiatric diagnosis, the more the patient differs from the average population regarding morbidity and contact rates.

The higher contact rate of DSM-IV patients is not restricted to a higher contact rate for psychological, social and vegetative symptoms; they have a higher contact rate for strictly somatic diseases as well (*see* Table 9.4). The proportion of contacts with a somatic diagnosis is 78% for DSM-IV-diagnosed patients, and 90% for the total population. Again, for patients with a more severe psychiatric diagnosis the differences from the total practice population are larger than for patients with a milder psychiatric diagnosis.

A relative difference in morbidity pattern is also visible when we inspect the top 10 most frequently encountered diagnoses (*see* Table 9.4). 'Depression or depressive feelings' is the most frequently encountered diagnosis for patients with a DSM-IV diagnosis, closely followed by 'nervous feelings, anxiety', 'sleeping problems' and 'stress, overworking'.On the other hand, hypertension, coughing, dermatophytosis and eczema are also found in the top 10 of psychiatric patients, while 'sleeping problems' and 'depression, depressive feelings' are part of the average practice's top 10 diagnoses as well.

In summary: patients with a psychiatric diagnosis differ clearly from the total practice population in their use of GP services, but the qualitative difference, regarding psychological or somatic diagnoses made by GPs, is more gradual. The psychiatric patient is more frequently seen as being depressed, anxious or with sleeping problems, but the majority of his illnesses concern hypertension, respiratory problems, or ordinary skin problems, whereas depression and sleeping problems are diagnosed frequently among patients without a psychiatric diagnosis as well.

What to think about it

Patients with a psychiatric disorder often have a combination of two or more psychiatric diagnoses. In particular, mood disorders and anxiety disorders are frequently found together in one person. Furthermore, depression or anxiety are often comorbid with alcohol addiction. This is known from previous studies in Australia, the Netherlands and the US, but it places the assignment of the GP in a different perspective.[13,14,15] Which psychiatric disorder should be diagnosed by the GP?

Psychiatric patients are extensive users of GP care. But they suffer from the same somatic problems as other patients.

Patients with a psychiatric disorder are more likely to visit their GP during one year than the average patient: 91% versus 76% (after controlling for age and sex). Only a minority of them are diagnosed with their specific diagnosis: 28% of the patients with a depressive disorder, 16% of those with anxiety and fewer than 5% of those with alcohol problems are diagnosed as such. However, more than half of them are diagnosed at least once with a psychological diagnosis, and between 10% and 15% of them are diagnosed with a social diagnosis (Chapter Z) or somatic symptoms indicative for anxiety or depression. However, about 40% of those with a DSM-IV diagnosis will never get any psychological, social or psychosomatic diagnosis during one year, despite having visited their GPs. These figures are more positive (more specific recognition, more general psychological diagnoses) for patients with severe psychopathology than for patients with milder diagnoses (single, not recurrent, mild). In general, these findings are comparable with figures from cross-sectional surveys in which GP diagnoses were compared with standardised psychiatric assessments, including the conclusion that recognition by the GP improves when a continuous scale is used instead of a categorical one.[16,17]

Although patients with a DSM-IV diagnosis receive significantly more psychological diagnoses than average patients, the vast majority of their diagnoses are somatic by nature. Depression, sleeping problems, nervousness and anxiety are observed in this subgroup indeed, but they are to a greater extent suffering from hypertension, diabetes, warts and climacterium problems, like all other patients. As a group, they are more easily distinguished from the average population by their more frequent contact rate and their larger number of diseases, than by the nature of their morbidity.

Limitations

Our results are based on a substantial sample of 376 respondents with at least one psychiatric DSM-IV diagnosis. It is not possible to assess the representativeness of the sample, because the CIDI was only applied to a preselected population of patients who already scored high on a screening instrument. We cannot therefore calculate a prevalence figure to compare with other studies. The aim of the study, however, was not to calculate prevalence or incidence of psychiatric disorder, which has already been done in the Netherlands, on a larger scale too. Our aim was to assess psychiatric morbidity on a large enough scale to study comorbidity in general practice of this sample.

Another limitation is our restriction of the CIDI interview to anxiety disorders, mood disorders and alcohol abuse. This restriction was made on purpose, because these disorders make up the vast majority of psychiatric disorders encountered in primary healthcare in which we are primarily interested.[18]

A more problematic restriction in our design is the lack of a recording of the patients' reason to visit their GPs. We have to use GPs diagnoses to deduct the symptoms with which patients will have presented themselves. From earlier studies in which we observed videotaped consultations we know that patients presenting themselves with psychological symptoms will in almost all cases be given a psychological diagnosis.[19]

For more than one-third of the patients with a psychiatric disorder, psychological problems are not an issue during encounters with the GP.

A final restrictive remark needs to be made about our 'average' population which served as a kind of reference group. A random sample of about 4% of the population at risk has been subjected to a health interview. Respondents with high scores on the psychiatric screeners (GHQ-12 and CAGE) were further assessed by the CIDI, resulting in 376 'cases' with at least one DSM-IV diagnosis. If this result would be generalised to the whole population, our 'average' reference group will have counted 25×376 more persons with at least one DSM-IV diagnosis. These nearly 10 000 persons in a group of 300 000 will account for quite a number of depressive episodes from the top 10 of the 'average' group.

Are there any triggers for the GP to suspect psychiatric problems?

Taking all these restrictions into account we may conclude that about half to two-thirds of the patients with a DSM-IV diagnosis are known by their GPs to be suffering from any kind of psychiatric disorder. Patients with a severe disorder and patients with a mood disorder are more easily recognised than patients with a less severe disorder, anxiety disorder or alcohol abuse. On the other hand, more than one-third did not receive any diagnosis related to psychological distress. Assuming that GPs will have registered psychiatric diagnoses when patients present explicit psychological symptoms, we conclude that many patients with a DSM-IV diagnosis have not presented any psychological symptom during our one year of registration, or that they did this in such an implicit way that it could not be noticed by the GP. They often present other symptoms requiring attention rather than symptoms that might be indicative of their psychiatric disorder. Although it has been suggested that these might be somatic symptoms of anxiety or depression, such as lack of appetite, loss of weight or tiredness, these symptoms constitute only a few percent of all symptoms and diagnoses of psychiatric patients. Moreover, these symptoms are registered to the same degree for average patients as well. We have not learned much about usable triggers for the GP. These patients are hardly recognisable by the kind of symptoms they present, they are only recognisable by the frequency of their contacts with their GPs and by the number of different illnesses they seek help for. This may be a depressing finding for many a GP.

References

1 WHO World Mental Health Survey Consortium (2004) Prevalence, severity and unmet need for treatment of mental disorders in the world health organization world mental health surveys. *JAMA*. **291**: 2581–90.

2 Bijl RV, de Graaf RD, Hiripi E *et al*. (2003) The prevalence of treated and untreated mental disorders in five countries. *Health Aff*. **22**: 122–33.

3 Lamberts H (1990) *Het Huis van de Dokter. Cijfers uit het tranisitieproject*. [The house of the GP. Data from the Transition Project.] Huisartsenpers, Lelystad.

4 van der Linden MP, Westert GW, de Bakker DH and Schellevis FG (2004) *Klachten en Aandoeningen in de Bevolking en in de Huisartspraktijk*. [Complaints and illnesses in the population and in GP practice.] Nivel. Utrecht. *See also:* www.NIVEL.ul/nationalestudie

5 Bijl RV and Ravelli A (2000) Psychiatric morbidity, service use and need for care in the general population: results of the Netherlands Mental Health Survey and Incidence Study. *Am J Public Health*. **90**: 602–7.

6 Luber MP, Hollenberg JP, Williams-Russo P *et al*. (2000) Diagnosis, treatment, comorbidity, and resource utilization of depressed patients in a general medical practice. *Int J Psychiatry Med*. **30**: 1–13.

7 Wagner HR, Burns BJ, Broadhead WE *et al.* (2000) Minor depression in family practice: functional morbidity, co-morbidity, service utilisation and outcomes. *Psychol Med.* **30**: 1377–90.

8 Goldberg D (1972) *The Detection of Psychiatric Illness by Questionnaire.* Oxford University Press, London.

9 Mayfield D, McLeod G and Hall P (1974) The CAGE questionnaire: validation of a new alcoholism screening instrument. *Am J Psychiatry.* **131**:1121–3.

10 World Health Organization (1997) *Composite International Diagnostic Interview.* WHO, Geneva.

11 American Psychiatric Association (1994) *Diagnostic and Statistical Manual of Mental Disorders* (4e). APA, Washington DC.

12 Lamberts H, Wood M (1987) *International Classification of Primary Care.* Oxford University Press, Oxford.

13 Andrews G and Carter GL (2001) What people say about their general practitioners' treatment of anxiety and depression. *Med J Aust.* **175** (Suppl): S48–S51.

14 Bijl RV, Zessen GV and Ravelli A (1997) Psychiatrische morbiditeit onder volwassenen in Nederland: het NEMESIS-onderzoek II: Prevalentie van psychische stoornissen. [Psychiatric morbidity in adults in the Netherlands: the NEMESIS-study II: the prevalence of psychological disorders.] *Ned Tijdschr Geneeskd.* **141**: 2453–60.

15 Kessler RC, McGonagle KA, Zhao S *et al.* (1994) Lifetime and 12–month prevalence of DSM-III-R psychiatric disorders in the United States. *Arch Gen Psych.* **51**: 8–19.

16 Tiemens BG, Ormel J and Simon GE (1996) Occurence, recognition and outcome of psychological disorders in primary care. *Am J Psychiatry.* **153**: 636–44.

17 Thompson C, Ostler K, Peveler RC, Baker N and Kinmonth A (2001) Dimensional perspective on the recognition of depressive symptoms in primary care. *Br J Psychiatry.* **179**: 317–23.

18 Goldberg D and Huxley P (1992) Common mental disorders. Routledge, London.

19 Pasch MAA van der, Verhaak PFM (1998) Communication in general practice: recognition and treatment of mental illness. *Patient Education and Counseling* **33**: 97–111.

Chapter 10

Perceived health and consultation of GPs among ethnic minorities compared to the general population in the Netherlands

Walter Devillé , Ellen Uiters, Gert Westert and Peter Groenewegen

What is this chapter about?

We have studied differences between the major migrant groups and the native Dutch population related to self-rated health and its sociodemographic determinants, the use of general practitioner (GP) care and the incidence of diagnoses made by GPs.

Self-rated health differs significantly between all migrant groups and the native Dutch, and clusters in two groups: Surinamese/Antillean and Turkish/Moroccan patients, especially in Turkish/Moroccan females. Turks rate their health worst and a higher percentage visit the GPs at least once a year. Fewer Surinamese and Antillean patients visit their GPs than the Dutch do. People from ethnic minorities in good health visit their GPs more often than their Dutch peers. Ethnic minorities who do visit their GPs do it more often than the Dutch. Seven diagnoses in the top 10 of incidence rates were similar in all groups. The incidence rates of acute respiratory infections and chest complaints were significantly higher in all migrant groups than in the Dutch.

Ethnicity is independently associated with self-rated health. The higher use of GP care by ethnic minorities in general, especially females, and more specifically the ones in good health, points towards possible inappropriate use of resources. The diagnoses with a higher incidence and the use of prevention need specific attention in these migrant groups.

Introduction

In the past 10 years, policy makers and researchers have paid increasingly more attention to the health of ethnic minorities in the Netherlands. This was due to two factors. Primarily, during the same period, research groups have initiated extensive research about the still existing differences in health, more specifically about socio-economic differences in health.[1] Secondly, the changing composition of the population in the same period has generated more attention to differences in health according to age, sex and ethnicity. In the past decades, the Netherlands has increasingly become a multicultural society. In 2001, when the study took place, the percentage of non-western ethnic minorities was 9%, mostly resident in large cities like Amsterdam and Rotterdam.[2–4] As a consequence of decolonisation, active labour recruitment and better labour circumstances, large groups of immigrants came to live and work in the Netherlands. Later on, their numbers increased strongly because of family reunion and family formation. Moreover, political refugees and asylum seekers from more than 160 countries are living in the Netherlands.[5] Eventually, the recent increase is not only due to immigration but also to an increasing size of the so-called second generation of ethnic minorities.[4]

The large number of people from ethnic minorities has important consequences for general practice and public health. Ethnic minorities often end up in a deprived position, characterised by various kinds of social disadvantages. Also in ethnic minorities the socio-economic situation – reflected by education, occupation, income and working situation – may be an important determinant of their health.[6] But other factors may be equally relevant: the health status in the country of origin at the moment of migration, the epidemiological profile of that country, the ethnic or cultural origin (e.g. genetic disorders, nephew–niece intermarriage). Recent research into the health of migrant populations in European countries has shown that, compared to the native population, different health problems exist within migrant groups and that their health is worse in respect of certain aspects. Perceived health is often worse among ethnic minority groups. Furthermore, ethnic minorities seem to be more susceptible to illness and to suffer from a wider variety of ailments. However, with respect to other aspects of health, results are less straightforward. Certain health problems, like mortality due to cancer, seem to occur with the same frequency or less often within some minority groups compared to the native population.[7–13]

Explanations for ethnic differences in health may be related to differences in behaviour, physical and social environment and psychosocial stress. Another important determinant for ethnic differences in health is the use of care.[14] An adequate use of healthcare services is an important precondition for health. In the Netherlands, little is known about the healthcare utilisation of ethnic minorities. Assumptions are made that ethnic minorities have less access to healthcare services than the native Dutch population. While it is important to study differences in morbidity patterns and aetiology, it is equally important to study to what degree persons make use of healthcare services. Does the use of care correspond with the perceived needs of the migrant groups; what differences exist between various groups of ethnic minorities; which factors affect their use and which problems arise with respect to accessibility and quality of care? These questions are all worth further investigation. Information on these aspects will help to improve healthcare in such a way that the needs and wishes of migrant groups are taken into account, and that these groups will be less disadvantaged in this respect.

In the second Dutch National Survey of General Practice (DNSGP-2) attention has been paid to the explanation of ethnic differences in health and healthcare utilisation. The research questions that will be addressed in this chapter are the following:

- How do ethnic minorities rate their own health compared to the native Dutch population? Which sociodemographic variables are associated with ethnic differences in self-rated health?
- Do migrant groups differ in utilisation of GP care from the native population?
- Do prevalence and incidence of diagnoses recorded by GPs differ between the migrant groups and the native population?

How was it done?

For a description of the methods of the second Dutch National Survey of General Practice (DNSGP-2, 2001), *see* Chapter 2. Self-rated health and socio-demographic characteristics were recorded on a form sent to all patients registered in a national sample of 104 GP practices. All Surinamese, Antillean, Turkish and Moroccan responders and a random sample of 2% of the Dutch responders were included in the study. For one year, data about all contacts with GPs and the incidence of diseases were registered.

Population

Sociodemographic characteristics were assessed by means of a registration form sent in four languages (Dutch, English, Turkish, Arabic) to all patients of the 104 GP practices in the study. It provided information about the country of birth of the patient and his or her parents. Information about country of birth was used to indicate the ethnic background of the patients. If at least one parent was born abroad, a patient was indicated as having a foreign background.[2] A total of 271 388 patients returned the registration form (70%), 3.9% of which belonged to the four major migrant groups. This chapter will focus on these four minority groups coming from Turkey, Surinam, Morocco and the Netherlands Antilles.

As the numbers of elderly people in some migrant groups are still small, the results reported in this chapter are restricted to people aged from 18 to 65 years. We took a random sample of 2% of the Dutch patients who responded to the registration form to end up with a number comparable to the biggest group among the four migrant groups. The total number selected for the five ethnic groups together was 10 252: 3215 Dutch, 2801 Surinamese, 938 Antillean, 1833 Turkish and 1465 Moroccan.

Self-rated health

For the analysis of self-rated health we used data of the registration form. Self-assessed health is measured by means of a single item question, 'In general would you describe your health as: (1) very good, (2) good, (3) neither good, nor poor, (4) poor or (5) very poor'.[15] For the purpose of this analysis the five-point scale was dichotomised into (very) good and fair to (very) poor perceived health. We performed univariate and multivariate analyses of possible determinants of self-rated health.

GP care

To analyse the use of GP care we analysed whether the patients had had any contact with their GPs in 2001, and its determinants in a multivariate logistic regression analysis. On those who had had contact with their GPs we performed multivariate linear regression analyses on the number of contacts with GPs registered during one year in the various practices. To normalise the distribution, the number of contacts was transformed by natural log.

Diagnoses

For answering the third research question about ethnic differences in the incidence of diseases, we based our analyses on the registration of diagnoses during one year in GP practices. All diagnoses were registered with their International Classification of Primary Care (ICPC) codes in the electronic medical records (EMR) by the GP. As numbers were small and the age range limited, we did not control for age or sex in this analysis.

What was found?

The various ethnic groups in this study differ in certain sociodemographic characteristics (*see* Table 10.1). The four migrant groups are somewhat younger than the Dutch group and they have received less education, especially the Moroccan patients: 24% had had no education at all (28% of the women). Half or more from the Surinamese and Antillean groups were single and the rates of divorce were twice as high compared to the other groups. About 40% of Turks and Moroccans were working, compared to around 60% in the other groups. Six to ten per cent in the migrant groups were unemployed, compared to 1.3% in the Dutch group, and 9–13% of Surinamese, Turks and Moroccans were disabled for work compared to 6% in the other two groups. One-quarter of Turkish and Moroccan women were housewives, which is higher than in other groups.

Migrants rate their health worse

Unadjusted self-rated health of Surinamese and Antillean patients was twice as bad as that of the Dutch, while Moroccan and Turkish patients rated their health up to three times worse (*see* Table 10.2). Older age, female sex, lower education, various categories of civil status and of occupation were positively associated with poor health. In multivariate analysis, all these factors remained associated, but while their association decreased, the odds ratios of all migrant groups increased compared to the Dutch native group as reference group. The odds of adjusted poor self-rated health were 2.4 times higher in Surinamese and Antillean patients compared to the Dutch, and 3.8–4.7 times higher for Moroccan and Turkish patients respectively. Regarding interactions, the effect of sex was specifically significantly higher in Moroccan and Turkish female, and Moroccan and Turkish married patients.

Table 10.1 Characteristics of study population, self-rated health and contact with GP according to ethnicity (%)

	Dutch (n = 3215)	Surinamese (n = 2801)	Antillean (n = 938)	Turkish (n = 1833)	Moroccan (n = 1465)
Female	52	60	57	49	50
Age (years):					
18–24	11	16	17	18	23
25–44	45	53	54	59	53
45–65	45	31	28	23	24
Education:					
none	1	3	3	10	24
basic	10	16	13	36	22
secondary	67	66	67	46	45
high	22	16	17	9	9
Civil status:					
single	30	50	61	20	26
married	65	37	28	73	64
divorced	4	12	10	5	6
widowed	2	2	1	2	4
Occupational status:					
student	7	11	15	11	14
working	65	63	58	42	39
unemployed	1	6	9	8	10
housewife/-husband	16	9	12	24	25
disabled for work	6	9	6	13	11
retired	4	2	1	2	2
Poor self-rated health	15	29	27	45	39
Contact with GP in 2001	74	62	70	84	79

Contacting the GP: differences between migrants

Unadjusted, significantly more Turkish and Moroccan patients had had at least one contact with their GP in 2001, while significantly fewer Surinamese and Antillean patients had had contact with their GPs compared to Dutch patients. Female sex, older age, lower education, various categories of civil status and occupation, and poor self-rated health were positively associated with use of GP care. Adjusted for the remaining significant determinants (female sex, lower education, categories of civil status and self-rated health), only significantly more Turkish patients made use of GP care during the year 2001.

Fewer Surinamese and Antillean clients visit their GPs during one year.

Regarding interactions, significantly more female and married Turks contacted their GP, as well as divorced Moroccans. On the other hand, fewer female Surinamese patients contact their GPs. The overall effect of self-rated health as poor increases, as interaction analysis shows that this effect is significantly lower in Moroccans, Antilleans and Surinamese patients (*see* Table 10.3).

Table 10.2 Determinants of self-rated health as poor

	OR (95% CI) univariate	OR (95% CI) multivariate	OR (95% CI) multivariate with interactions
Ethnicity:			
Dutch	1	1	1
Surinamese	1.8 (1.6–2.0)	2.4 (2.0–2.8)	2.1 (1.3–3.2)
Antillean	1.6 (1.3–1.9)	2.4 (2.0–3.0)	2.0 (1.3–3.0)
Turkish	3.3 (2.9–3.8)	4.7 (3.9–5.6)	2.1 (1.3–3.3)
Moroccan	2.6 (2.3–3.0)	3.8 (3.1–4.6)	1.7 (1.2–2.3)
Sex:			
male	1	1	1
female	1.3 (1.2–1.4)	1.3 (1.1–1.5)	1.0 (0.8–1.3)
Age (years):			
18–24	1	1	1
25–44	2.4 (2.0–2.9)	2.3 (1.8–2.9)	2.2 (1.7–2.8)
45–65	4.8 (4.0–5.8)	4.4 (3.4–5.7)	4.3 (3.3–5.6)
Education:			
none	7.0 (5.7–8.7)	2.3 (1.7–3.0)	2.1 (1.6–2.8)
basic	4.4 (3.8–5.2)	1.9 (1.5–2.3)	1.8 (1.5–2.3)
secondary	1.6 (1.4–1.8)	1.4 (1.2–1.6)	1.4 (1.2–1.7)
high	1	1	1
Civil status:			
single	1	1	1
married	1.7 (1.5–1.9)	1.0 (0.8–1.1)	0.7 (0.6–1.0)
divorced	4.0 (3.4–4.7)	1.8 (1.4–2.2)	1.6 (1.0–2.7)
widowed	4.4 (3.6–4.7)	2.0 (1.4–2.8)	1.5 (0.7–3.0)
Occupational status:			
student	1	1	1
working	1.4 (1.1–1.7)	0.9 (0.7–1.2)	0.9 (0.7–1.1)
unemployed	5.4 (4.4–7.4)	2.7 (2.0–3.6)	2.7 (2.0–3.6)
housewife/-man	4.0 (3.2–5.0)	1.5 (1.1–2.0)	1.4 (1.1–1.9)
disabled for work	26.3 (20.4–34.0)	12.0 (8.0–16.4)	11.6 (8.5–15.8)
retired	4.9 (3.9–6.1)	1.2 (0.8–1.8)	1.1 (0.7–1.7)
Interactions:			
Moroccan female (n = 738)			1.4 (1.0–2.0)
Turkish female (n = 906)			1.5 (1.1–2.1)
Married Moroccans (n = 923)			1.7 (1.1–2.7)
Married Turks (n = 1321)			2.1 (1.3–3.3)

OR: odds ratio.

Table 10.3 Determinants of contacting GP at least once in 2001

	OR (95% CI) univariate	OR (95% CI) multivariate	OR (95% CI) multivariate with interactions
Ethnicity:			
Dutch	1	1	1
Surinamese	0.6 (0.5–0.6)	0.5 (0.5–0.6)	0.7 (0.5–0.9)
Antillean	0.8 (0.7–0.96)	0.9 (0.7–1.0)	0.9 (0.6–1.2)
Turkish	1.8 (1.6–2.1)	1.5 (1.3–1.8)	0.7 (0.5–1.0)
Moroccan	1.3 (1.2–1.6)	1.1 (0.9–1.3)	0.9 (0.7–1.3)
Sex:			
male	1	1	1
female	1.8 (1.7–2.0)	2.0 (1.8–2.2)	2.1 (1.8–2.5)
Age (years):			
18–24	1	ns	ns
25–44	1.3 (1.2–1.5)		
45–65	1.5 (1.3–1.7)		
Education:			
none	2.5 (2.0–3.1)	1.5 (1.2–2.0)	1.5 (1.2–2.0)
basic	1.9 (1.6–2.2)	1.4 (1.2–1.7)	1.4 (1.2–1.6)
secondary	1.3 (1.1–1.4)	1.2 (1.1–1.4)	1.3 (1.1–1.4)
high	1	1	1
Civil status:			
single	1	1	1
married	1.9 (1.7–2.0)	1.5 (1.3–1.6)	1.2 (1.0–1.5)
divorced	1.8 (1.5–2.2)	1.5 (1.2–1.9)	1.3 (0.8–2.1)
widowed	2.0 (1.4–2.9)	1.3 (0.9–1.9)	2.2 (0.9–5.8)
Occupational status:			
student	1	ns	ns
working	1.3 (1.1–1.5)		
unemployed	1.2 (0.9–1.4)		
housewife/-man	2.7 (2.2–3.1)		
disabled for work	1.8 (1.5–2.2)		
retired	1.5 (1.1–2.0)		
Self-rated health:			
good	1	1	1
poor	1.5 (1.4–1.7)	1.3 (1.1–1.4)	2.1 (1.6–2.8)
Interactions:			
Turkish female (n = 906)			1.4 (1.0–2.0)
Surinamese female (n = 1664)			0.7 (0.6–0.9)
Divorced Moroccans (n = 85)			2.7 (1.0–6.9)
Married Turks (n = 1321)			2.3 (1.5–3.3)
Moroccans in poor health (n = 471)			0.6 (0.4–0.9)
Antilleans in poor health (n = 226)			0.7 (0.4–0.9)
Surinamese in poor health (n = 712)			0.4 (0.3–0.6)

ns: not significant

Once they have started contacting a GP, women (5.1, 95% confidence interval (CI) 5.0–5.2) contact their GPs more frequently than men do (3.6; 95% CI 3.4–3.7). People who rate their health as poor also had more contacts per year (6.0; 95% CI 5.8–6.2) than people who rated their own health as good (3.9; 95% CI 3.7–4.0) (*see* Table 10.4). Multiple linear regression analysis demonstrated that poor self-rated health and sex were the strongest determinants for the number of contacts per year, followed by age. All ethnic minorities had a higher number of contacts compared to the Dutch population in the following order of importance: Surinamese, Moroccan, Turkish and Antillean patients. Antillean patients differed significantly from Surinamese and Moroccan patients, Turkish from Surinamese patients. Adjusted for age, all ethnic minorities who rate their health as good had significantly more contacts with their GP than the Dutch, men as well as women (but Antillean men). Of the patients who rated their health as poor, Surinamese men as well as women, and Turkish women had significantly more contacts per year compared to the general population (data not shown).

Migrants have more diagnoses

The number of various diagnoses differed between the ethnic groups. While the Dutch had 0.17 different diagnoses per person, Surinamese had 0.30, Antilleans 0.35, Turkish 0.22 and Moroccans 0.14 different diagnoses per person. The top 10 diseases varied among the different ethnic groups; however, seven diagnoses appeared on each top 10 (*see* Table 10.5). Looking at the top 10 in the various groups, the incidence rates of acute respiratory infections (ARI) among Surinamese, Turkish and Moroccan patients are significantly higher compared to the Dutch. The diagnoses with lower incidence rates are as follows: earwax was lower in all groups; urinary tract infections (UTI) and dermatomycosis lower in Surinamese; and sinusitis lower in Surinamese, Antilleans and Moroccans. The incidence rates of the following diagnoses were higher: chest complaints was higher among all groups; back complaints in Antilleans, Turks

Table 10.4 Mean number of contacts with GP per year per ethnic group, once clients are contacting GP (adjusted for age) (mean, 95% CI)

	Dutch	Surinamese	Antillean	Turkish	Moroccan
Overall	3.7 (3.5–3.8)	4.9 (4.7–5.1)	4.4 (4.1–4.7)	4.8 (4.6–5.0)	4.9 (4.7–5.1)
Good self-rated health	3.4 (3.2–3.6)	4.3 (4.1–4.5)	4.0 (3.6–4.4)	3.9 (3.6–4.2)	4.4 (4.0–4.7)
male	2.8 (2.5–3.1)	3.6 (3.2–3.9)	3.3 (2.7–3.9)	3.2 (2.7–3.6)	3.6 (3.2–4.1)
female	3.8 (3.6–4.1)	4.7 (4.5–5.0)	4.5 (4.0–5.0)	4.7 (4.3–5.2)	5.0 (4.6–5.5)
Poor self-rated health	5.7 (5.3–6.1)	6.7 (6.4–7.1)	5.5 (4.9–6.1)	5.8 (5.5–6.1)	6.0 (5.6–6.4)
male	4.5 (3.9–5.1)	5.5 (4.9–6.2)	4.2 (3.2–5.2)	4.3 (3.9–4.8)	5.1 (4.5–5.6)
female	6.5 (6.0–7.0)	7.3 (6.9–7.8)	6.1 (5.4–6.8)	6.8 (6.4–7.2)	6.8 (6.3–7.3)

Table 10.5 Ten most frequently diagnosed diseases in general practice by ethnic group in 2001 (incidence rates per 1000 persons)

Dutch		Surinamese		Antillean		Turkish		Moroccan	
ARI	45.7	ARI	56.5	ARI	59.3	ARI	83.5	ARI	77.1
Ear smear	43.5	Low back pain	37.3	UTI	33.6	Low back pain	50.2	Low back pain	56.0
UTI	42.6	Contact eczema	36.2	Low back pain	31.8	Coughing	45.3	Dermatomycosis	45.1
Dermatomycosis	37.3	Dermatomycosis	30.9	Coughing	29.6	UTI	42.0	UTI	41.0
Coughing	36.7	Coughing	30.9	Contact eczema	28.9	Dermatomycosis	41.5	Contact eczema	32.1
Low back pain	32.7	UTI	27.7	dermatomycosis	25.7	Muscle pain	32.7	Back complaints	29.4
Sinusitis	31.4	Fatigue/weakness	26.7	Chest complaints	24.3	Contact eczema	30.0	Fatigue/weakness	28.7
Contact eczema	31.1	Chest complaints	25.6	Back complaints	24.3	Back complaints	27.8	Neck complaints	28.0
Fatigue/ weakness	27.4	Neck complaints	23.5	Neck complaints	20.7	Throat complaints	27.3	Coughing	25.9
Neck complaints	24.9	Other abdominal complaints	23.5	Knee complaints	20.3	Neck complaints	26.2	Other abdominal complaints	25.3

ARI: acute respiratory infections; UTI: urinary tract infections.

and Moroccans and low back pain in Turks and Moroccans; muscle pain in Turks and Moroccans; throat complaints in Surinamese and Turks; and other abdominal complaints in Moroccans. Incidence rates of coughing were lower in Surinamese and Moroccans. Incidence rates of contact eczema, fatigue/weakness, neck and knee complaints did not differ from the Dutch patients.

The higher incidence of ARI and chest complaints in most groups needs special attention.

What to think about it

It seems clear from the various analyses that the four ethnic minorities in the Netherlands rate their health worse compared to the Dutch patients. Self-rated health is associated with various patient characteristics, e.g. education. Taking these characteristics into account, and controlling for socio-economic differences, the difference in poor health between the various ethnic groups and the Dutch increases. Ethnicity seems to be independently associated with self-rated health, as it was in other research.[16,17] These differences seem to cluster in two groups, a Caribbean one (Surinamese and Antillean) and a Mediterranean one (Turkish and Moroccan). Different ethnic groups may rate their health in a different way and use different references. Also, the distances between the various cut-off points may differ and certainly the use of the moderate category may differ between populations. Fair health was included in poor health for this analysis.[18] But we see that in the Mediterranean cluster poor self-rated health seems to be concentrated in female and/or married respondents.

The Turkish people rate their health the worst of all five ethnic groups, which is consistent with a significantly higher proportion consulting their GPs during 2001, even when controlled for all other associated factors. Also, Turkish females visit their GPs most of all. Additionally, poor self-rated health remains an independent factor for visiting the GP, validating this measurement as a predictor for use of care. On the other hand, a significantly smaller proportion of Surinamese and Antillean patients have visited their GPs, especially Surinamese females. These data do not explain this finding, as these patients rated their health twice as badly compared to the Dutch patients. Contrary to what could be expected, Moroccan, Antillean and Surinamese patients in poor health seem less prone to consult their GP than the general population.

When patients visit their GP, all ethnic minorities overall visit their GP more often than the Dutch do. But these differences remain more pronounced among people with good self-rated health. Of the patients who rate health as poor, only Surinamese people visit their GPs more often.

Women rate their health worse than men, twice as many women visit their GP at least once in a year, and women of all ethnic groups visit the GP more often. Differences between ethnic groups are similar for both sexes.

The findings above show a heterogeneous picture in the use of GP care. Turkish and Moroccan populations signify a higher workload for GPs, as a higher proportion visit their GPs, and when they visit their GPs they do it more often. For the other groups the message is different, as a smaller proportion use care, but when they do, they do it more often than the Dutch. The same differences exist for men and women. It seems that efforts in education and information about GP care should focus on the Moroccan and Turkish populations. Information about self-care for minor complaints has to be addressed for all ethnic groups, because people in good health of all ethnic minorities visit their GPs more often, particularly the Surinamese and Moroccan people.

All ethnic minorities should be educated about possibilities of self-care, in order to decrease the number of GP contacts.

The incidences of specific diseases and complaints are difficult to summarise, as the picture is quite heterogeneous over the four groups. Three of the four groups visit their GPs with a larger number of different complaints. Only Moroccan people present a smaller number of different diagnoses and complaints to their GPs. It should be investigated whether this means that this group has difficulties in presenting some health problems to their GPs, although they are already making more use of GP care. Regarding specific diagnoses and complaints, when incidences are higher than those of the Dutch, it often concerns Turkish and/or Moroccan patients. This again is consistent with the outcome of self-rated health and the use of GP care. The higher incidences of ARI in almost all groups, and chest complaints in all, and the lower incidence of sinusitis in three groups might ask for further research into the specific causes and factors related to these diagnoses.

References

1 Mackenbach JP and Stronks K (2002) A strategy for tackling health inequalities in the Netherlands. *BMJ.* **325**: 1029–32.
2 Netherlands Bureau of Statistics (2002) *Statistical Yearbook of the Netherlands.* Netherlands Bureau of Statistics, Voorburg/Heerlen.
3 Wissen van L and Huisman C (1998) *Regionale Prognose Allochtonen.* [Regional prognosis of immigrants.] DEMOS. NIDI, Den Haag.
4 de Jong de A and Hoefnagel J (2001) Verdubbeling van het aantal allochtonen in de afgelopen kwart eeuw. [Doubling of the number of immigrants during the last century] *Mndstat bevolking.* [The population's monthly statistics] **49**(9): 11–15.
5 Castles S and Miller MJ (2003) *The Age of Migration: international population movements in the modern world.* Palgrave Macmillan, Basingstoke.
6 Uitenbroek DG and Verhoeff AP (2002) Life expectancy and mortality differences between migrant groups living in Amsterdam, The Netherlands. *Soc Sci Med.* **54**: 1379–88.
7 Reijneveld SA (1998) Reported health; lifestyles, and use of health care of first generation immigrants in the Netherlands: do socioeconomic factors explain their adverse position? *J Epidemiol Community Health.* **52**: 298–304.
8 Uniken Venema HP, Garretsen HF and van der Maas PJ (1995) Health of migrants and migrant health policy, The Netherlands as an example. *Soc Sci Med.* **41**: 809–18.
9 Bollini P and Siem H (1995) No real progress towards equity: health of migrants and ethnic minorities on the eve of the year 2000. *Soc Sci Med.* **41**: 819–28.
10 Sundquist J (1995) Ethnicity, social class and health. A population-based study on the influence of social factors on self-reported illness in 223 Latin American refugees, 333 Finnish and 126 south European labour migrants and 841 Swedish controls. *Soc Sci Med.* **40**: 777–87.

11 Stronks K, Uniken-Venema P, Dahhan N and Gunning-Schepers LJ (1999) Allochtoon, dus ongezond? Mogelijke verklaringen voor de samenhang tussen etniciteit en gezondheid geïntergreerd in een conceptueel model. [Immigrant, meaning in poor health? Possible explanations for the association between ethnicity and health status integrated into a conceptual model.] *Tijdschr Gezondheidswet.* **77**: 33–40.

12 Weide M and Foets M (1997) Migranten en de huisarts. bevindingen uit twaalf onderzoeken in kaart gebracht. [Immigrants and general practioners: findings from twelve studies summarised.] *Tijdschr Soc Gezondheidsz.* **75**: 4–12.

13 Razum O, Zeeb H, Akgun HS and Yilmaz S (1998) Low overall mortality of Turkish residents in Germany persists and extends into a second generation: merely a healthy migrant effect? *Trop Med Int Health.* **3**: 297–303.

14 Wersch van SFM, Uniken-Venema HP and Schulpen TWJ (1997) De gezondheidstoestand van allochtonen. [The health of immigrants.] In: Mackenbach JP, Verkleij H (eds) *Volksgezondheid Toekomst Verkenning II, gezondheidsverschillen.* RIVM, Bilthoven, pp. 199–223.

15 Gandek B, Ware JE, Aaronson NK *et al.* (1998) Cross-validation of item selection and scoring for the SF-12 Health Survey in nine countries: results from the IQOLA Project. International Quality of Life Assessment. *J Clin Epidemiol.* **51**: 1171–8.

16 Pudaric S, Sundquist J and Johansson SE (2003) Country of birth, instrumental activities of daily living, self-rated health and mortality: a Swedish population-based survey of people aged 55–74. *Soc Sci Med.* **56**: 2493–503.

17 Franks P, Gold MR and Fiscella K (2003) Sociodemographics, self-rated health, and mortality in the US. *Soc Sci Med.* **56**: 2505–14.

18 Salomon JA, Tandon A and Murray CJ (2004) Comparability of self rated health: cross sectional multi-country survey using anchoring vignettes. *BMJ* **328**: 258. http://bmj.bmjjournals.com/cgi/content/full/328/7434/258 (accessed 14 September 2005).

Chapter 11

Respiratory tract infections in general practice according to age, sex and high-risk comorbidity

Eelko Hak, Maroeska Rovers, Marijke Kuyvenhoven and Theo Verheij

What is this chapter about?

This contribution shows the incidence rates of episodes of respiratory tract infections according to age, sex and common high-risk diseases presented to the Dutch general practitioner (GP). Over the last decades, demographic changes, such as ageing and increase in comorbid conditions, the introduction of respiratory vaccination programmes, as well as change in illness behaviour, have made the sparse reports on the occurrence of acute respiratory tract infections in primary care out of date for most western countries. Incidence rates of upper respiratory tract infections were highest among children and an U-shaped association was observed between age and lower respiratory tract infections. Also, patients with chronic medical conditions like pulmonary and cardiac disease run more than two times higher risks for respiratory tract infections episodes. Our study emphasises the importance of knowledge on diagnosis and prognosis of respiratory tract infections and the potential impact of preventive and therapeutic measures among children, elderly persons and patients with chronic lung and cardiovascular disease and diabetes mellitus in general practice, because of the high incidence rates among these groups.

Introduction

Acute respiratory tract infections (RTI) have long been recognised as the major cause of morbidity and they rank among the most frequent causes of death among the elderly and very young. Accordingly, epidemiological studies on the occurrence of such illnesses have been abundant. Milestone studies include, for instance, the Hagerstown morbidity studies in 1926 and Tecumseh study by Monto *et al.* in 1971.[1,2] The majority of studies were set in communities or families. Most persons are affected by infections without any complications from them and recover without medical treatment, as shown by the authors. Individuals that experience more severe, prolonged, recurrent or complicated illnesses, however, need to come to the attention of the general practitioner (GP).

In the Netherlands, where antibiotic prescribing is low, up to 50% of the prescriptions for RTIs are not indicated by guidelines.

Among children, upper respiratory tract infections (URTI) such as rhinosinusitis or acute otitis media are common reasons for encounter in the medical practice. Since most such episodes are of viral origin, notably during epidemics, empirical treatment of such illnesses is usually symptomatic and antibiotics have not been demonstrated to be beneficial to these patients. Elderly patients are mostly affected by lower respiratory tract infections (LRTI), like acute bronchitis, exacerbations of pre-existent chronic obstructive pulmonary disease (COPD) or, less often, pneumonia. Although Dutch antibiotic prescription rates are relatively low compared to other European countries and the USA; even in the Netherlands up to 50% of antibiotics prescribed for RTIs can be assumed to be not indicated by national guidelines.[3] Careful differential diagnosis of these entities is important for evidence-based treatment by antibiotics.

Reports on occurrence of RTIs are rare, although they belong to the most frequent reasons for encounter.

Over the last decades, demographic changes, such as ageing and increase in comorbid conditions, the introduction of respiratory vaccination programmes, as well as changes in illness behaviour, have made the sparse reports on the occurrence of acute RTIs in primary care out of date for most western countries including the Netherlands.[4] Prevention of at least part of RTI by vaccination against influenza virus or *S. pneumoniae*, for example, has been an option for decades now. It can be expected that new and improved respiratory vaccines will become available in the next few years. Since most of the burden by these respiratory agents is present in primary care, knowledge is required on the occurrence of URTI and LRTI among different groups of primary care patients that are relatively easy to identify. The second Dutch National Survey of General Practice (DNSGP-2) provided the opportunity to determine the incidence of upper and lower (recurrent) RTI according to age, sex and common high-risk comorbidity in primary care nationwide.

How was it done?

For a description of the methods of the DNSGP-2, *see* Chapter 2 of this book. The following is specific for the study described in this chapter.

Study population

From the DNSGP-2 we have analysed data from a sample of 90 computerised general practices with 358 008 patients (mid-time population).[5]

Incidence rates of episodes of disease

GPs were trained to record new episodes of illness according to the International Classification of Primary Care (ICPC). The presence of common high-risk comorbid conditions was determined on the basis of diagnoses, medical drug prescriptions and tags integrated in an accurate search algorithm in the general practitioner information system (GPIS).[6] We defined URTI diagnoses as the occurrence of acute otitis media (ICPC code H71), acute rhinitis (R74), acute sinusitis (R75), acute tonsillitis (R76) and acute laryngitis (R77). LRTI diagnoses were defined as acute bronchitis (R78), influenza (R80), pneumonia (R81) or exacerbations of asthma or chronic obstructive pulmonary disease (COPD). Asthma/COPD exacerbations were recorded by the use of R78 for those with asthma or COPD. We calculated incidences per 1000 person-years using the mid-year population in the denominator and the occurrence of a new or first-time RTI episode as the numerator.

What was found?

In all, 15 106 patients (4.2% of the patient population) had three episodes of RTI illnesses per patient on average with a total of 51 538 GP visits for RTIs in one year. In approximately 50% of the cases an antibiotic was prescribed and 4% led to a referral to the specialist. The median age of the patient population with RTI was 31 years (range 0 to 105 years) and 44% were male. The top five highest incidences of the RTIs described were acute rhinitis, acute sinusitis, acute bronchitis, acute otitis media and acute tonsillitis (51, 23, 20, 16 and 10 per 1000, respectively) (*see* Table 11.1). Incidence rates of URTI were higher for females than for males, except for acute otitis media.

4% of the patient population had three episodes of RTI illnesses per patient on average.

URTI were more than twofold more common among patients with chronic lung disease than in the total patient population (209 and 104 per 1000, respectively). LRTI was significantly more common among patients with diabetes mellitus, cardiovascular and lung diseases than in the total patient population (67, 70 and 156 versus 30 per 1000, respectively). In all, incidence rates of URTI were significantly higher among children than in other year-cohorts (*see* Figure 11.1). An U-shaped association was observed between age and LRTI with highest incidences among children and the elderly.

What to think about it

RTI workload for GP

This contemporary study among a large representative patient population in primary care showed that only a small part of the patient population (4%) accounted for these RTI-related GP visits with a high average number of

Table 11.1 Incidence rates of first episodes of respiratory tract infections per 1000 person years

	All	Sex		Age (years)						Comorbidity[a]		
		♂	♀	0–4	5–14	15–49	50–64	65–74	>74	CV	Lung	DM
URTI												
H71 acute otitis media	15.6	16.3	15.0	135.9	33.5	5.4	3.2	2.7	1.6	3.8	33.4	3.6
R74 rhinitis	51.0	45.1	57.5	211.5	47.6	40.3	39.3	41.7	41.9	54.1	107.6	52.9
R75 acute sinusitis	22.7	15.7	29.9	2.9	7.4	29.7	25.8	17.2	9.6	27.7	42.4	23.0
R76 acute tonsillitis	10.2	8.7	11.7	25.8	13.6	12.0	3.2	2.3	0.8	4.2	13.3	3.5
R77 acute laryngitis	4.5	4.0	5.1	16.2	2.6	3.5	5.2	4.5	3.7	6.6	12.5	5.5
LRTI												
R78 acute bronchitis	19.9	18.6	21.5	55.4	14.0	12.8	21.8	31.8	42.0	43.2	–[b]	41.5
R80 influenza	2.2	2.2	2.2	1.8	1.9	2.4	2.3	1.6	2.4	3.1	3.3	2.3
R81 pneumonia	6.4	6.7	6.2	16.6	4.8	3.2	6.1	12.5	21.6	18.9	32.1	18.2
R78 asthma/COPD exacerbation[b]	1.4	1.4	1.5	3.7	1.0	0.7	1.5	3.5	3.7	5.0	120.6	4.8

[a]CV: cardiovascular disease including angina pectoris (ICPC code K74), acute myocardial infarction (K75), ischaemic heart disease (K76), decompensatio cordis (K77), atrial fibrillation (K78), paroxysmal tachycardia (K79), ectopic beats or extrasystole (K80), cor pulmonalis (K82), non-rheumatic valve disease (K83), cerebral vascular disease (K89, K90), peripheral artery disease (K92) and heart disease not specified (K84), in this group also persons who use endocarditis prophylaxis and chronic medications for heart disease (ATC codes: C01, C02, C03, C07 and B01) were included: Lung: chronic lung disease including malignancies of bronchus, lung or respiratory tract (R84, R85), asthma (R96) and COPD (R91,R95), in this group also persons who use lung medication were included (R03); DM: diabetes type I and type II (T90), in this group persons who used anti-diabetic drugs (A10) were included.
[b]R78 was encoded for exacerbations of asthma or chronic obstructive pulmonary disease (COPD).

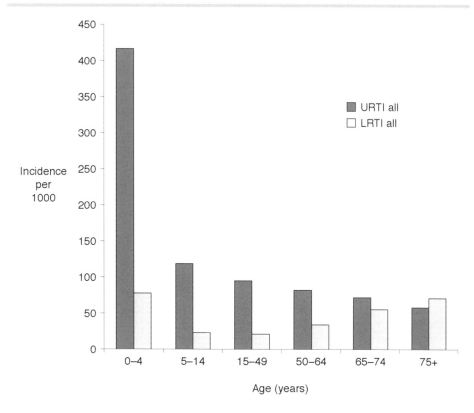

Figure 11.1 Incidence rates of URTI and LRTI according to age (in years). URTI = ICPC codes: H71, R74, R75, R76, R77; LRTI = ICPC codes: R78, R80, R81 and asthma/COPD exacerbations. See methods section for ICPC codes.

episodes per year. In addition to these visits GPs are visited for minor RTI illness such as ear complaints, cough, sinus and throat complaints and for medical control of health status and repeat medication in the case of patients with chronic respiratory disease. Totally, about 15% of all episodes in general practice relate to RTI illness (*see* Chapter 5).

High-risk groups for RTI

Young children were at highest risk for URTI, whereas both young children and the elderly were at increased risk for episodes of LRTI. Patients with chronic medical conditions run more than two times higher risks for RTI episodes, notably those with chronic lung disease. As we have recently shown, both groups visit the GP much more often than adults, but in proportion they do not receive more antibiotics.[7] These patient populations should therefore be prioritised in therapeutic and preventive strategies as well as in patient education programmes.

International decline of RTI incidence

The presented data refer to physician-diagnosed RTI, hence incidence rates of community-acquired RTI might be many times higher than observed in our study. Fleming and colleagues have conducted a general practice-based survey in the UK and they observed similar figures and trends in increased RTI occurrence among children and elderly persons.[8] For the UK and the Netherlands, a lowered incidence of RTIs has been shown for children as well as for adults in the last decade,[8,9] while it is unclear whether this decrease has been caused by a real reduction of incidence or by a reduced inclination of patients to present respiratory illness to the GP.

Fleming and colleagues have conducted a general practice-based survey in the UK and they observed similar figures and trends in increased RTI occurrence (2002).

What this study adds

Information on RTI among patients with comorbid conditions was not available until now, whereas a large proportion of general practice resources is consumed by such patient groups at high risk for RTI. In the Netherlands with approximately 16 million inhabitants, for example, 800 000 (5.0%) persons have chronic lung disease, 500 000 (3.0%) diabetes mellitus and 400 000 (2.5%) cardiovascular disease. The results of our study emphasise the importance of knowledge on diagnosis and prognosis of RTI and the potential impact of preventive and therapeutic measures among these high-risk groups in general practice.[10]

References

1 Stebbings JH Jr (1971) Chronic respiratory disease among nonsmokers in Hagerstown, Maryland. I. Design of the study and prevalence of symptoms. *Environ Res.* **4**: 146–62.

2 Monto AS and Cavallaro JJ (1971) The Tecumseh study of respiratory illness. II. Patterns of occurrence of infection with respiratory pathogens, 1965–1969. *Am J Epidemiol.* **94**: 280–9.

3 Akkerman AE, Kuyvenhoven MM, van der Wouden H and Verheij JTM (2004) *Het Voorschrijven van Antibiotica door de Huisarts bij Luchtweginfecties, Astma en COPD* [Prescribing antibiotics by general practitioners in cases of RTIs, asthma and COPD.] A confidential report for the Health Care Insurance Board, Diemen, the Netherlands, Utrecht.

4 Janssens JP and Krause KH (2004) Pneumonia in the very old. *Lancet Infect Dis.* **4**: 112–24.

5 Westert GP, Schellevis FG, de Bakker DH *et al.* (2005) Monitoring health inequalities through general practice: the second Dutch National Survey of General Practice. *Eur J Public Health.* **15**: 59–65.

6 Hak E, van Essen GA, Stalman W and de Melker RA (1998) Improving influenza vaccination coverage among high-risk patients: a role for computer-supported prevention strategy? *Fam Pract.* **15**: 138–43.

7 Akkerman AE, van der Wouden JC, Kuyvenhoven MM, Dieleman JP and Verheij TJ (2004) Antibiotic prescribing for respiratory tract infections in Dutch primary care in relation to patient age and clinical entities. *J Antimicrob Chemoth*. **54**: 1116–21.

8 Fleming DM, Smith GE, Charlton JR and Nicoll A (2002) Impact of infections on primary care greater than expected. *Commun Dis Public Health*. **5**: 7–12.

9 Kuyvenhoven MM, van Essen GA, Schellevis F and Verheij TJM (2004) Differences in prescribing antibiotics and incidences of upper respiratory tract infections (URTIs) in Dutch general practice between 1987–2001; have national guidelines changed practice and consequently patients' inclination to consult their GP? WONCA abstract book, Amsterdam.

10 Verheij TJM (2001) Diagnosis and prognosis of lower respiratory tract infections: a cough is not enough [Editorial]. *Br J Gen Pract*. **51**: 174–5.

Part 3

Use of care

Chapter 12

The activities of general practitioners: are they still gatekeepers?

Mieke Cardol, Dinny de Bakker and Gert Westert

What is this chapter about?

This study shows a change in the activities of general practitioners (GPs) between 1987 and 2001, to meet an increasing demand of care. The most striking changes are a drop in the percentage of home visits from 17% to 9% of all contacts with GPs and the fact that more work is done by telephone and more tasks are performed by assistants. Nevertheless, GPs and their assistants still are efficient gatekeepers of the Dutch healthcare system: they deal with 96% of all contacts themselves, whereas for nearly 80% of all health complaints, patients only consult their GPs once.

Introduction

Gatekeeping refers to a role as a guide for patients in healthcare and as a person who decides which ailments are minor and which are looking suspicious and need referral to specialists. As far as the latter part of the role is concerned, the rate of new referrals best shows the ability of GPs to deal with requests for treatment themselves.[1] Both nationally and internationally, Dutch GPs are highly regarded as gatekeepers of the healthcare system because of their contribution to the effectiveness of healthcare.[2–4] Nevertheless, a proposed reorganisation of primary healthcare in the Netherlands has given rise to the question of whether GPs should be the only gatekeepers in the healthcare system.

The challenge for general practice in the years ahead is how to continue as efficient gatekeepers and a focal point for patients' health complaints in times of an increasing demand for care.

Furthermore, in the last decades, changes have taken place with regard to the sociodemographic composition of the population in the Netherlands and in other European countries. For example, people are getting older. Consequently, more elderly patients with chronic illness and comorbidity consult their GP. Also general practices are faced with various changes. In the Netherlands, a possible shortage of GPs is a current topic. Other changes include an increasing number of group practices, more female practitioners, and the introduction of clinical guidelines. As a result of these changes, the activities of the GPs and practice assistants will probably have changed too.

This contribution intends to provide a descriptive overview of the activities of Dutch GPs and assistants in 2001 and to show the most remarkable changes compared to 1987. The main questions to be answered are:

- what are the activities in general practice and have these activities changed since 1987?
- as a consequence, can GPs still be considered to be the gatekeepers of health-care?

How was it done?

During one year all contacts of patients with general practices were recorded, including a diagnosis code (International Classification of Primary Care, ICPC), type and number of prescriptions and referrals. For a description of the methods of the second Dutch National Survey of General Practice (DNSGP-2, 2001), *see* Chapter 2 of this book. The following is specific for the study described in this chapter. In 90 practices the type of contact of all patients was recorded during a period of six weeks, whereas diagnostic activities were recorded in 78 practices. The following types of contact were registered: consultation, home visit, telephone call, and other contacts. Other contacts include for example administrative activities. For the registration of diagnostics a list of common activities had to be filled in.

The following activities are considered a 'contact': consultation, home visit, telephone call, and other contacts such as administrative activities.

The duration of contacts with GPs was calculated based on video observations of consultations of 142 GPs, about 20 observations per GP ($n = 2784$). The duration was measured in minutes from the first verbal utterance until the last; interruptions were subtracted from the total duration in minutes.

Furthermore, information from the patient census was used. Finally, the results of the DNSGP-2 were compared with the results of the first national survey in general practice in the Netherlands, which took place in 1987.[5]

What was found?

Contacts with the GP's surgery

The demand for general practice care has risen compared to 1987. In 2001, over three-quarters of the population had one or more contacts with the GP's surgery. While this fraction has remained unchanged since 1987, the number of annual contacts per patient has increased. This increase is particularly striking among older patients.

In 2001, patients had an average of six contacts on an annual basis with their GP's surgery (GPs and/or assistants), whereas in 1987 patients had an average of 4.5 contacts on an annual basis. The variables that determine the frequency of contacts have not changed over the years; they still include age, sex, and cultural origin. Patients aged over 75 years had an average of 16 contacts with their GP's surgery. Women have a higher number of contacts than men. With the exception of the 15–24 years age group, the frequency of contacts for those of non-western origin is higher than for those of western origin in the same age category.

Health problems

On an annual basis, patients consult the GP's surgery for an average of four different health problems. For nearly 80%, patients only consult their GP once. The number of health problems presented to the GP in one year increases with age. Patients consult their GP with many different health problems. Ten health problems account for 19% of all registered problems presented to the GP. Top of this list are upper respiratory tract infections (including coughing: 4.5%), followed by eczema (3.8%), the contraceptive pill (2.5%), hypertension (2.3%), urinary tract infection (1.8%) and low back pain (1.6%). Of course, this list changes with age. From the age of 45 years, hypertension is at the top of the list, and other chronic illnesses such as diabetes mellitus enter the list. Those who rate their health as poor or bad attend their GP more often for mental health problems. Of all the conditions under review, patients with mental health problems and/or chronic conditions have the highest number of contacts with their GP's surgery.

Type of contact

Most contacts take place in the GP's surgery. A distinction can be made between contacts with assistants and contacts with GPs. Some 70% of contacts with the practice assistants consist of telephone or other contacts, and 30% consist of contacts with patients in the practice. Of all GP contacts, 74% take place in the surgery; 9% are home visits. The remaining 18% of GP contacts are telephone calls or other contacts. Figure 12.1 shows that the percentage of home visits has dropped from 17% to almost 9% of all contacts with GPs compared to 1987. The number of telephone contacts has increased from 4% to 11%. Overall, GPs pay fewer home visits to patients of non-western origin than to patients of western origin. Patients of non-western origin also have fewer telephone contacts with the GP's surgery; they attend their GP more frequently in person.

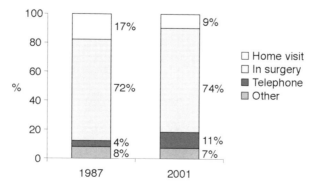

Figure 12.1 Types of contact with GPs in 1987 and in 2001.

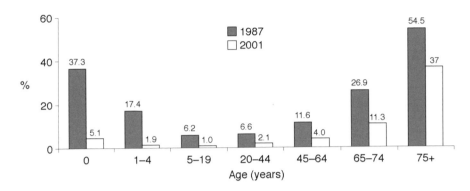

Figure 12.2 Home visits in 1987 and 2001 as a percentage of consultations at the surgery and at the patients' homes by age.

A hypothesis was formulated referring to a possible sharpening of criteria for home visits in 2001. If indeed criteria have sharpened, it was expected to find more home visits to elderly patients and more home visits related to serious health problems. Figure 12.2 shows the percentage of home visits in 1987 and 2001 by patient age group. In 2001, in all age groups the percentage of home visits is lower. The difference between 1987 and 2001 is the most noticeable in the youngest age groups (0–4 years). In 1987, as well as in 2001, the highest percentages of home visits are found related to elderly patients.

In addition, Table 12.1 shows ten diagnoses with the highest home visit to consultation ratio in 1987 and in 2001. In 1987 and also in 2001, the highest ratio is found related to obstetric care. However, in 2001, fewer GPs were involved in obstetric care (not in the table). Furthermore, in 2001 almost all diagnoses referred to life-threatening disease or chronic illness, whereas in 1987 acute health problems such as a fractured leg were also a motive for a home visit.

Table 12.1 Ten diagnoses with the highest home visit to consultation ratio in 1987 and 2001

1987: Top 10 diagnoses home visit to consultation ratio (%)			2001: Top 10 diagnoses home visit to consultation ratio (%)		
	1987	2001		2001	1987
1 Child delivery	91.1	82.6	1 Child delivery	82.6	91.1
2 Fractured leg	88.9	34.4	2 Cancer of the lung	79.9	82.7
3 Myocardial infarction	88.5	34.1	3 Cancer of the stomach	77.6	86.6
4 Disease of the digestive organs	88.2	31.4	4 Cancer of the breast (females)	69.5	69.0
5 Dementia / psychosis	86.7	63.8	5 Loss of partner	67.9	76.2
6 Cancer of the stomach	86.6	77.6	6 Stroke	65.7	70.7
7 Urine retention	86.5	30.4	7 Dementia	63.8	84.1
8 Cancer of the lung	82.7	79.9	8 Heart failure	59.4	64.9
9 Stroke	77.8	65.7	9 Parkinson's disorder	57.7	47.0
10 Loss of partner	76.2	67.9	10 Cancer of the prostate	56.2	72.9

Note: diagnoses are included in analysis only if the number of cases ≥50.

Duration of consultations with GPs

Although, compared to 1987, the average length of GP consultation remained unchanged in 2001, more consultations took longer than 10 minutes (*see* Figure 12.3). In 2001, 40% of GP consultations took longer than 10 minutes, whereas in 1987 only 25% were longer than 10 minutes. Consultations involving social or mental problems take the longest time on average. Young people aged up to 18 years had shorter average consultations. The average duration of a consultation does not increase significantly with age.

Diagnostics

In addition to physical examinations, GPs conduct diagnostic tests in 13% of all contacts. Diagnostic tests are carried out mainly for patients aged over 45 years. As a percentage, most diagnostic testing conducted in the surgery relates to contacts with patients aged over 65 years (8–9% of all contacts); requests for diagnostic testing outside the surgery are more often for patients aged between 20 and 64 years (3–4% of all contacts).

Measuring blood pressure is the most common intervention of all registered diagnostic interventions. It takes place in 8% of all contacts; it is usually related to a diagnosis of hypertension and often conducted by assistants.

Since 1987, the number of requests for blood testing outside the practice has slightly increased (from 2 to 3% of all contacts); at the same time, fewer blood tests have been registered within the practice (from 2 to 1% of all contacts). From the age of 45 years, blood tests are most often conducted in connection with the diagnosis of diabetes mellitus, whereas for younger patients (less than 45 years), 'tiredness' is often the reason.

Prescribing medication

Of the interventions reviewed, the most common is prescribing medication: in 57% of all contacts, GPs issue one or more prescriptions. The number of prescriptions per patient has increased since 1987, particularly for patients aged over 75 years.

In 1987, the average number of prescriptions per patient per annum was four. In 2001, the average per patient is almost six, but more often for a shorter

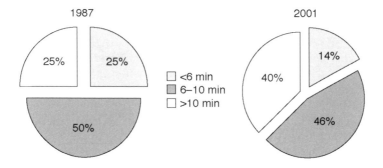

Figure 12.3 Duration of consultations with GPs in 1987 and in 2001.

period. In first consultations GPs prescribe less often than in subsequent visits. Women aged over 75 years are prescribed the most medication – almost 18 prescriptions per person per annum, compared to 15 for men in this age group. Drugs for the cardiovascular system are among the most frequently prescribed for both men and women, although these are prescribed at a later age for women.

Referrals within primary care and to secondary care

In contrast to the prescribing of medicines, referrals mainly take place during first contacts. GPs and their assistants deal with 96% of all contacts themselves; in 4% of all contacts referrals are made. Per 1000 registered patients, GPs make 99 referrals annually within primary care (1.6% of all contacts). Most referrals within primary care are for physiotherapy, with a rate of over 80 per 1000 registered patients. The number of new referrals to secondary care is 153 per 1000 registered patients (2.5% of all contacts). The most frequent new referrals to secondary care concern dermatology (12% of all referrals to secondary care), surgery (11%), ear, nose and throat (11%), ophthalmic (10%) and orthopaedics (10%). Patients with a non-western background are more frequently referred, both within primary care and to secondary care. In general the number of referrals to specialists appears to have dropped since 1987. Referrals for physiotherapy have remained fairly stable.

What to think about it

The results show that GPs continue to play their role as gatekeepers. There has been a rise in the care demand by patients, as expressed in contact frequency with the GP's surgery. However, GPs are not making more referrals to specialist care or to other practitioners in primary care. In addition, the number of minor surgical interventions has remained virtually unchanged but a shift has taken place in type of surgery from treating cuts and wounds to treating benign warts.[6]

Changes have taken place in GP care, which contribute to meet the increased demand. The second national survey has shed light on these changes. For instance, GPs pay far fewer home visits, and they get more work done by telephone. A closer look shows that GPs mainly pay fewer home visits to patients with acute health problems, such as a fractured leg. Another part of the decline in home visits in 2001 may be explained by altered insights regarding the care of newborn and young children. Furthermore, surgery assistants have taken over some of the GPs' work, which is visible in a slight decrease in the 'other' GP contacts, including administrative contacts (from 8% in 1987 to 7% in 2001), and a decrease in the number of blood pressure readings conducted by GPs. The tendency towards a changing 'product' of general practice care is in line with other publications about general practice care in the Netherlands. For example, it was shown that in 2002 the number of births assisted by GPs was much lower than before,[7] and interview data showed that the task scope of GPs has narrowed as far as psychosocial care is concerned.[8]

Bypassing the gatekeeper?

Nevertheless, as stated before, GPs still can be considered to be the gatekeepers of healthcare. The following needs to be added. In contrast to the referral figure registered in practice, the percentage of people who self-reported to have contact with a medical specialist in 2001 shows a slight increase. In particular, those with a high level of education and people in paid employment have more contacts with specialists.[9] This may be an indication of a small group of contacts with specialists that have taken place without referrals from GPs. On the other hand, this discrepancy may also be related to the fact that in the registration data collected in the general practices only new referrals to secondary care were counted.

Why more contacts?

The increase in the number of GP contacts can partly, but not fully, be explained by an increase in the number of older people in the population. The higher contact frequency is most striking among those aged over 75 years, which also applies to the increased number of prescriptions; however, in other age groups too, the contact frequency and the number of prescriptions has risen.

The results show that specific groups of patients receive intensive GP care: older patients and those suffering from chronic illnesses or mental conditions, such as heart disease, diabetes mellitus or depression.

The number of new referrals to specialists or other healthcare workers shows that GPs can still be considered to be the gatekeepers of healthcare.

Another explanation for the finding of increased average contact frequency is that it is a result of the policy implementation on care substitution in the home situation. This policy encourages ill and elderly people to remain at home for as long as possible, and to be treated if possible as outpatients. The existence of waiting lists for secondary care has put increased pressure on primary care. It is not clear from this study whether this factor plays a part in the increased contact frequency.

To conclude, the demand for GP care has increased. Changes have taken place in the organisation of care in order to meet this increasing demand, such as fewer home visits, more telephone calls, fewer obstetric tasks and assistants who have taken over former GP activities such as reading blood pressure. The number of new referrals to specialists or other healthcare workers shows that GPs can still be considered to be the gatekeepers of healthcare. However, waiting lists and continuing care substitution in the home situation might further intensify the already intensive GP care needed for specific groups.

References

1 Stokx LJ, De Bakker DH, Delnoij DMJ, Gloerich ABM and Groenewegen PP (1992) *Verwijscijfers Belicht* [Referral figures highlighted]. NIVEL, Utrecht.

2 Boerma WGW (2003) *Profiles of General Practice in Europe. An international study of variation in the tasks of general practitioners* [Dissertation]. University Maastricht.

3 Starfield B (1994) Is primary care essential ? *Lancet.* **344**: 1129–33.

4 Ministerie van Volksgezondheid, Welzijn en Sport (VWS) (2003) *De Toekomstbestendige Eerstelijnszorg* [The future persistent primary care]. Den Haag, Ministerie van Volksgezondheid, Welzijn en Sport, Sdu Uitgevers, Den Haag.

5 van der Velden K (1999) *General Practice at Work. Its contribution to epidemiology and health policy* [Dissertation]. Erasmus University Rotterdam.

6 Marquet R (2003) Kleine chirurgische verrichtingen in de huisartsenpraktijk in 1987 en 2001: meer aandacht voor huidtumoren [Small surgical interventions in GP practice in 1987 and 2001: more attention for skin tumors]. *Huisarts en Wetenschap.* **46**: 661.

7 Wiegers TA (2003) General practitioners and their role in maternity care. *Health Policy.* **66**: 51–9.

8 van den Berg MJ, Kolthof ED, de Bakker DH and van der Zee J (2004) *Tweede Nationale Studie naar Ziekten en Verrichtingen in de Huisartspraktijk. De werkbelasting van huisartsen* [Second Dutch National Survey of General Practice. The work of general Practitioners]. NIVEL, Utrecht. *See also* www.NIVEL.nl.nationalestudie

9 van Lindert H van, Droomers M and Westert GP (2004) *Tweede Nationale Studie naar Ziekten en Verrichtingen in de Huisartspraktijk. Een kwestie van verschil: verschillen in zelfgerapporteerde leefstijl, gezondheid en zorggebruik* [Second Dutch National Survey of General Practice. A matter of difference: differences in self-reported life style, health and use of care]. NIVEL/RIVM, Utrecht/Bilthoven. *See also* www.NIVEL.nl.nationalestudie

Chapter 13

Prescription in Dutch general practice

Liset van Dijk

What is this chapter about?

The second Dutch National Survey of General Practice (DNSGP-2) has combined registration data on morbidity and prescription, making it possible to unravel diagnosis-specific prescription behaviour of general practitioners (GPs). Prescription rates for different disorders vary considerably, especially in first consultations. Dutch GPs are known for being reluctant to prescribe medication, compared to doctors in other European countries. This is confirmed by lower prescription rates in first consultations compared to follow-up consultations. Moreover, for unspecified symptoms such as 'general disorders', prescription rates are considerably lower than for other disorders. But in the case of prescribing for some specific disorders, such as sleeping disorders, GPs do not comply with the guideline of the Dutch College of GPs. Although this guideline advises preferably not to prescribe medication, GPs do so in 74% of first consultations and 96% of follow-up consultations.

Behind a single figure such as '5.8 prescriptions per patient per year' there is a world of differences between patients, drugs, and disorders.

Dutch people are reluctant users of medication

'Patients are relieved when medication turns out to be unnecessary after a consultation with their doctor.'[1] Dutch experts made this statement in a study on Europeans and their medicines. It puts strikingly well into words the reluctant attitude the Dutch have towards the use of medication. Compared to other European countries, the use of medication in the Netherlands is low and the Organization for Economic Cooperation and Development (OECD) data showed that the Netherlands has almost the lowest expenditure on prescribed medication.[1]

'Patients are relieved when medication turns out to be unnecessary after a consultation with their doctor.'

Nevertheless, the use of medication in the Netherlands has increased substantially over the last decade. This increase can partly be attributed to the increasing age of the population.[2] Also, the use of medication is becoming more accepted in the Netherlands. It is part of a cultural trend in which drugs are being increasingly considered as part of a lifestyle.[3] In 2001, the year of the second National Survey of General Practice (DNSGP-2), expenditures on medication delivered in public pharmacies increased by 11% compared to 2000.[2]

This chapter seeks to answer the following questions:

- What is the volume and type of medication GPs prescribe?
- What are the indications for which GPs do prescribe most?
- For what indications are frequently used drugs prescribed by GPs?
- What are the prescription rates for a series of commonly presented diseases in general practice?

How was it done?

For a description of the methods of the DNSGP-2, 2001, *see* Chapter 2 of this book. The following is specific for the study described in this chapter.

Next to the data on contacts and morbidity, data on prescribing were used. General practitioners (GPs) recorded every single prescription. Ninety-two per cent of these prescriptions were coded according to the Anatomical Therapeutic Chemical classification (ATC). Almost two-thirds of all prescriptions (62%) were labelled with an International Classification of Primary Care (ICPC)-coded indication. The registration data only included prescriptions made within the general practices and did not provide information on prescriptions of medical specialists, unless repeated in general practice or prescribed to patients in a dispensing practice. Data from the morbidity registration were linked to the prescription registration data.

What was found?

Number of prescriptions

In 2001, Dutch GPs prescribed medication in 57% of all consultations (including face-to-face consultations, telephone consultations and visits). GPs prescribed 5.8 prescriptions per patient per year. Women in all age categories received more prescriptions than men, however, between the ages of 15 and 45 years; this is partly due to the prescription of contraceptive pills. Women of 75 years and older received 18 prescriptions on average in 2001, their male peers 15.

Type of medication

Drugs for cardiovascular diseases were the most prescribed drugs for men, followed by drugs classified under 'nervous system' (hypnotics, antidepressants), the respiratory system, the gastrointestinal and the metabolic system. For women, drugs classified under nervous system were prescribed most frequently, followed by drugs for the cardiovascular system, urinogenital/sex hormones, and drugs for the gastrointestinal and metabolic system.

Table 13.1 Top five most frequently registered diagnoses on prescriptions for men, according to age (% of ICPC- and ATC-coded prescriptions)

0–19 years (n = 48 457)[a]	%	20–44 years (n = 99 792)	%	45–64 years (n = 152 134)	%	65–74 years (n = 80 023)	%	75+ (n = 72 702)	%
Asthma	10.4	Dermatomycosis	4.9	Hypertension	11.3	Hypertension	11.7	Hypertension	8.0
Constitutional eczema	6.4	Asthma	4.6	Diabetes mellitus type 2	6.5	Diabetes mellitus type 2	7.7	Diabetes mellitus type 2	6.6
Allergic conjunctivitis	5.5	Allergic rhinitis	4.5	Hypercholesterolaemia	3.6	COPD	6.0	COPD	6.1
Coughing	5.3	Depression	3.8	Depression	2.7	Ischaemic heart disease with angina	3.5	Heart failure	4.6
Allergic rhinitis	5.2	Contact eczema	3.1	Sleeping disorder	2.4	Hypercholesterolaemia	3.3	Sleeping disorder	4.1

[a]n: number of ICPC- and ATC-coded prescriptions.

Indications for prescriptions

Men

For young men (<20 years), prescriptions were mainly for respiratory or dermatological problems (*see* Table 13.1). Asthma was the most common reason to prescribe medication for men in this age group (10% of all prescriptions). For men aged 20 to 45 years, respiratory symptoms were again the most common reason to prescribe. After the age of 45 years, heart diseases and related problems occurred, with hypertension being the most frequently registered indication (8–12%). Another important reason to prescribe medication for older men was chronic obstructive pulmonary disease (COPD), while depression was one of the more frequent reasons to prescribe medication for men aged 20 to 64 years.

Women

Until the age of 45 years, contraception was the most frequent reason for a prescription (13–14%) (*see* Table 13.2). Apart from this, women under 45 years resembled men with respect to frequently registered diagnoses. For women aged 20 to 65 years, as for men, depression was an important reason for prescribing medication. Hypertension was the most frequent diagnosis on prescriptions for women, as was the case for men from 45 years onwards. For women over the age of 45 years, the indications for a prescription were more varied than for men. Heart diseases and related problems were reasons to prescribe, but their role was less prominent than in men. For women, diagnoses related to psychological problems were more often a reason to prescribe medication than for men.

Drugs and their indication range

For the 10 most frequently prescribed categories of drugs (classified according ATC-4 level) we analysed for what indications they were mostly prescribed (*see* Table 13.3). In some of these categories of drugs, one indication was predominant and included over half of the prescriptions in that particular category. This was true for hypnotics, where sleeping disorders accounted for 60% of all prescriptions. For both selective beta-blocking agents and angitensin-converting enzyme (ACE) inhibitors, hypertension was predominant (60% and 58% respectively). Selective serotonin reuptake inhibitors (SSRIs) were prescribed mainly for depression (54%), and lipid-lowering medication for hypercholesterolaemia (67%). Asthma and COPD accounted for 63% of the prescriptions of selective adrenergic inhalants. Other groups of drugs showed a much wider indication range: even the top five did not include half of the prescriptions. This was the case for anxiolytics and non-steroidal anti-inflammatory drugs (NSAIDs). Both for anticoagulants and proton pump inhibitors, the top five included over half of the prescriptions, but there is not one clearly predominant indication.

In five out of the ten most prescribed groups of drugs one indication was predominant.

Table 13.2 Top five most frequently registered diagnoses on prescriptions for women, according to age (% of ICPC- and ATC-coded prescriptions)

0–19 years (n = 63 666)[a]	%	20–44 years (n = 214 008)	%	45–64 years (n = 225 792)	%	65–74 years (n = 121 021)	%	75+ (n = 160 187)	%
Contraception	12.9	Contraception	14.4	Hypertension	10.3	Hypertension	14.0	Hypertension	10.7
Asthma	5.9	Depression	4.1	Depression	4.0	Diabetes mellitus type 2	6.6	Sleeping disorder	5.9
Constitutional eczema	4.6	Allergic rhinitis	3.3	Menopausal symptoms	3.8	Sleeping disorder	4.7	Diabetes mellitus type 2	5.7
Coughing	4.1	Asthma	3.1	Diabetes mellitus type 2	3.8	COPD	2.5	Heart failure	3.5
Allergic conjunctivitis	3.5	Contact eczema	2.7	Sleeping disorder	3.3	Hypercholesterolaemia	2.4	Constipation	2.8

[a]n = number of ICPC- and ATC-coded prescriptions.

Table 13.3 Top five most frequent registered diagnoses on prescriptions for 10 most prescribed drugs (ATC-4 level, % of ATC- and ICPC-coded prescriptions)[a]

Drug prescribed and diagnosis	% of coded prescriptions
1 Non-steroidal anti-inflammatory drugs (two main groups: M01AB and M01AE) (n = 76 086)	
Low back pain without irradiation	11.3
Symptoms of the back	5.2
Shoulder syndrome, periarthrytis humero-scapularis (PHS)	4.9
Low back pain with irradiation	4.6
Symptoms shoulder	4.3
Total top 5	*30.3*
2 Anxiolytics (N05BA) (n = 56 522)	
Anxious feelings	25.7
Sleeping disorder	8.5
Depression	5.9
Anxiety	5.4
Post-traumatic stress disorder	4.6
Total top 5	*50.1*
3 Hypnotics (N05CD) (n = 41 620)	
Sleeping disorder	60.0
Depression	3.4
Anxious feelings	3.0
Drug abuse	2.9
Hypertension	1.8
Total top 5	*71.1*
4 Selective beta-blocking agents (C07AB) (n = 39 064)	
Hypertension without organ damage	59.7
Angina pectoris	6.7
Hypertension with organ damage	6.0
Other ischaemic heart diseases	3.2
High blood pressure	2.0
Total top 5	*77.6*
5 Anticoagulants (B01AC) (n = 28 940)	
Angina pectoris	12.7
Cerebrovascular disease	10.1
Transient ischaemic accident	9.8
Hypertension	9.3
Other ischaemic heart disease	8.7
Total top 5	*50.6*
6 Selective beta-2-sympatheticomimetic agents (R03AC) (n = 30 876)	
Asthma	43.9
Chronic obstructive pulmonary disease (COPD)	19.0
Acute bronchitis	7.9
Cough	4.9
Dyspnoea	4.3
Total top 5	*80.0*

Drug prescribed and diagnosis	% of coded prescriptions
7 Selective serotin reuptake inhibitors (N06AB) (n = 33 787)	
Depression	53.9
Anxiety	11.4
Down/depressed feeling	7.3
Anxious feeling	4.2
Overwork	1.8
Total top 5	*78.6*
8 Lipid-lowering drugs (C10AA) (n = 24 456)	
Hypercholesterolaemia	66.5
Hypertension without organ damage	5.8
Diabetes mellitus	4.5
Angina pectoris	2.3
Other ischaemic heart disease	2.2
Total top 5	*81.3*
9 Proton pump inhibitors (A02BC) (n = 27 566)	
Oesophagal disease	19.5
Stomach disorder	15.4
Pain of the stomach	14.3
Dyspepsia	11.1
Hernia diafragmatica	5.3
Total top 5	*65.6*
10 Angiotensin-converting enzyme inhibitors (C09AA) (n = 26 698)	
Hypertension	57.7
Hypertension with organ damage	9.2
Heart failure	6.7
Diabetes mellitus	5.1
Other ischaemic heart disease	2.0
Total top 5	*80.7*

[a]In total 62% of all prescriptions were ICPC-coded. However, drugs differed in the percentage of coded prescriptions. For example, anticoagulants had a lower percentage of ICPC-coded prescriptions compared to SSRIs. Although anticoagulants are prescribed more often than SSRIs , the n in this table is lower than for SSRIs. The reason is that this table only includes ICPC-coded prescriptions.

Prescription rates for specific disorders

Although Dutch GPs are reluctant to prescribe medication, Table 13.4 shows that prescription was a common action for almost all of the 13 categories of disorders selected. GPs were more reluctant to prescribe in first consultations compared to follow-up consultations. Many symptoms disappear without medication and some have to become more specific or clear before the GP decides whether or not to prescribe medication and what to prescribe. There was considerable variation in prescription rates between different disorders. Looking at first consultations, prescription rates were highest for asthma/COPD and eczema. High prescription rates in first consultations were also found for upper respiratory tract infections and mental disorders. GPs often wrote prescriptions in follow-up consultations for all chronic diseases and mental disorders, as well as for upper respiratory tract infections. In particular GPs tend to prescribe for sleeping disorders: this occurred in 96% of the follow-up contacts.

Table 13.4 Prescription rates for 13 diseases or symptoms (% of all consultations with a prescription and most prescribed type of medication)

Disease/complaint	First consultations		Follow-up consultations	
	Prescription rate (%)	Most prescribed drug	Prescription rate (%)	Most prescribed drug
Somatic disorders:				
general disorders	9	Acetaminophen	44	Acetaminophen
children's disorders	24	Antibiotics	33	Antibiotics
upper respiratory tract infections (adults)	63	Antibiotics	74	Antibiotics
gastrointestinal infections	28	Antidiarrhoeics	53	Antidiarrheoics
Mental disorders:				
depression	52	SSRIs	81	SSRIs
anxiety	50	Anxiolytics	85	Anxiolytics
sleeping disorder	74	Hypnotics	96	Hypnotics
Chronic diseases:				
diabetes mellitus	31	Oral antidiabetics	70	Oral antidiabetics
coronary heart diseases and heart failure	39	Cardiac drugs	81	Antithrombotics
asthma and COPD	72	Sympathomimetics for inhalation	85	Sympatho-mimetics for inhalation
eczema	81	Corticosteroids	86	Corticosteroids
Dorsopathies:				
shoulder and back disorders	37	NSAIDs	56	NSAIDs
osteoarthritis	26	NSAIDs	63	NSAIDs

COPD: chronic obstructive pulmonary disease; NSAID: non-steroidal anti-inflammatory drug; SSRI: selective serotonin reuptake inhibitor.

Dutch GPs are reluctant to prescribe during first consultations.

What to think about it

Dutch patients receive almost six prescriptions per year. But behind this single figure is a world of differences between groups of patients, categories of drugs, and diseases. There are, for example, differences between men and women. It was well known that medicines are prescribed more often for women than for men. But within the group of female patients, there is much more variation in type of prescriptions compared to men, especially after the age of 45 years. This can partly be explained by the fact that women report different and more disorders than men.[4]

With respect to differences between drugs it became clear that indications widely vary. Obviously, this variation is related to the indication(s) for which the drug has been developed. Painkillers can be prescribed for a dozen types of pain, whereas lipid-lowering drugs can mainly be used to lower lipid levels. Nevertheless, this finding is important. Other studies with the same data showed, for example, that the level of off-label prescribing is higher in those medicines that have a wide or unspecified range of indications. Off-label prescribing means that a drug is prescribed for other indications than the ones for which it is formally registered.[5,6]

Another conclusion that can be derived from the top five indications for which drugs were prescribed is that sometimes GPs prescribe frequently, while guidelines advise to prescribe sparingly. An example is the guideline concerning sleeping disorders of the Dutch College of GPs, which advises to be reluctant in prescribing sleep medication: 'when information and sleep hygienic advices are consequently followed, a minority of sleeping complaints needs to be treated with hypnotics'.[7] In three-quarters of initial consultations, however, GPs prescribe medication, mostly hypnotics. A reason for this might be that GPs only register sleeping disorders if they prescribe medication. However, GPs in the National Survey were asked to register a diagnosis in every consultation, including when they did not prescribe medication or refer a patient. Also, with repeat prescriptions for sleeping disorders GPs do not seem to comply with the guideline. While the guideline states that sleeping medication should not be repeated, GPs prescribed hypnotics in 96% of the follow-up consultations for sleeping disorders. This was also confirmed by the findings of the questionnaire about repeat prescriptions filled out by all GPs who participated in the National Survey: 80% allow their practice assistant to repeat sleeping medication, and half of them allow it even more often than twice.[8]

GPs do not follow Dutch guidelines on sleep medication.

Prescription rates differ considerably across disorders, especially when it comes to first consultations. For some chronic diseases, such as diabetes mellitus and ischaemic heart disease or heart failure, GPs are reluctant to prescribe when they establish the diagnosis for the first time. This cannot be explained by the fact that the GP refers the patient to a medical specialist.[9] In the case of diabetes mellitus only 8.5% of all patients were referred after their first consultation and almost half of them were referred to a dietician. For ischaemic heart disease (IHD) and heart failure only 11% of all patients were referred after their first consultation. For all disorders prescription rates are higher in follow-up consultations.

From the single figures one could conclude that Dutch GPs are reluctant to prescribe: the number of prescriptions per patient is 5.8 per year and patients received a prescription in only 57% of all contacts, which is lower than in other countries (*see* also Chapter 26 of this book). However, our analyses showed that behind these figures, there is a world of difference depending on what the disorders are and which patients they concern.

References

1 Kooiker S and van der Wijst L (2003) *Europeans and their Medicines. A cultural approach to the utilization of pharmaceuticals.* The Hague: SCP/Gfk, Den Haag.

2 Stichting Farmaceutische Kengetallen (2002) *Data en Feiten 2002.* [Data and facts 2002.] SFK, Den Haag.

3 Kooiker S (2002) Geneesmiddelen en de consumptiegeneigdheid van de bevolking [Medicines and the consumption tendency of the population]. In: Timmerman H and van den Berg Jeths A (eds) *Geneesmiddelen nu en in de Toekomst.* [Medicines now and in the future.] Volksgezondheid Toekomst Verkenning. Achtergrondstudie. RIVM, Bilthoven, pp. 543–53.

4 van Lindert H, Droomers M and Westert GP (2004) *Tweede Nationale Studie naar Ziekten en Verrichtingen in de Huisartspraktijk. Een kwestie van verschil: verschillen in zelfgerapporteerde leefstijl, gezondheid en zorggebruik.* [The Second Dutch National Survey of General Practice. A matter of difference: variations in self reported life style, health and use of care.] NIVEL/RIVM, Utrecht/Bilthoven. *See also* www.NIVEL.nl.nationalestudie

5 van Dijk L, de Jong A, Florentinus S and Verheij R (2004) Therapeutisch probleem of academisch probleem? Off-label voorschrijven in de huisartspraktijk. [Therapeutic problem or academic problem? Off-label prescribing in general practice.] *Pharmaceutisch Weekblad.* **139**: 902–5.

6 Jabaaij L, Stokx LJ and de Bakker DH (2001) Artrosemiddel in de lift: huisartsen schrijven rofecoxib breder voor dan geïndiceerd is. [Increase in arthritis medication: doctors prescribe rofecoxib beyond indicated applications.] *Medisch Contact.* **56**: 1493–6.

7 Knuistingh Neven A, Lucassen PLBJ, Bonsema K (2005) *et al. NHG-Standaard Slaapproblemen en Slaapmiddelen.* [NHG-standard sleeping problems and sleeping medication 2005.] http://nhg.artsennet.nl. Accessed 23 December 2005.

8 van Dijk L, Dijkers F and Schellevis F (2003) Gecontroleerd voorschrijven. Monitoring herhaalreceptuur verdient meer aandacht. [Controlled prescribing. Monitoring repeat prescriptions should get more attention.] *Medisch Contact.* **58**: 1306–9.

9 Cardol M, van Dijk L, de Jong JD *et al.* (2004) *Tweede Nationale Studie naar Ziekten en Verrichtingen in de Huisartspraktijk. Huisartsenzorg: wat doet de poortwachter?* [The second Dutch National Survey of General Practice. GP care: what does the gatekeeper do?] NIVEL/RIVM, Utrecht/Bilthoven. *See also* www.NIVEL.nl.nationalestudie

Medical practice variation: does it cluster within general practitioners' practices?

Judith de Jong, Peter Groenewegen and Gert Westert

What is this chapter about?

In the ideal situation a patient receives treatment, independent of the general practitioner (GP) or the practice where this GP is working. But this is far from everyday reality. Patients are not alike. GPs are not alike. Practices are not alike. And this leads to sometimes huge variation in medical practice between GPs. Insurance companies, patient organisations, physicians and policy makers are all interested in this phenomenon. We have studied whether visibility of a doctor's clinical behaviour and the use of shared resources influence decisions on prescription, referrals, diagnostics, treatment, and advice. We have found that when behaviour is visible to colleagues, or shared resources are used, GPs working in the same practice behave more alike. The other way around, when behaviour is less visible or no shared resources are used, GPs are less inclined to behave in the same way.

Introduction

It is known that there is variation in medical practice between general practitioners (GPs). This variation has been found for the frequency of contacts,[1] registration of diagnoses,[2,3] diagnostic test ordering,[3-7] referral,[1,8] prescription,[3] and return visits.[3,9-11] Variation is due to differences in patient characteristics and morbidity, but also to GPs who differ in the treatment of similar patients.[12,13] These variations have primarily been studied between individual GPs. GPs used to work in single-handed practices, but by now, more than half of the Dutch GPs work in partnerships or groups.[14] Working in partnerships or groups implies mutual dependency and influence on treatment decisions.[15] In this chapter we will study to what extent GPs working in the same practice behave alike and to what extent GP practices differ from one another.

What is the relevance of understanding variations in treatment?

The observation that similar patients are not treated similarly raises a number of questions that are of central concern in healthcare. Do patients receive the treatment that works best? Is the relationship between costs and effects acceptable? Do all people have equal access to healthcare? These questions are of importance to all stakeholders in the healthcare system, and concern effectiveness, efficiency and equity. Policy makers, insurance companies and patient organisations generally aim at decreasing variation in medical practice. Their questions are whether behaviour of physicians can be influenced and, if it is possible to do so, how. Before these questions can be answered it is important to measure the extent of variation and understand its causes.

Why do GPs in the same practice behave more alike?

Freidson already argued that professional behaviour was more related to the (social) circumstances in which physicians work than to their professional education.[16] Westert found similarities among physicians working in the same hospital in the use of hospital care, while there was variation between the hospitals.[17] De Jong, Groenewegen, and Westert found that GPs working in the same partnership showed similarities in attitudes and stated medical behaviour, while there were differences between GPs working in different partnerships.[18] Apparently, sharing a work environment is related to similarities in behaviour.

The idea is that variation in medical practice between physicians is related to differences in incentives and circumstances between their work environments, providing opportunities and constraints on behaviour. An important aspect of working in the same environment, the same practice, is that GPs use shared resources, like assistants and equipment. The work environment serves as a social system in which decisions take place, and this social system may cause physicians to make similar medical decisions. Visibility of behaviour is an important precondition for similarities to come into being. When behaviour is visible, norms may develop. Similarities in clinical behaviour can be caused by more or less conscious processes. GPs run the risk of being criticised by other GPs working in the same partnership, because they see each others' behaviour. This risk can be minimised by showing similar behaviour. Colleagues develop an informal system to help protect their common interests and to overcome free-riding and maintain solidarity.[19]

This study

We have studied how visibility of clinical behaviour and the use of shared resources influence variation in medical practice between GPs working in different practices. Some of the clinical activities that are studied are more visible for colleagues than others, some use shared resources, and others not (*see* Table 14.1). We expect more variation between practices than between GPs working in the same practice for clinical activities in the least visible situation, e.g. prescription, referrals, diagnostic tests performed in an external laboratory, and advice. When clinical behaviour is visible and/or uses shared resources, similarities are expected between GPs working in the same practices. Examples are diagnostic tests performed in the GP's practice, and treatment.

Table 14.1 Clinical activities of general practitioners included in the analyses

Clinical activity	Description	Visible/using shared resources	Expectation
Prescription	Prescription of medicines	No/no	Variation primarily within practices
Referrals:			
primary care	Referral to e.g. physical therapy, mental healthcare	No/no	Variation primarily within practices
secondary care	Referral to medical specialists	No/no	Variation primarily within practices
Diagnostics performed in the GP's practice	Blood test, urine test, blood pressure, weight, breast examination	Yes/ yes	Similarities primarily within practices
Diagnostics performed in a laboratory	Ordering blood test, ordering urine test, X-rays, electrocardiogram, echoscopy, endoscopy	No/ no	Variation primarily within practices
Treatment	Wound care, removal of earwax, surgery, bandage, catheterisation, intrauterine device (IUD) insertion	Yes/ yes	Similarities primarily within practices
Advice	Advice about work, over-the-counter medication	No/ no	Variation primarily within practices

How was it done?

For a description of the methods of the second Dutch National Survey of General Practice (DNSGP-2, 2001), *see* Chapter 2 of this book and the work of Westert *et al.*[20]

Multilevel analyses

Multilevel models are used to analyse hierarchical structured data.[21–23] With multilevel analysis total variation in clinical activity is separated into three parts: a part due to differences between patients, a part due to differences between GPs and a part due to differences between practices.[21,24] In the analyses, a model with three levels is used: practices, GPs, and patient diagnoses.

Based on the patient list of the GP, patients are attributed to GPs. Besides the intercept and the variance components, we will present two coefficients of correlation: the intra-class correlation (ICC), measured in two different ways. The ICC is a measure of homogeneity within practices, or, in other words, the degree of resemblance within the same practice. It measures the extent to which, for instance, referral rates for patients are similar in the same practice. A higher ICC means that there is homogeneity within the same practice, patients within the same practice are treated similarly. The ICC shows us how much of the variation is due to the combined effect of practices, and GPs; the ICC2 tells us whether this variation is primarily situated between practices or between GPs. In other words: a higher ICC2 means that GPs working in the same practices are more alike and that practices differ from one another, without the 'disturbing' effect of different patient diagnoses.

The model

As dependent variables we used whether (*see* Table 14.2):

- drugs were prescribed for a selected number of diagnoses
- a patient was referred within primary care, or to secondary care
- diagnostic tests were ordered
- diagnostic tests were performed in the GP's practice
- treatment was given
- advice was given.

To control for differences in data collection we included a variable for the type of electronic medical record (EMR) system. To make patient populations comparable we adjusted for medically relevant characteristics of the patient: age, sex, subjective health status, and as an additional indicator of health status, the number of contacts with the GP per year.[25] For the analysis in which prescription was studied we also included a variable that indicates whether a practice is a dispensing practice. Single-handed practices were excluded.

In the general model we did not take into account the diagnoses of the patients. Due to too many diagnoses, no model could be fitted in which the diagnoses were taken into account. In a second analysis seven diagnoses were selected that frequently occur in the GP's practice: hypertension, lower back pain, insomnia, depression, cough, respiratory tract infection, and diabetes mellitus (*see* Table 14.2). For these diagnoses we performed the same analyses as described for the general model. Treatment was not included in this analysis, because treatment, as we defined it (*see* Table 14.1), was less relevant for these diagnoses and consequently occurred in only a few cases.

For the analyses the MLwiN software package was used. All variables included in the models were centred around their means.[22]

Table 14.2 Description of the variables (numbers) included in the analyses

Variable	Prescription		Referral		Diagnostics	
Practices	29		31		36	
General practitioners	56		63		68	
Age (years)	Patients		Patients		Patients	
0–19 (n (%))	11 057 (12.5)		12 054 (12.5)		13 414 (12.5)	
20–44 (n (%))	23 826 (26.9)		26 175 (27.2)		29 171 (27.1)	
45–64 (n (%))	28 262 (31.9)		30 655 (31.9)		34 670 (32.2)	
65–74 (n (%))	12 923 (14.6)		13 974 (14.5)		15 694 (14.6)	
>75 (n (%))	12 485 (14.1)		13 216 (13.8)		14 790 (13.7)	
All	88 553		96 074		107 739	
Number of contacts (mean per patient and standard deviation)	16.2 (14.2)		16.2 (14.5)		15.9 (14.2)	
Health status:	Patients		Patients		Patients	
very good/good (n (%))	58 668 (66.3)		64 308 (66.9)		71 991 (66.8)	
moderate (n (%))	25 164 (28.4)		26 703 (27.8)		30 086 (27.9)	
bad/very bad (n (%))	4 721 (5.3)		5 063 (5.3)		5 662 (5.3)	
all	88 553		96 074		107 739	
EMR:	p	c	p	c	p	c
Microhis	5	14 796	5	14 796	5	14 796
Promedico	4	15 581	4	15 834	7	24 595
Elias	2	4 820	3	6 576	4	8 164
Arcos	3	3 683	3	5 221	4	6 537
Machis	15	49 673	16	53 647	16	53 647
Pharmacy:	5 practices, 16 029 cases					
ICPC diagnoses:						
					number of contacts	
hypertension (K86)					3690	
lower back pain (L03)					1006	
insomnia (P06)					1198	
depression (P76)					1055	
cough (R05)					1434	
respiratory tract infection (R74)					990	
diabetes mellitus (T90)					1318	

p = number of practices; c = number of contacts

What was found?

General model: analysis with all diagnoses

There is significant variation both between and within practices for prescription, and diagnostics performed in the GP's practice (*see* Table 14.3). For referral to primary care, referral to secondary care, diagnostics performed in a laboratory, and giving advice there is significant variation between GPs only, while for treatment there is significant variation between practices. The ICC varied from 0.04 to 0.20, for giving advice, which means that from 4% to 20% of the total variation is located between practices. Based on the ICC2 we conclude that there is more variation between practices than between GPs for diagnostics performed in the GP's practice, and treatment. Prescription, referral to primary care, referral to secondary care, diagnostics performed in a laboratory, and advice show more variation between GPs than between practices. Following Table 14.1 (final column) our expectations are confirmed for all clinical activities (*see* Table 14.3).

Analysis with selected diagnoses

For the analysis with the selected diagnoses, in which we took into account data collection variables, patient characteristics and diagnoses, we found significant variation between and within practices for diagnostics performed in the GP's practice (*see* Table 14.3). For prescription, referral to secondary care and advice, the variation between GPs was significant, as there was no significant variation between practices. Referral to primary care and diagnostics performed in a laboratory show no significant variation between practices or between GPs. The ICC varies from 0.03 to 0.19 for diagnostics performed in the GP's practice. Based on the ICC2 we conclude that there is clustering of variation within practices for diagnostics performed in the GP's practice. Our expectations are confirmed for all clinical activities.

What to think about it

The treatment by physicians is assumed to be based on theoretical knowledge and the medical condition of the patient only. Patients, and other lay persons, are not able to judge the decision of physicians, and this gives the profession its special social and legal status.[26] The existence of variation, even if clinically relevant variables are taken into account, undermines this position: if physicians do what is best for their patients, based on evidence, how come there is variation in treatment between similar patients? Existing explanations are based on individual preferences or (social) circumstances.[27,28]

Most patients will get different treatment elsewhere.

In this chapter we found that clustering of variation within practices depends on the clinical activity studied. GPs working within the same practice differed more from colleagues in other practices than from their colleagues in the same practice, for activities like treatment and diagnostics performed in the GP's practice. It was the other way around for prescription, referral to primary care, referral to secondary care, diagnostics performed in the laboratory, and advice. For these activities, practices looked more alike than GPs working in the same practice. These clinical activities are less visible to colleagues, and do not make use of shared resources. When only diagnoses that occur frequently are selected and these diagnoses are taken into account in the analyses, these conclusions do not change. Our hypothesis, that there is less variation within practices when shared resources are used and when behaviour is visible for colleagues, was confirmed.

Table 14.3 Intercept and variance components for several clinical activities for all diagnoses, and for selected diagnoses

	All	Selected diagnoses
Prescription		
Intercept	0.15 (0.08)	1.22 (0.12)
Practice level variance	0.06 (0.03)[a]	0.17 (0.10)
GP level variance	0.09 (0.03)[a]	0.22 (0.07)
ICC	0.02	0.05
ICC2	0.41	0.44
Referral within primary care		
Intercept	−4.44 (1.21)[a]	−6.20 (0.31)[a]
Practice level variance	0.05 (0.04)	0.13 (0.18)
GP level variance	0.09 (0.04)[a]	0.35 (0.21)
ICC	0.04	0.11
ICC2	0.34	0.27
Referral to secondary care		
Intercept	−3.72 (0.08)[a]	−5.10 (0.22)[a]
Practice level variance	0.03 (0.03)	0.00 (0.00)
GP level variance	0.11 (0.04)[a]	0.76 (0.26)[a]
ICC	0.04	0.13[a]
ICC2	0.19	0.00
Diagnostics in practice		
Intercept	−3.06 (0.08)[a]	−2.87 (0.12)[a]
Practice level variance	0.07 (0.03)[a]	0.24 (0.09)[a]
GP level variance	0.06 (0.02)[a]	0.12 (0.06)[a]
ICC	0.04	0.19
ICC2	0.54	0.66
Diagnostics in lab		
Intercept	−3.59 (0.08)[a]	−3.84 (0.10)[a]
Practice level variance	0.00 (0.00)	0.00 (0.00)
GP level variance	0.15 (0.04)[a]	0.09 (0.05)
ICC	0.04	0.03
ICC2	0.00	0.00
Treatment		
Intercept	−4.50 (0.11)[a]	–
Practice level variance	0.14 (0.06)[a]	–
GP level variance	0.05 (0.03)	–
ICC	0.05	–
ICC2	0.75	–
Advice		
Intercept	−4.52 (0.18)[a]	−4.45 (0.14)[a]
Practice level variance	0.00 (0.00)	0.00 (0.00)
GP level variance	0.81 (0.17)[a]	0.41 (0.14)[a]
ICC	0.20	0.11
ICC2	0.00	0.00

Values in parentheses are standard errors.
[a] $P < 0.05$.
ICC: a higher ICC means that there is more homogeneity within practices; patients are treated alike in a practice.
ICC2: a higher ICC2 means that there is more homogeneity between GPs within the same practice; GPs act alike in a practice.

Visibility of behaviour

In this study, we assumed that behaviour is either visible or not. In reality this is not an on/off phenomenon: some behaviour is more visible than others. We did not make such distinctions in our study, but it might be useful in explaining the difference in the amount of variation between the clinical activities. Furthermore, we used a very narrow definition of visibility: actual behaviour that can be seen by colleagues. Using a more broad definition, behaviour is also 'visible' when colleagues talk about it. We could think of meetings, which a small number of GPs attend, and in which prescription is discussed. In these meetings, prescribing behaviour of individual GPs can be evaluated, and is therefore 'visible'. This could have an influence on when and what to prescribe. Attending GPs can become more alike in their prescribing behaviour.

Limitations of this study

In the analysis in which all diagnoses (the general model) were included, we did not take into account the specific diagnoses. This was not possible, because there were too many diagnoses, and a model could not be fitted. Differences in diagnoses in a GP's practice are an important source of variation in clinical activities. This, however, would be reflected in all clinical activities. If differences in diagnoses were an explanation of the remaining variation, all clinical activities should show patterns of variation by practice (if diagnoses differ between practices) or by GP (if diagnoses differ between GPs). That is not what we found.

Guidelines have been developed for diagnoses that frequently occur, and this could result in less variation between and within practices. However, our conclusions did not differ between the analyses in which all diagnoses are included, and the diagnoses in which only seven diagnoses were included.

Our hypothesis was about variation and not about characteristics of patients, GPs or practices that might explain variation. Often research jumps to explaining variation without carefully examining variation in the first place. For instance, there is extensive empirical literature about the effects of the introduction of guidelines on physician behaviour. However, we almost never see the obvious hypothesis tested that the introduction of guidelines reduces variation between physicians. An exception is Verstappen *et al.*, who reported a larger decrease of variation in the experimental group after an intervention in laboratory test ordering.[29]

The current study gives insight into whether or not medical practice variation occurs within or between practices. A next step is to search more specifically for the causes of patterns of medical practice variations, and how these variations should be dealt with. Multilevel analyses help us identify the appropriate level at which interventions for changing GPs' behaviour should be targeted.

References

1 Groenewegen PP, de Bakker DH and van der Velden J (1992) *Basisrapport Verrichtingen in de Huisartspraktijk. Nationale Studie naar ziekten en verrichtingen in de huisartspraktijk.*

[Basic report on actions in GP practice. Dutch National Survey of General Practice.] NIVEL, Utrecht.

2 Marinus AMF (1993) Inter-dokter Variatie in de Huisartspraktijk [dissertation]. [Inter-GP variation in GP practice.] University of Amsterdam, Amsterdam.

3 Davis P, Gribben B, Lay-Yee R and Scott A (2002) How much variation in clinical activity is there between general practitioners? A multi-level analysis of decision-making in primary care. *J Health Serv Res Policy.* **7**: 202–8.

4 Zaat JOM (1991) *De Macht der Gewoonte; over de Huisarts en Zijn Laboratoriumonderzoek* [dissertation]. [By force of habit; about GPs and their laboratory research.] University of Amsterdam, Amsterdam.

5 Peterson S, Eriksson M and Tibblin G (1997) Practice variation in Swedish primary care. *Scand J Prim Health Care.* **15**: 68–75.

6 Guthrie B (2001) Why do general practitioners take blood? *Eur J Gen Pract.* **7**: 138–42, 160.

7 Verstappen WHJM (2004) *Towards Optimal Test Ordering in Primary Care* [dissertation]. Universiteit Maastricht, Maastricht.

8 O'Donnell CA (2000) Variation in GP referral rates: what can we learn from the literature? *Fam Pract.* **17**: 462–71.

9 Verhaak PFM (1993) Analysis of referrals of mental health problems by general practitioners. *Br J Gen Pract.* **43**: 203–8.

10 Davis P and Gribben B (1995) Rational prescribing and interpractitioner variation. *Int J Technol Assess Health Care.* **11**: 428–42.

11 Taroni F, Stiassi R, Traversa G *et al.* (1990) The nature content and interpractice variation of general practice: a regional study in Italy. *Eur J Epidemiol.* **6**: 313–18.

12 Mulder HC (1996) *Het Medisch Kunnen: technieken, keuze en zeggenschap in de moderne geneeskunde* [dissertation]. [Medical ability; technics, choice and power of control in modern medical science.] Van Gorcum, Assen.

13 Delnoij DMJ and Spreeuwenberg PMM (1997) Provider practices: variations in GPs' referral rates to specialists in internal medicine. *Eur J Public Health.* **7**: 427–35.

14 Boerma WGW and Fleming DM (1998) *The Role of General Practice in Primary Health Care.* World Health Organization. The Stationery Office, London.

15 Groenewegen PP, Dixon J and Boerma WGW (2002) The regulatory environment of general practice: an international perspective. In: Saltman RB, Busse R and Mossialos E (eds) *Regulating Entrepreneurial Behaviour in European Health Care Systems.* Open University Press, Buckingham, pp. 200–14.

16 Freidson E (1975) *Profession of Medicine. A study of the sociology of applied knowledge.* Dodd, Mead and Company, New York.

17 Westert GP (1992) Variation in Use of Hospital Care [dissertation]. Van Gorcum, Assen.

18 de Jong JD, Groenewegen PP and Westert GP (2003) Mutual influences of general practitioners in partnerships. *Soc Sci Med.* **57**: 1515–24.

19 Lazega E (2000) *The Collegial Phenomenon. The social mechanisms of cooperation among peers in a corporate law partnership.* Oxford University Press, Oxford.

20 Westert GP, Schellevis FG, de Bakker DH *et al.* (2005) Monitoring health inequalities through General Practice: the Second Dutch National Survey of General Practice. *Eur J Public Health.* **15**: 59–65.

21 Leyland AH and Groenewegen PP (2003) Multilevel modelling and public health policy. *Scand J Public Health.* **31**: 267–74.

22 Snijders TAB and Bosker RJ (1999) *Multilevel Analysis. An introduction to basic and advanced multilevel modelling.* Sage Publications Ltd, London.

23 Hox JJ (1995) *Applied Multilevel Analysis.* TT-Publicaties, Amsterdam.

24 Diez Roux AV (2002) A glossary for multilevel analysis. *J Epidemiol Community Health.* **56**: 588–94.

25 Powell A, Davies H and Thomson R (2004) Using routine comparative data: understanding and avoiding common pitfalls. In: Grol R, Baker R and Moss F (eds) *Quality Improvement Research. Understanding the science of change in health care.* BMJ Books, London, pp. 29–50.

26 Evans RG (1990) The dog in the night-time: medical practice variations and health policy. In: Andersen TF and Mooney G (eds) *The Challenges of Medical Practice Variations.* The Macmillan Press Ltd, London, pp. 117–52.

27 Wennberg JE and Gittelsohn A (1975) Health care delivery in Maine I: patterns of use of common surgical procedures. *J Maine Med Assoc.* **66**: 123–49.

28 Westert GP and Groenewegen PP (1999) Medical practice variations: changing the theoretical approach. *Scand J Public Health.* **27**: 173–80.

29 Verstappen, WHJM, van der Weijden T, Sijbrandij J *et al.* (2003) Effect of a practice-based strategy on test ordering performance of primary care physicians. *JAMA* **289**: 2407–12.

Chapter 15

Social networks and receiving informal care

Alice de Boer, Mirjam de Klerk, Mieke Cardol and Gert Westert

What is this chapter about?

In 2001, roughly half a million people (4% of the Dutch population) received informal care from family members living outside their home, and a quarter of a million (2% of the Dutch population) received this care from acquaintances, such as friends, neighbours and work colleagues. The potential supply of informal care – indicated by the number of people in one's network – was shown to be of less importance than the actual frequency of contacts with network members. Furthermore, adults aged up to 44 years receive informal care from family members relatively frequently. Membership of labour organisations, churches and recreational associations showed no additional correlation with the receipt of informal care from acquaintances.

Introduction

Informal care is an important resource for those in need of support for health problems. Informal carers are said to provide four to five times more help than home care professionals.[1] Expectations regarding the availability of this care in the near future are bleak.[1-3] Demographic changes will lead to an increase in the number of people requiring help. At the same time, the sources of informal care are becoming scarcer, as the number of people without a partner or without children rises, and family members increasingly live further apart. This chapter sets out to describe the present situation. It examines the relationship between characteristics of social networks and receipt of informal care.

Expectations regarding the availability of informal care in the near future are bleak.

What do we know?

Having a partner is a characteristic of the social network that correlates with the probability of receiving informal care. The research findings are not entirely unambiguous, however. For example, it is found that people living alone are over-represented among older recipients of informal practical help, but also that people living with a partner more frequently receive practical help and emotional support from their informal network.[4-6]

Having children also influences the receipt of informal care. Thomése showed that having a large number of relatives in a network does not automatically lead to receiving practical help from this network: in fact, the probability that older persons will receive informal care from family members is actually smaller when more family members are present in the network.[7] Thomése states that the same applies for friends and acquaintances: the larger the number of acquaintances in local networks, the lower the chance of receiving informal care. Other authors, by contrast, have found a positive correlation between network size and informal care.[8]

Most research on informal care focuses on older persons.

Another important aspect of the social network which correlates with informal care is contact frequency: older persons in need of support who have frequent contact with their children more often receive help from these children.[9] When it comes to emotional support, the frequency of contact appears to make no difference.

The mutual provision of informal care also plays a role in receiving this care.[8,10] Among 60–85 year olds living independently, a strong correlation is found between practical support they have given in the past and the frequency of the practical support they receive today.

The travel distance between children and parents in need of support is found not to be a relevant factor in the receipt of practical or emotional support.[9] Travel time is, however, a determinant in the giving of informal care.[11] Several studies have focused explicitly on the effect of urbanisation on informal care: older residents of urban areas receive domestic help and/or personal care from their informal network less frequently than people living in rural areas in the Netherlands.[5,7] Verheij and others studied the correlation between informal care and (local) social integration.[5] People who participate in local associational life and those with children living nearby receive more informal care than those who do not meet these criteria. In the literature, other factors are of course also cited which correlate with receiving informal care: need for support,[7–9,12–14], socio-economic status,[7,12,15] and professional help or care.[5,16]

In summary, little is known of the influence the social network has on the receipt of informal care. In the first place, research is often focused on older persons,[17] whereas people aged under 55 years also obviously receive informal care from their social network.[12,18] Secondly, many studies examine only a limited number of network characteristics.

Do characteristics of social networks associate with receipt of informal care?

We address two questions in this chapter:

- what proportion of the adult Dutch population receives informal care from family members and acquaintances for health problems?
- to what extent do differences in the receipt of informal care correlate with differences in characteristics of the social network, taking into account the need for help, socio-economic status and receipt of professional care?

In this study, informal care is defined as the practical help (help with household activities, personal care and/or nursing care) given to a person with health problems by family members and acquaintances who do not form part of the household of the person receiving that help. Family members are children, brothers, sisters and parents; acquaintances include friends, acquaintances, work colleagues and neighbours. In addition, informal care is restricted to help in one year's time and given for a minimum of two weeks.

How was it done?

For a description of the methods of the second Dutch National Survey of General Practice (DNSGP-2, 2001), *see* Chapter 2 of this book. The following is specific for the study described in this chapter. A random sample of the total study population was interviewed about their social network, need for help, socio-economic characteristics and take-up of professional care. The database used here consists of 4814 persons aged over 18 years. The measurement instruments used are presented in Table 15.1.

Table 15.2 contains a description of characteristics of the respondents, their sociodemographic characteristics, their social network, need for help, and receipt of professional care.

The descriptive analysis of the receipt of informal care focused on people aged over 18 years; the findings for this group were compared with the receipt of informal care by older persons (*see* Table 15.3). The percentages were extrapolated to absolute numbers of recipients of informal care in the Dutch population. Logistic regression was applied to investigate the extent to which receiving informal care from family members (model 1) and acquaintances (model 2) correlates with relevant characteristics of the social network, need for care, socio-economic status and receipt of other help (*see* Table 15.4). Table 15.4 presents odds ratios (OR) that express the unique correlation between the receipt of informal care and the factors entered in the empirical model.

What was found?

Receipt of informal care and age

The number of over-18s receiving informal care in 2001 is presented in Table 15.3. By way of comparison, figures are also included for the over-55s and over-75s.

Just under 6% of people aged over 18 years received informal care from family members or acquaintances. The figure for the subpopulation aged over 75 years is 12%. For the 18+ group, the care is provided almost exclusively by family members. Among the oldest group, 7% receive informal care only from family members, followed by 4% who receive informal care only from acquaintances, and fewer than 1% who receive informal care from both sources simultaneously. If informal care provided by family members was considered separately (i.e. not in conjunction with the care provided by acquaintances), it was found that 4% of people aged over 18 years received informal care from

Table 15.1 Instruments used in the questionnaire

Measurement instruments	Response categories
Number of family members outside home[a]	Continuous
Contact frequency with family member outside home per week[b]	Continuous
Contact frequency with acquaintances per week	Continuous
Number of times support given[19,c]	Continuous
Degree of urbanisation[20]	Very highly -, highly -, moderately -, not very -, not urbanised
Number of times attended religious service	Never, <once/year, once/year, 4×/year, once/week, >once/week
Number of memberships of recreational associations[21,d]	Continuous
Labour market position[e]	No paid work; paid work

[a]Children, grandchildren, brothers and sisters, father, mother.
[b]Contact with children, grandchildren, other family members (not telephone contact).
[c]Such as someone to talk to, help with practical matters or consolation or help in special cases (illness, moving house, babysitting).
[d]Such as choral, music or amateur dramatic society, women's association or union, youth association, clubhouse, scouts, sports association.
[e]Regardless of the number of hours worked.

Table 15.2 Population characteristics (n = 4814)

	%	Mean (±SD)
Mean age (years)		46.2 (16.6)
Women	52	
No education or primary school	13	
Household income of less than €2259[a]	37	
Use of home care and/or private help[b]	5	
Paid work	52	
No (cohabiting) partner	22	
Very high degree of urbanisation	18	
Moderate or severe long-term motor limitations[c]	11	
GHQ score of 4 or higher[d]	13	
Moderate or poor perceived health	18	
At least one chronic disorder[e]	63	
Three or more family members living outside the home	88	
Mean contact frequency with family members per week		3.1 (1.3)
Mean contact frequency with acquaintances per week		3.0 (1.5)
Mean number of times support given		9.5 (2.3)
Never attending religious service	60	
At least one membership of one or more recreational associations	45	

[a]An equivalent income was used which took into account the composition of the household.
[b]In the 12 months prior to the interview, on account of health problems.
[c]The limitations relate to three activities: carrying 5 kg, bending, walking 400 m without stopping.[22]
[d]A score at the General Health Questionnaire (GHQ) of more than 4 indicates the presence of psychological problems.[23,24]
[e]List of 20 disorders.[25]

Table 15.3 Receipt of informal care[a] by age of recipient, in percentages and extrapolated to the Dutch population (2001)

| | Age (years) | | | | | |
| | 18+ | | 55+ | | 75+ | |
	%	n	%	n	%	n
No care	94.4		94.3		88.3	
Only from family members	3.5	435 000	3.5	135 000	7.4	65 000
Only from acquaintances	1.3	155 000	1.6	60 000	3.5	30 000
From both family members and acquaintances	0.8	100 000	0.6	25 000	0.7	6 000
Total number		12 000 000		3 800 000		850 000
From family members	4.3	540 000	4.1	160 000	8.2	70 000
From acquaintances	2.1	260 000	2.2	85 000	4.2	35 000
From family members and/or acquaintances	5.6	690 000	5.7	220 000	11.7	100 000
(n)	(4 814)		(1 656)		(356)	

[a]Care received during health problems for more than two weeks during the 12 months prior to the interview.

this network. Slightly more than 2% received informal care from acquaintances. Extrapolated to the whole country a total of 690 000 adults received informal care during health problems from family, acquaintances or a combination of these two (in 2001).

When do people receive informal care from family members and acquaintances

Table 15.4 shows the correlation between characteristics of the social network and the receipt of informal care from family members and from acquaintances.

People without a partner received informal care for health problems more frequently than people with a partner. This is not due to their receiving care from other members of the nuclear family, since both models correct for this.

The number of family members a person has does not correlate with receiving informal care from others. However, the intensity of social contacts was found to be relevant. People with a higher contact frequency with family members, friends, acquaintances or neighbours receive informal care more frequently. People who receive informal care from immediate family members have a higher chance of receiving care from members of the extended family and acquaintances as well. The same applies for care provided by extended family members, which correlates closely with informal care received from acquaintances.

No correlation was observed between support given to others, the frequency of attending religious services, membership of recreational associations, labour market position and receiving informal care from acquaintances.

The degree of urbanisation does have an influence on receiving informal care from family members: people living in non-urban areas are more likely to receive informal care from relatives than town-dwellers.

Table 15.4 Determinants of receipt of informal care,[a] OR and 95% confidence intervals (CI),[b] n = 4456 over-18s, 2001

	Help from family		Help from acquaintances	
	OR	95%-CI	OR	95%-CI
Social network				
no cohabiting partner	**1.89**	**1.31–2.73**	**2.95**	**1.79–4.84**
number of family members	0.97	0.93–1.00	–	–
contact frequency with family members	**1.57**	**1.36–1.81**	–	–
contact frequency with acquaintances	–	–	**1.45**	**1.23–1.69**
number of times support given	1.01	0.95–1.08	0.98	0.89–1.07
degree of urbanisation[c]	**1.18**	**1.04–1.34**	0.93	0.77–1.10
number of times attends religious service	–	–	1.00	0.89–1.11
number of memberships of recreational associations	–	–	1.15	0.79–1.67
paid work (yes)	–	–	1.28	0.71–2.29
Need for care				
severity of long-term motor limitations	**1.41**	**1.19–1.66**	**1.43**	**1.13–1.80**
GHQ score[d]	**1.11**	**1.06–1.18**	**1.16**	**1.08–1.23**
perceived health	**1.46**	**1.18–1.79**	**1.51**	**1.12–2.02**
chronic disorders (yes)	**2.91**	**1.75–4.85**	1.47	0.71–3.02
Age (years)				
18–34 years	**3.55**	**1.80–6.99**	1.41	0.55–3.61
35–44 years	**2.23**	**1.13–4.37**	1.74	0.69–4.40
45–54 years	0.94	0.48–1.84	1.19	0.48–2.96
55–74 years	0.56	0.31–1.02	0.85	0.38–1.89
75+ (ref)	1		1	

[a]Care received during health problems for more than two weeks during the 12 months prior to the interview. Corrected for sex, highest educational level, household income, home care/private help, help from nuclear family members, help from extended family.
[b]The odds ratios and reliability intervals printed in bold are significant ($P < 0.05$).
[c]The higher the score, the lower the degree of urbanisation.
[d]The higher the score, the worse the problem.

Surprisingly, the type of health problems does not seem to matter for receiving informal care from family members and acquaintances. One striking finding is that people in the 18–34-year and 35–44-year age groups relatively frequently receive informal care from family members. This is not due to differences between 'younger' adults and older persons in terms of network characteristics, severity of the need for help, socio-economic status or other sources of help, since the model corrected for all these factors.

What to think about it

This study investigates what proportion of the adult Dutch population receives informal care and the role of their social network. The available studies focus mainly on older people. The present study looks at informal care given to people aged over 18 years.

In 2001, 4% of the Dutch population aged over 18 years received informal care from family members living outside the home for at least two weeks because of health problems, while 2% received such care from acquaintances. The total number receiving informal care was almost 6%, or just under 700 000 persons.

An important finding is that people who have frequent contact with members of their network receive care relatively frequently from that network. This result corresponds with findings on care given by children to their parents.[9] The causality in this relationship may run in two directions, with contact being both a determinant and a result of the receipt of informal care. In the first case, the informal care ensues from the social contacts; in the second case, informal care leads to an intensification of contacts within the network.

Not the availability but the quality of relationships seems important for receiving informal care.

In this study no correlation was found between network size and the receipt of informal care from family members. Evidently, the intensity of relationships is more important in determining the receipt of informal care than the potential supply of this care. Also striking is the effect of age on informal care. Although most researchers demonstrate that the very oldest people receive informal care more frequently than others,[4,7] in this study we found that people aged under 44 years (after adjusting for the severity of the need for care) receive care frequently from family members. One study reported a comparable result.[14] The explanation must be sought in the nature of the network of 18–44 year olds. 'Younger' adults will generally still have both parents, who are moreover likely to be still relatively healthy and therefore able to care for their children during illness. For older people this type of care is often no longer available. In addition, people aged under 44 years may also have several close family members who are still young and healthy (e.g. brothers and sisters) and who are consequently able to provide informal care more easily than older persons. It is also possible that younger people need extra care because of pregnancy and/or childbirth.

This study demonstrates that adults with few social contacts receive care from their informal network less frequently. It is known from care for the elderly and care for psychiatric patients and for people with a learning disability that people can successfully be introduced to new contacts.[26] It is argued that this not only improves the feelings of wellbeing of those concerned, but may also increase the chance of care being provided by the enlarged social network.

Who will take care of us in the future?

We have stated that informal care could be jeopardised in the future by demographic changes; recent research suggests that the average number of relatives per older person will decline in the near future.[27] This prediction needs to be qualified in two ways. First, the demographic changes have already begun. For example, the average number of children per family has fallen in recent years and the age at which women have children has increased.

Informal care not only comes from social networks but also helps to maintain them.

So far, however, this has not led to a decrease in receiving informal care.[26] Moreover, the research findings described here suggest that it is not so much the size of the informal network as the frequency of contacts which influences the receipt of care. People may have a small network, but if contacts within the network are intensive, there is a high probability that members of that network will provide informal care when needed. The converse argument can also apply, however: the mutual provision of informal care strengthens the social contacts. Viewed in this way, informal care not only comes from social networks but also helps to maintain them.

References

1 Raad voor Maatschappelijke Ontwikkeling en Raad voor Volksgezondheid en Zorg (1999) *Zorgarbeid in de Toekomst. Gevolgen van demografische ontwikkelingen voor de zorg.* [Providing care in the future. Consequences of demographic developments for care.] SDU, Den Haag.

2 Timmermans J (1997) Tehuizen voor ouderen: een verouderde oplossing? [NL Homes for the elderly: an old-fashioned solution?] In: de Boer A, Heering L and Faessen W (eds) *Pakhuizen of Paleizen? (Boekaflevering bevolking en Gezin).* [Warehouses or palaces? (Book issue of Population and Family).] NIDI, Den Haag.

3 Dykstra PA (2001) Netwerken van informele steun en sociaaldemografische veranderingen. [Networks of informal support and sociodemographic changes.] In: Vrooman JC (ed) *Netwerken en Sociaal Kapitaal (SISWO/NSV-reeks).* [Networks and social capital (SISWO/NSV-series)]. NSV, Amsterdam.

4 de Boer A, Hessing-Wagner J, de Klerk M and Kooiker S (2001) Gebruik van dienstverlening en zorgvoorzieningen. [Using services and care.] In: de Klerk MMY. *Rapportage Ouderen 2001; veranderingen in de leefsituatie.* [Report on the elderly 2001; changes in the living situation.] SCP, Den Haag.

5 Verheij R, de Boer AH and Westert GP (1998) Stad-plattelandverschillen in het Gebruik van Informele Zorg door Ouderen. [Urban–rural differences in the use of informal care by elderly people.] *TSG.* 76: 2–9.

6 Broese van Groenou M (2002). Het persoonlijk netwerk van ouderen. [The personal network of the elderly.] In: Alsum FM, Ubels GM, de Coole MPO, Penninx CCM and Voermans HW (eds) *Handboek Lokaal Ouderenwerk.* [Handbook local care for the elderly.] Elsevier Gezondheidszorg, Maarssen.

7 Thomése F (1998) *Buurtnetwerken van Ouderen; een wetenschappelijke onderzoek onder zelfstandig wonende ouderen in Nederland.* [Local networks of elderly people; a study amongst independent living elderly people in the Netherlands.] Thela Thesis, Amsterdam.

8 van Tilburg T, van Broese and van Groenou M (2002) Network and health changes among older Dutch adults. Network and health. *J Soc Issues.* 58: 697–713.

9 Broese van Groenou MI and Knipscheer CPM (1999) Onset of physical impairment of independently living older adults and support received from sons and daughters in the Netherlands. *Int J Aging Hum Dev.* 48: 263–78.

10 Klein-Ikkink CE (2000) *If I Scratch your Back ... ? Reciprocity and social support exchanges in personal relationships of older adults* [PhD thesis]. VU, Amsterdam.

11 Timmermans JT, de Boer AH, van Campen C *et al.* (eds) (2001) *Vrij om te helpen; verkenning betaald langdurig zorgverlof.* [Free to help; survey of long-term paid care leave.] SCP, Den Haag.

12 de Klerk MMY (2002) *Rapportage Gehandicapten 2002; maatschappelijke positie van mensen met lichamelijke beperkingen of verstandelijke handicaps.* [Report on the Disabled 2002; social position of physical or mentally disabled people.] SCP, Den Haag.

13 Deeg DJH (2003) *Ontwikkelingen in het gebruik van informele en professionele zorg in Nederland, 1992–2002* (presentatie op 20 november 2002 Centrum voor Veroudering Onderzoek 'Grenzen aan woonzorgzones: pretenties en perspectieven'). [Developments in the use of informal and professional care in the Netherlands, 1992–2002 (presentation on 20 November 2002 Centre for Research into Ageing.] VU, Amsterdam.

14 Riemsma RP, Klein G, Taal E *et al.* (1998) The supply of demand for informal and professional care for patients with rheumatoid arthritis. *Scand J Rheumatol.* 27: 7–15.

15 Deeg DJH, Bosscher RJ, Broese van Groenou MI, Horn L and Jonker C (eds) (2000) *Ouder Worden in Nederland; Tien Jaar Longitudinal Ageing Study Amsterdam.* [Ageing in the Netherlands; ten years of Longitudinal Ageing Study Amsterdam.] Thela Thesis, Amsterdam.

16 de Boer AH (1999) *Housing and Care for Older People; a Macro–micro Perspective* [dissertation]. NGS, Utrecht.

17 Timmermans JM, Schellingerhout R and de Boer AH (2004) Wat heet mantelzorg? Prevalentie van verschillende vormen van mantelzorg in Nederland. [What encompasses informal care? Prevalence of several kinds of informal care in the Netherlands.] *Tijdschr voor gezondheidswetenschappen.* 82: 230–6.

18 de Boer AH (2003) Relatie tussen mantelzorg en thuiszorg. The relationship between informal care and home care. In: Timmermans JT (ed) *Mantelzorg; over de Hulp van en aan Mantelzorgers.* [Informal care; help from and those behind informal care.] SCP, Den Haag.

19 van Sonderen E (1995) Sociale steun en sociale netwerken. [Social support and social networks. In: Sanderman R, Hosman CMH and Mulder M (eds) *Het Meten van Gezondheid: een overzicht van beschikbare meetinstrumenten.* [Measuring health: a survey of available measuring instruments.] Van Gorcum, Assen.

20 den Dulk CJ, van den Stadt H and Vliegen JM (1992) Een nieuwe maatstaf voor stedelijkheid: de omgevingsadressendichtheid. [A new standard for urbanicity: address density in the environment.] *Maandstatistiek Bevolking.* 7: 14–27.

21 de Klerk MMY and Timmermans JT (1999) *Rapportage Ouderen 1998.* [Report on the elderly 1998.] SCP, Den Haag.

22 McWhinnie JR (1981) Disability assessment in population surveys: results of the OECD common development effort. *Rev Epid Sante.* 29: 413–19.

23 Goldberg DP (1972) *The Detection of Psychiatric Illness by Questionnaire.* Oxford University Press, London.

24 Goldberg DP, Gater R, Satorius N *et al.* (1997) The validity of two versions of the GHQ in the WHO study of mental illness in general health care. *Psychol Med.* 27: 191–7.

25 Foets M and van der Velden J (1990) *Nationale Studie naar Ziekten en Verrichtingen in de Huisartspraktijk. Basisrapport; meetinstrumenten en procedures.* [Second Dutch National Survey of General Practice. Basic report; measuring instruments and procedures.] NIVEL, Utrecht.

26 de Hart J (2002) *Zekere Banden; Sociale Cohesie Leefbaarheid en Veiligheid.* [Secure ties; social cohesion quality of life and security.] SCP, Den Haag.

27 van Imhoff E (2004) *Ouderen en Vergrijzing: heden, verleden en toekomst.* [Elderly people and ageing: present, past and future.] RIVM, Bilthoven. www.rivm.nl/vtv/data/site_kompas/index.htm versie 2.8 (accessed 16 September 2005).

Part 4

Organisation and communication

Chapter 16

The workload of general practitioners in the Netherlands: 1987 and 2001

Michael van den Berg, Esmée Kolthof, Dinny de Bakker and Jouke van der Zee

What is this chapter about?

Like in many other countries, it has often been stated that the workload of general practitioners (GPs) in the Netherlands has increased in the past few years. However, empirical evidence for this statement is lacking. Additionally, most previous research has focused on only one or a few aspects of workload, e.g. the number of working hours or the consultation frequency. In this study we describe changes in objective and subjective workload using a range of workload measures. Compared to 1987, GPs have to deal with an increasing number of medical problems within a shorter time frame. This is mainly due to a 10% increase in demand for care, combined with a shorter working week on average for GPs, i.e. a decline of nine hours per week. Approximately three-quarters of the GPs were satisfied or very satisfied with their work in 2001. In comparison with 14 years ago, this represents a distinct decline.

Although workload is partly determined by care demand, it can be influenced by the GP. An increasing workload requires creative solutions and can often be managed by organisational measures, e.g. task delegation.

Doctors' workload

Especially in healthcare systems in which general practitioners (GPs) are paid per capita, workload is an important issue. Morrison and Smith (2001) summarised in an editorial contribution to the *British Medical Journal* the situation as follows: 'Across the globe doctors are miserable because they feel like hamsters on a treadmill. They must run faster just to stand still'.[1] Morrison and Smith claimed that in many countries, healthcare systems were inefficient and especially unfair on doctors, who have to keep on working harder without making any progress. In the same year, dissatisfaction reached a climax among Dutch GPs, which resulted in a series of nationwide campaigns and even a one-day strike. Although many GPs perceive an increase in their workload, there is hardly any substantial evidence to justify this observation. Reacting to the above-mentioned editorial, Mechanic has shown findings of the UK and the USA that are in contrast with the idea of an increasing workload.[2]

'Across the globe doctors are miserable because they feel like hamsters on a treadmill. They must run faster just to stand still.'[1]

Workload is a complicated concept and can be defined and measured in many ways. In our study we distinguish between objective workload, which is the volume of work, the amount of time that certain activities consume or the frequency in which they take place, and job satisfaction, which can be seen as a subjective aspect of workload.[3] The aim of this study was to investigate the current workload of Dutch GPs, to determine whether their workload has changed in the course of time, and, if so, to explain these changes. The central question of this chapter is

- did the objective and subjective workload of Dutch GPs change between 1987 and 2001?

How was it done?

For a description of the methods of the first and second Dutch National Survey of General Practice (DNSGP-1, 1987 and DNSGP-2, 2001), *see* Chapter 2 of this book and previous publications.[4–6] The following is specific for the study described in this chapter.

Objective workload measures were derived from consultation registration, video observations and diaries (kept by GPs). Subjective workload measures were derived from questionnaires filled out by GPs. Data about explanatory factors on patient level were collected via consultation registration and registration of sociodemographic characteristics. We have compared the results of 2001 with data of the DNSGP-1 (1987).

Table 16.1 shows the workload measures we have used, the sources and the number of valid cases in both years.

What was found?

More patients per GP and higher consultation rates

The number of registered patients per full-time equivalent (fte) GP increased by 10% between 1987 and 2001 (*see* Table 16.2).

Also, the number of consultations per patient increased by 10% in these years (*see* Figure 16.1). This rise is seen in all age groups, except for the youngest patients between 0 and 4 years. The oldest cohorts show the highest increase. This means that the demand of care has increased considerably since 1987.

Although the average list size per fte has increased, the GP density – the number of GPs divided by number of Dutch citizens – has stayed more or less the same in this period. The rise in list size per fte is mainly due to a decrease in the number of weekly working hours. Table 16.2 shows a distinct decline in the average number of weekly working hours from approximately 53 to 44 hours a week.

Obviously, this decline is partly related to the rise in GPs working part-time. In 2001, part-time working has become very common. Over 40% of all GPs work part-time, while in 1987 approximately 10% of the GPs worked part-time. However, this is not the only explanation for the decreased number of working

Table 16.1 Operationalisation, data sources and number of observations

	Source	1987	2001
Objective workload:			
number of weekly working hours	Diaries, (registration of activity at 15 min intervals, during 24 h a day, 7 consecutive days)	157 GPs	157 GPs
consultation rate	Patient survey (random sample of study population)	13 014 patients	12 699 patients
list size	Data practice registration	154 GPs	189 GPs
fte	Data practice registration	159 GPs	188 GPs
consultation length	Video registration	442 consultations, 17 GPs	2111 consultations, 142 GPs
proportion of house calls/ practice consultations/ telephone contacts	Contact registration	418 219 contacts	387 033 contacts
Subjective workload:			
overall job satisfaction (one item)	GP survey	161 GPs	164 GPs
satisfaction with material and financial circumstances (3 items)	GP survey	161 GPs	164 GPs
satisfaction with available time (4 items)	GP survey	161 GPs	164 GPs
satisfaction with intercollegial contacts (3 items)	GP survey	161 GPs	164 GPs

hours. Figure 16.2 shows the average number of working hours in 1987 and 2001 for all GPs. The figure shows a decline for both full-timers and part-timers.

GPs are less satisfied

The question: 'How satisfied are you with your job in general?' was answered with 'satisfied' or 'very satisfied' by approximately three-quarters in 2001. Compared with the situation 14 years earlier, a distinct decline is noticeable: in 1987 88% were satisfied or very satisfied. The number of GPs dissatisfied with material and financial circumstances, such as practice costs and income, has increased respectively by 24% and 17% (*see* Figure 16.3). The number of GPs dissatisfied with contacts with others, like specialists and colleagues, seems to have decreased, but these changes are not statistically significant. Fewer GPs are

Table 16.2 Workload in 1987 and 2001 (mean, mean difference and observed significance level)

	1987 Mean	2001 Mean	Difference
Consultation rate	3.59	3.94	0.35*
List size per fte	2297	2529	232*
Weekly working hours	52.9	44.1	−8.8*
Direct patient-related working hours	37.0	31.0	−6.0*
fte	0.94	0.84	−0.10*
Weekly working hours per fte	58.6	53.4	−5.2*
Consultation length (minutes)	9.93	9.81	−0.12

*$P < 0.05$.

dissatisfied with the time available for continuous medical education (CME), leisure time and time with the family. This is in sharp contrast with the number of GPs dissatisfied with time for the practice, which has increased by almost 17%. In general, in 2001 GPs are less satisfied about their work and more satisfied with the time available for private activities compared to 1987. Most of the dissension is related to a lack of time and money.

What to think about it

Morrison and Smith expect a firm increase in workload, and the decline of satisfaction among Dutch GPs could be regarded as an indication of this increase.[1] However, our findings show that there is not a single and simple answer to the

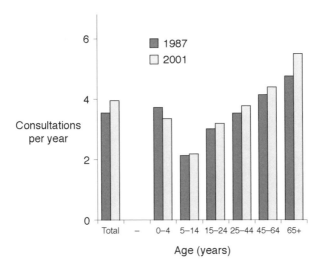

Figure 16.1 GP consultation rate of Dutch citizens, total and by age in 1987 and 2001.

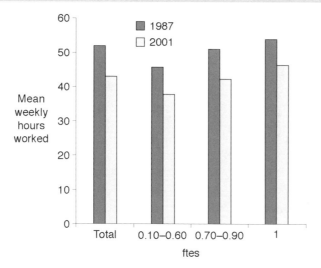

Figure 16.2 Mean number of weekly working hours of Dutch GPs, total and divided by fte categories in 1987 and 2001.

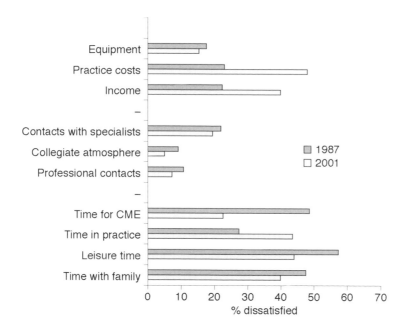

Figure 16.3 Proportions of GPs that were (very) dissatisfied with different aspects of their job, 1987 and 2001.

question whether or not workload has increased. Considering workload in terms of demand for care and list size per fte, we observe an increase. On the other hand, this increase of list size per fte is mainly due to GPs' own choice to reduce their number of working hours. GPs have found many effective strategies to handle more contacts within a shorter time frame. The picture of GPs developing strategies to improve their situation is in sharp contrast to the metaphor of rather passive hamsters that keep on running without making progress.

As other researchers has shown before, these results indicate that workload not just depends on the level of care demand, but is also affected by the supply side.[3,7] That is to say, workload is affected by the way this demand is managed. Focusing on only one of these aspects, e.g. the number of working hours or the consultation rate, can easily lead to false conclusions.

Looking for an explanation of how GPs manage to see more patients in fewer working hours, we have found five important developments affecting workload in this period.[5,8] These will be discussed under separate headings.

The nature of contacts has changed

The first, most likely, explanation was found in the nature of patient contacts. A clear shift has taken place towards less labour-intensive and time-consuming contacts. In 1987, over 16% of all contacts were house calls; in 2001 this percentage had dropped to 9%. At the same time, the proportion of telephone contact has increased from 4.4% to 10.8% of all contacts. GPs have gained much time by these changes. Another possible way to attend to a greater number of patients in less time would be to reduce the consultation time. However, this turned out not to the case: the average duration of a consultation remains the same: almost 10 minutes.

Access to the GP has become more regulated

Walk-in consultations are being increasingly replaced by consultations-by-appointment; some 50% of GPs adopt a policy of phone consultations by return phone call, and over half of the practice assistants independently advise by phone for a number of problems. These two aspects have contributed to a reduction in the number of telephone calls between GPs and their patients. Assistants almost always ask the reason for requesting a house call. They also do so for less than half of the requests for an appointment at the surgery. Increasingly, patients cannot see their GPs on the same day of their requests. However, waiting times for an appointment in the Netherlands remain very short compared to international standards. For instance, data from the mid 90s show that in the Netherlands only 6% of the GPs reported more than two days between appointment and consultation. In Denmark, Belgium, the UK, and France this percentage is 45, 21, 31 and 12 respectively.[9]

Task delegation

Task delegation continues to be an important means to contain the workload of GPs and possibly to address the consequences of a future shortage of GPs. There has been a particularly significant increase in the number of technical medical tasks delegated to practice assistants. These include conducting cervical smears, reading blood pressure and treating warts.

Reorganisation of out-of-hours work

GP co-operatives greatly alleviate the workload outside surgery hours. The emergence of GP co-operatives with centres for healthcare outside surgery hours is certainly one of the most spectacular organisational developments in GP care of the past 14 years. From the perspective of reducing the workload, the GP co-operatives have certainly been a success. The number of shifts worked has been significantly reduced. GPs who participate in a co-operative spend up to 70% less time on shifts than GPs who operate an on-call rota (a difference of 5 hours versus 19 hours per week). GPs are also very satisfied with the co-operatives: they experience their services as less onerous, and are generally happy with the organisation of the services.

Task restriction

GPs can also respond to the increasing work burden by restricting the tasks they reckon among their duties. Care for psychosocial problems is one of these. In 2002, fewer GPs reckoned psychosocial care to their duties than 14 years previously. This does not mean that patients can no longer can consult their GPs for psychosocial problems: GPs are now less likely to treat people who have, for instance, relationship problems, or problems at work. What is actually taking place here is task delegation, mainly delegation to primary care psychologists and social workers. It reduces the GPs' work burden, because patients with psychosocial problems usually have frequent contacts with their GPs, and consultations of this nature tend to take up a lot of time.

GPs on strike: how dissatisfied must you be?

The national strike of GPs in 2001 was the first in Dutch history. This event led us to infer that job satisfaction had decreased. The findings lent support to this assumption but not on all aspects of work. While GPs became less satisfied with financial aspects, like practice costs and income, they became more satisfied with the time available for professional education and leisure time. This seems to reflect the changes in the objective workload that took place. GPs spend less time on working but still handle a bigger care demand. Although they are more satisfied with the time available for other things than working, many of them apparently feel that improvements on the organisational level remain financially unrewarded.

In contrast to previous research, a range of workload aspects in this study were analysed by relating them to each other, instead of relating them to one outcome measure. One shortcoming of this study is that trends were described on the basis of only two moments in time. Also, the GPs in 1987 and those in 2001 were not the same group, but both samples were representative for the Dutch GP population.

An increase in care demand forces GPs to work more efficiently. The question arises as to how quality and accessibility of care may have suffered under the pressure of developments, such as increased task delegation, the emergence of GP co-operatives and the shift from house calls to surgery appointments and from surgery appointments to telephone consultations. Although this was beyond the scope of this study, results from other studies carried out in the framework of the DNSGP-2 indicated that Dutch GPs remain low prescribers, show a great adherence to professional guidelines and have low referral rates.[10,11] Patient satisfaction with the content of care has increased slightly, although there are concerns about the accessibility of care outside surgery hours and about the willingness of GPs to make house calls.[11] There are only a few signs that the quality of care has suffered.

Finally, this study did not address the question how organisational changes and workload affect the quality of care. Further research into the relationship between quality indicators (derived from professional guidelines) and workload indicators (as described in this study) will provide a deeper insight into this matter. We intend to continue along this path in the period ahead of us.

References

1 Morrison I and Smith R (2000) Hamster health care. *BMJ.* **321**: 1541–2.

2 Mechanic D (2001) How should hamsters run? Some observations about sufficient patient time in primary care. *BMJ.* **323**: 266–8.

3 Groenewegen P and Hutten JBF (1991) Workload and job satisfaction among general practitioners: a review of the literature. *Soc Sci Med.* **32**: 111–19.

4 van den Berg MJ, Kolthof ED, de Bakker DH and van der Zee J (2004) *De Werkbelasting van Huisartsen.* [The workload of general practitioners.] NIVEL, Utrecht.

5 Schellevis FG, Westert GP, de Bakker DH and Groenewegen PP (2004) Vraagstellingen en methoden. [Research questions and methods.] In: *Tweede Nationale Studie naar Ziekten en Verrichtingen in de Huisartspraktijk.* [Second national study into diseases and actions in GP practice.] NIVEL, Utrecht. *See also* www.NIVEL.nl/nationalestudie.

6 Westert GP, Schellevis FG, de Bakker DH de *et al.* (2005) Monitoring health inequalities through general practice: the second Dutch National Survey of General Practice. *Eur J Public Health.* **15**: 59–65.

7 Hutten JBF (1998) *Workload and Provision of Care in General Practice.* NIVEL, Utrecht.

8 van den Berg MJ, de Bakker DH, Kolthof ED, Cardol M and van den Brink-Muinen A (2003) De werkdruk van de huisarts, Zorgvraag en arbeidsduur in 1987 en in 2001. [The workload of the general practitioner, care demand and working hours in 1987 and 2001.] *Medisch Contact.* **58**: 1054–6.

9 Boerma WGW (2003) *Profiles of General Practice in Europe, an International study of Variation in the Tasks of General Practitioners.* NIVEL, Utrecht.

10 Cardol M, van Dijk L, de Jong JD, de Bakker DH and Westert GP (2004) Huisartsenzorg: wat doet de poortwachter? [GP care: what does the gatekeeper do?] In: *Tweede Nationale Studie naar Ziekten en Verrichtingen in de Huisartspraktijk.* [Second Dutch National Survey of General Practice.] NIVEL, Utrecht, Part two.

11 Braspenning JCC, Schellevis FG and Grol RPTM (eds) (2004) Kwaliteit huisartsenzorg belicht. [Quality of GP care in focus.] In: *Tweede Nationale Studie naar Ziekten en Verrichtingen in de Huisartspraktijk.* [Second Dutch National Survey of General Practice.] NIVEL, Utrecht, Part four. *See also* www.NIVEL.nl/nationalestudie.

Chapter 17

'Doing better but feeling worse'. Changes in the workload of general practitioners in the United Kingdom

Michael Calnan

What is this chapter about?

This paper examines changes in the workload of general practitioners (GPs) in the UK over the last 25 years and compares these changes to some of the evidence from the second national Dutch survey of general practice. The lack of a regular national survey of workload in the UK limits comparison and data had to be drawn from a range of different sources. Both countries saw a decline in job satisfaction, an increase in the delegation of tasks to nurses and other primary care workers and a decline in home visits. However, in the Netherlands, while list sizes increased, the number of hours worked declined. The UK experienced the opposite trend with list sizes decreasing dramatically but hours worked remaining the same. One implication is that list size is no longer a sensitive indicator of workload. There was also evidence to suggest that while doctors working in general practice may have better working conditions their subjective experience of their work is negative.

What is new?
Job satisfaction amongst GPs in both the Netherlands and the UK has declined markedly over the last 25 years but there is little evidence of an increase in volume of work.

Implications for general practice
This pattern suggests that dissatisfaction in general practice is an international phenomenon, which implies that policies should focus on GPs' expectations of their work in addition to its organisation.

Comparing workload: aspects to consider

The aim of this chapter is to provide a broader perspective on the trends identified in the second Dutch National Survey of General Practice (DNSGP-2) on the workload of Dutch GPs by comparing these patterns with the experience of general practice in the UK. However, before the trends and patterns of GP workload in the UK are outlined, two issues need to be emphasised and taken into account when making comparisons between the UK and the Netherlands.

First, comparisons can be made because there are similarities between the two healthcare systems. Both countries have GP gatekeeping and co-ordinating systems, and general practice is usually the first point of access for patients seeking professional medical care[1].

The second issue is methodological. No equivalent of the second Dutch national survey and database currently exists in the UK and thus direct comparisons are not straightforward. Therefore, the analysis of the UK experience is derived from a range of different data sources using different definitions and measures geographical areas and time periods. Hence, caution must be used in interpreting any differences.

Changes in workload: evidence from the UK

Workload can be operationalised in a number of different ways, although three different dimensions have been identified which are: (1) volume of work; (2) complexity of work; and (3) psychological burden of work.[2,3]

Most research on workload focused on 'volume of work'

The bulk of evidence available focuses on volume of work and there is baseline information available on which to assess changes. For example, a national cross-sectional survey was carried out in 1984 in the UK which provides information about different aspects of volume of work.[4] GPs reported that the average number of hours spent each week on general medical services (surgery consultations, home visits, administration, training) was 38.8, with 20 of these hours spent on surgery consultations, 10.5 hours on home visits and 3.2 hours (8%) on practice administration. A further 4.7 hours per week were spent on non-general medical services such as hospital appointments or insurance work.

Evidence from this survey also showed that consultation lengths (booking intervals) were on average 6.9 minutes with annual consultation rates and home visits being 2.7 and 0.6 respectively.[4] The major focus of this study was to examine the relationship between GPs' list sizes and allocation of time.[1]

In 1984 'list size' was a strong predictor of allocation of time.

Average list sizes were estimated as 2308 patients and the statistical analysis showed that list sizes were a strong predictor of allocation of time. GPs with larger list sizes spent more time on both general medical services and non-general medical services activities. GPs with smaller list sizes reported higher rates of consultation and home visiting and longer consultations. However, it was concluded that the effects of further reductions in list sizes would be haphazard, being differentially distributed across the range of list sizes. Longer consultation rates would result, but most of the extra time would probably be used in higher rates of consultation in surgeries and home visits, and some would be taken as free time.

Have there been significant changes in the volume of GP work since then? Robust evidence from longitudinal studies and regular surveys is in short supply. However, reviews have been carried out examining the impact of organisational changes on workload such as the impact of a primary care-led NHS or shifts from secondary to primary care.[3,5] The evidence is inconsistent and contradictory and no clear conclusions can be drawn apart from an increase in the volume of administration and paperwork rather than in clinical work.[2]

There are, however, some data available that suggest some changes in volume of work or at least allocation of time have taken place. First, in terms of hours worked in 1997, GPs spent on average 39.21 hours per week on general medical services' duties (excluding on-call) which is slightly above the 37 hours per week reported in 1989–1990 and 38.8 hours reported in 1992–1993,[6] and also the 1984 figure of 38.8 hours.[4] This might be explained by GPs spending more time with patients as consultation lengths have increased (the average length of consultation in the surgery was 9.36 minutes in 1997 compared with 8.33 minutes in 1990) as have consultation rates (each person saw their GP on average four times during 1998).[6] However, there has been a decline in home visiting (6% of patient consultations per week in 1998 compared with 14% in 1989) and there is now a more efficient organisation of out-of-hours care with approximately 12 000 GPs (approximately 40%) belonging to co-operatives in 1997.[6]

There are now doubts about 'list size' as an indicator of workload.

The more plausible explanation is that GPs are spending the extra time on practice management and administration (20% of time in 1998 compared with only 8% in 1984).[6] Certainly, there has been a dramatic decline in list sizes and an increase in the supply of GPs (allowing for the shift towards part-time work). For example, in England between 1986 and 2000 there was a 9% fall in list size from 2042 to 1859 in 2000 per full-time equivalent (fte) and between 1985 and 2003 there was 24% increase in the number of GPs. The implication is that GPs would have to work fewer hours but have more time to invest in patient care, hence the longer consultation length. However, this is based on the assumption that list size is still, in spite of recent changes in the structure and organisation of general practices, a strong indicator of workload.

In summary, there is no consistent objective evidence that there has been a major change (increase or decrease) in volume of work. Working hours on general medical service activities may have slightly increased, possibly due to an increase in administrative and managerial workload, but this has probably been compensated for by a major decrease in list sizes and increase in support for on-call working.

Workload increased because the complexity of the work increased

The evidence about whether the workload complexity of GPs has changed is in even shorter supply. However, a recent study examining increases in job weight amongst GPs concluded that the range and complexity of GPs' work was likely to have increased from 1990, particularly in the areas of clinical knowledge and mental demands.[7]

Job satisfaction and stress in general practice

The third dimension of workload relates to the psychological burden of work. There is, according to Sibbald and Young, consistent evidence from GPs who report substantial increases in the (psychological) burden of work.[2]

This latter finding is reflected in the trends in GP job satisfaction. General practice as an occupation and branch of medicine traditionally had a relatively high level of job satisfaction and was at its peak during the 1980s when general practice was experiencing rapid growth in its professional development.[8] Since then, job satisfaction has decreased, although the decrease has not been linear. Sibbald and colleagues, using the same scale, examined levels of job satisfaction in 1989, 1990, 1998 and 2001 (see Figure 17.1) and found a marked drop between 1989 and 1990 after the introduction of the new GP contract[9,10] (see also Calnan and Corney 1994[8]), when GPs reported increasing administration workloads.[9,10] The 1990 contract was viewed by GPs as an attack on their independent contractor status and professional autonomy.[11] Yet by 1998 satisfaction levels had partially recovered, although not reaching the higher levels of the 1980s,[8] illustrating that satisfaction can be a trade-off between the positive and negative aspects of the job. There then followed a further series of organisational reforms and developments including the introduction of primary care trusts, clinical governance, personal medical service contracts, walk-in centres, NHS Direct and, more recently, the introduction of a new national GP contract with its emphasis on financial incentives to improve quality.[2,12]

Traditionally, GPs had a high job satisfaction – till the tide turned in the 1980s.

Sibbald and colleagues[10] found that in 2001 (see Figure 17.1) job satisfaction was at its lowest recorded level. Doctors were least satisfied with their hours of work and pay and most stressed by increasing workloads. Paperwork coupled with changes imposed by health authorities and primary care groups and primary care trusts and the overall pace of change in general practice were also perceived an important source of stress.

It cannot be assumed that job stress and job dissatisfaction go hand-in-hand, and some occupations are stimulating and rewarding but also stressful or perceived as stressful. There is also a difference between self-reports of stress which may indicate low morale and those experiences of stress which manifest themselves in physiological signs and symptoms.[13] There is some debate about whether GPs experience higher levels of job stress than other members of the workforce.[2] Calnan and Wainwright[13] examined stress levels amongst different members of the general practice workforce (doctors, nurses, managers, administrators and clerical staff). The results showed that practice managers (see Figure 17.2) had the highest level of stress followed by GPs. This mirrored findings in hospitals where hospital managers experienced elevated levels of stress, compared with their colleagues. One explanation for this, at least in general practice, is that practice managers experience high levels of job demands but low levels of control and support.

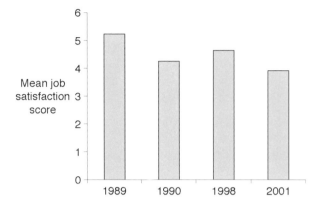

Figure 17.1 Changes in GP job satisfaction in the United Kingdom: 1989–2001.[10]

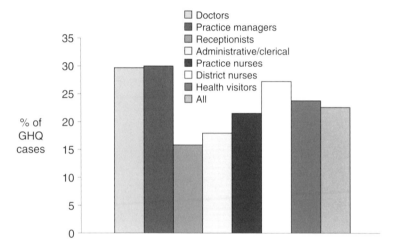

Figure 17.2 Stress in the general practice workforce: mental health by occupation.[13] GHQ cases: respondents reporting four or more symptoms on the General Health Questionnaire.

Changes in the general practice workforce in the UK

Over the past decades there has been a marked shift towards part-time working among men as well as women. For example, 25% of GPs in the UK, in 2003, worked part-time compared with 9% in 1992.[6] Coupled with this there has been a demand for greater job flexibility – hence the attraction of the new personalised medical services contracts – and a shift away from the traditional systems of permanent full-time employment with partners owning the practices.[2,14]

Working part-time became immensely popular during the past decade.

Two strategies have been adopted by the government to try to compensate for these changes. These are an increase in the size of the GP workforce and a shift in workload from GPs to other healthcare workers, notably practice nurses. For example, the number of staff working in general practice in England rose by around a fifth between 1994 and 2002. More specifically, between 1992 and 2002 there was a 32% increase in the number of practice nurses, 35% increase in administrative and clerical staff and 108% increase in practitioners providing direct patient care such as physiotherapy and counselling.[6]

Changes in public and patient views of general practice in the UK

Data on trends in public and patients' views of general practice are also in short supply. However, evidence from regular, national public attitudes' surveys since 1983 (*see* Figure 17.3) shows levels of public satisfaction with GPs remain high despite an overall decline in public satisfaction with the NHS over this period.[15] These percentages are probably under-estimates as those with more recent experience of general practitioner care tend to report significantly higher levels of satisfaction.[16]

Patients remain satisfied with GP care.

Evidence about long-term changes in patient perceptions is scarce. However, a national survey of general practice patients carried out in 1998 was repeated in 2002 and showed that, in the great majority of aspects of primary care, the situation is largely unchanged from that reported in 1998.[17,18] The views held by patients about their GPs were generally very favourable. However, patients' views about a few aspects such as waiting times and response to out-of-hours calls were more critical.

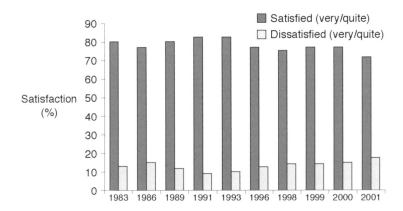

Figure 17.3 Public satisfaction with general practice: 1983–2001. Source: British social attitudes data.[15]

Conclusions: doing better, feeling worse?

This brief outline of patterns of change in the workload of GPs in the UK over the last two decades has showed some similarities to the Dutch experience and some differences (*see also* Chapter 16). First, the similarities. Both countries saw a decline in job satisfaction amongst GPs. There was also an increase in the delegation of tasks to nurses and other primary care workers in both countries. Finally, general practice in both countries experienced a decline in home visits and increase in telephone contacts, and the setting up of organised systems such as GPs' co-operatives to alleviate the burden out-of-hours work.

There were, however, distinct differences. List size, at least in previous decades, was used as a proxy indicator of workload. Yet, list size in the UK decreased markedly but in the Netherlands list sizes increased, implying differences between the countries in changes in patterns of workload. Certainly, in the UK an expected increase in consultation length and consultation rates took place, although hours worked increased slightly. In the Netherlands, consultation lengths did not change but average numbers of hours worked declined. This might suggest that list size is no longer a sensitive indicator of workload. For example in the UK, reimbursement systems in general practice have changed which may have influenced the relationship between hours worked and list size.[12,19]

Decreasing job satisfaction as an indicator of broader changes in society: people get more dissatisfied.

Finally, the 'doing better but feeling worse' hypothesis implies that even though working conditions improve there is a deterioration in satisfaction with work. This argument has some explanatory power in general practice in both the UK and the Netherlands, in that while hours worked in both countries decreased or did not increase and there was increasing support from practice staff, there was a marked decline in job satisfaction and possibly morale. This pattern suggests that it might reflect a broader social change in attitudes and that expectations about medical work now far exceed experience and rewards from the work.[20] The alternative explanation is that the reduction in volume of workload and the implication that GPs 'have never had it so good' has been counterbalanced by increases in the complexity of work and psychological burden of work, e.g. the need to be patient-centred and be expected to deal with a range of psychosocial problems.[21] In the Netherlands, GPs narrowed their task orientation with respect to treating psychosocial problems, although they are increasingly expected to 'manage' their practice which is a major source of stress. The plethora of organisational changes in primary care, at least in the UK, may have brought with them an increased administrative and managerial burden and a reduction in professional and clinical autonomy, manifested in the introduction of clinical governance. In addition to challenges and controls from the new public management, patient expectations and demands may have also risen.[22] Further analysis is required to understand this relationship between objective and subjective indicators of workload. Moreover, one specific question which needs exploration is how far low job satisfaction and morale influence the performance of practitioners and the quality of care provided.

References

1 Calnan M (2000) The NHS and private health care. *Health Matrix.* **10**: 3–19.

2 Sibbald B and Young R (2001) *The General Practitioner Workforce: workload, job satisfaction, recruitment and retention.* NPCRDC, Manchester.

3 Scott A and Vale L (1998) Increased general practice workload due to a primary care led NHS. *Br J Gen Pract.* **48**: 1085–8.

4 Butler J and Calnan M (1987) List sizes and use of time in general practice. *BMJ.* **295**: 1383–6.

5 Pederson IL and Leese B (1997) What will a primary care led NHS mean for GP workload? *BMJ.* **314**: 1337–41.

6 Royal College of General Practitioners (2001, 2004) *General Practitioner Workload.* RCGP information sheets no 3, May 2001 and no 1, June 2004. Royal College of General Practitioners, London.

7 Doctors' and Dentists' Remuneration Board (1998) *Twenty-seventh Report of the Review Body on Doctors' and Dentists' Remuneration.* HMSO, London.

8 Calnan M and Corney R (1994) Job satisfaction in general practice: a longitudinal study. *Int J Health Sci.* **5**: 51–8.

9 Sibbald B, Enser I, Cooper C *et al.* (2000) Job satisfaction in 1989, 1990 and 1998: lessons for the future? *Fam Pract.* **17**: 364–71.

10 Sibbald B, Gravelle H and Bojke C (2001) *General Practitioner Job Satisfaction.* Unpublished paper. NPCRDC, Manchester.

11 Calnan M and Williams S (1995) Challenges for professional autonomy in general practice. *Int J Health Serv.* **25**: 219–41.

12 Roland M (2004) Linking physicians pay to the quality of care – a major experiment in the UK. *N Eng J Med.* **351**: 1448–53.

13 Calnan M and Wainwright D (2002) Is general practice stressful? *Eur J Gen Pract.* **8**: 5–17.

14 Sibbald B, Shen J and McBride A (2004) Changing the skill-mix of the health care workforce. *J Health Serv Res Policy.* **9**: 28–38.

15 Exley S and Jarvis C (2003) *Trends in Attitudes to Health Care (1983–2001).* National Centre for Social Research, London.

16 Appleby J and Alvarez-Rosete A (2003) The NHS: keeping up with public expectations. In: Park A, Curtice J, Thompson K *et al.* (eds). *British Social Attitudes: The 20th report.* Sage, London, pp. 29–44.

17 Airey C and Erens B (eds) (1999) *The National Surveys of NHS Patients, General Practice 1998.* NHS Executive, London.

18 Boreham R, Airey C, Erens B and Tobin R (2003) *The National Surveys of NHS Patients, General Practice 2002.* NHS Executive, London.

19 Calnan M, Groenewegen P and Hutten J (1992) Professional reimbursement and the management of time in general practice: An international comparison, *Soc Sci Med.* **35**: 209–16.

20 Mechanic D, McAlpine D and Rosenthal M (2001) Are patient's office visits with physicians getting shorter? *N Engl J Med.* **344**: 198–204.

21 Wainwright D and Calnan M (2002) *Work Stress: the making of a modern epidemic.* Open University Press, Buckingham, pp. 122–3.

22 Mechanic D (2001) How should hamsters run? Some observations about sufficient time in primary care. *BMJ.* **323**: 266–8.

Chapter 18

Professionalisation of the practice assistant enables task delegation: 1987–2001

Michael van den Berg, Esmée Kolthof, Dinny de Bakker and Jouke van der Zee

What is this chapter about?

In times of a rising shortage of GPs, task delegation is in the centre of attention. We have investigated the role of practice assistants nowadays and how this role has been changing since the late 1980s. In addition, we studied the relationship between delegation to practice assistants and workload. Results indicated that the occupation of practice assistants has professionalised since 1987. Practice assistants are better educated and carry out more medical tasks. General practitioners (GPs) regard their practice assistants as competent and would prefer to delegate more to them. There appears to be room for expansion of the tasks of practice assistants: the GPs and the assistants are in favour of it, the assistants are sufficiently competent, and according to GPs, patients find delegation acceptable. However, according to the GPs, task delegation is hampered by lack of time of the practice assistant, room and funds.

Introduction

Under pressure of a rising demand for care and a growing shortage of GPs, policy makers and GPs develop strategies to improve the efficiency in general practice. Delegation of tasks is generally considered as a suitable strategy. Reduction of GPs' workload is one of the most important reasons to delegate tasks and, in addition, delegation can improve the quality of care.[1] By delegating routine activities, GPs can concentrate on more complicated tasks.

Which tasks may be delegated to whom and under what circumstances? This depends on the complexity of the tasks on the one hand and the expertise of the person who has to carry out these tasks on the other hand. This expertise can be achieved by education, but for effective delegation it is also important that GPs and patients acknowledge the need for delegation and accept it.

The days that the doctor's wife fulfilled the role of practice assistant are bygone.

Fifty years ago, the organisational structure of an average Dutch general practice was fairly simple: a single-handed practice with a GP, assisted by his wife or practice assistant with no specific education. Nowadays, the practice becomes more and more an organisation with a range of disciplines with different tasks and responsibilities.

The practice assistants have been the GPs' right hand since the 1960s. In recent times they have received an education at intermediate vocational level and their tasks are widely ranged: routine medical work (such as treating warts, removing stitches, blood pressure readings), administration, intake/counter activities, making appointments, cleaning instruments, management activities and triage. Table 18.1 summarises the tasks and educational level of the GP, the practice nurse and the practice assistant.

Although the practice assistant has the least complex tasks, he or she is, quantitatively, still by far the most important person next to the GP. Every Dutch general practice employs one or more practice assistants; around 40% employs a practice nurse. In this study we have investigated the role the practice assistants play in the practice nowadays: in what respect this role has been changing since the late 1980s, and which factors determine task delegation to practice assistants. In addition, information about practice nurses will be presented.

Table 18.1 Staff in Dutch general practice, 2001

Function	Tasks	Education
General practitioner	• Responsibility for the care process • Important decisions regarding prescriptions, referrals, etc • Gatekeeper in Dutch healthcare system	University, medical training 9 years
Practice nurse (since late 1990s)	• Taking care for chronically ill (diabetes, asthma/COPD) check-ups, instructions and information (about use of drugs, smoking, drinking and eating habits)	Higher vocational
Practice assistant (since 1960s)	• Routine medical activities (such as treating warts, removing stitches, blood pressure readings) • Administration, intake/counter activities, making appointments, cleaning instruments, management activities	Intermediate vocational

COPD: chronic obstructive pulmonary disease.

How was it done?

For a description of the methods of the first and second Dutch National Survey of General Practice, DNSGP-1 (1987) and DNSGP-2 (2001), *see* Chapter 2 of this book. Specific for the study described in this chapter is the following. To investigate task delegation and attitude towards delegation, surveys were carried out amongst all participating GPs and practice assistants (*see* Table 18.2). The response rate was 95% for the GPs and 91% for assistants in 2001. We have compared the results of the DNSGP-2 with comparable data of the DNSGP-1 (1987) and data from Nijland which were collected in 1990.[2,3] Response rates in these surveys were 96% in 1987 (only assistants) and 76% in 1990 (only GPs). Practice nurses did not participate in these surveys. Instead, GPs were questioned about their opinion on delegation to a practice nurse (only 2001). To test the statistical reliability of our findings, we have used Student's *t*-test for two independent samples, tests for two proportions and linear regression analysis. The operationalisations, data sources and numbers of valid cases are summarised in Table 18.2.

What was found?

In general, it appears that practice assistants have professionalised over the period studied. The number of practice assistants with vocational training

Table 18.2 Survey of GP staff, variables, data sources and number of cases

	Operationalisation	Source	DNSGP-1, (*n*)	DNSGP-2, (*n*)
Practice assistant				
profile	Age, education, fte, number of working hours	Questionnaires among assistants	158	246
tasks	List of (medical) tasks			
General practitioner				
attitude towards delegation and hampering factors	Statements about delegation, workload, quality	Questionnaire among GPs	436[a]	185
workload	Number of working hours a week	Diaries; registration of activities every quarter of an hour during one week		157
list size	Total list size, distributed by fte	DNSGP-2 practice database	154	189

[a]Data Nijland *et al.*, 1991.[3]

increased, and a rising number of practice assistants have a contract, a separate working area and a clearly defined package of responsibilities.

Education

The proportion that was trained as a practice assistant increased from 56% in 1987 to 79% in 2001. Figure 18.1 shows the number of practice assistants with an official vocational training in 2001. There is a clear relationship between the assistants' age and education: from the oldest assistants (45 years and older) nearly 60% took part in vocational training while in the youngest category, practice assistants without vocational training have become an exception. In 1987 only one-third of the oldest cohort had received vocational training (not shown).

Performance of medical tasks

From a list of 23 medical tasks, derived from the official occupational profile of the practice assistants, 15 were significantly more frequently performed by practice assistants in 2001 than in 1987. Figure 18.2 shows the 10 tasks with the largest shifts. The proportion of practice assistants that conducts cervical smears has increased from 3% to 53%. However, in 2001 smears were usually taken in the GP's practice which was not yet the case in 1990. The proportion of practice assistants that measure blood pressure has risen from 41% to 88%. Other remarkable shifts were those in treating warts and removing earwax. In 2001, 53% of the practice assistants had their own consulting hour (not shown).

GPs' attitude towards delegation

Most GPs had a favourable opinion about delegation. Eight out of ten GPs saw task delegation as a means to reduce their workload. In addition, 70% believed

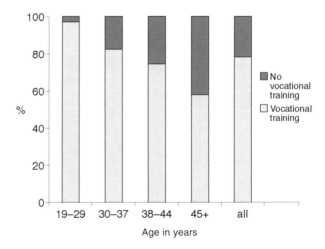

Figure 18.1 Percentage of assistants with/without vocational training classified by age quartiles (2001) ($n = 246$).

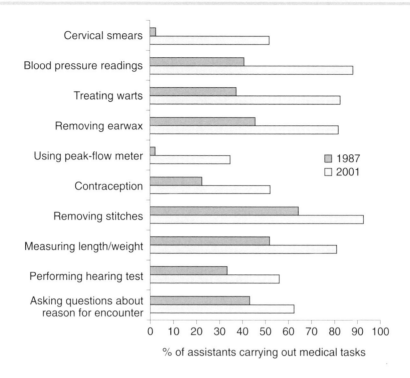

Figure 18.2 Ten medical tasks and the percentage of assistants that carried out these tasks in 1987 (*n* = 158) and 2001 (*n* = 246).

that task delegation increases their job satisfaction. Moreover, 77% assumed it saves time. The proportion of GPs that believe delegation increases their job satisfaction increased from 1990 to 2001 by 16% (*P* < 0.01).

Most GPs would prefer to delegate more to their practice assistants; more than half of the GPs (52%) were dissatisfied with the amount of assistance, they wanted more assistance, if this were possible. Approximately the same percentage was found in 1990.[2] However, GPs mention some factors that hamper task delegation (*see* Figure 18.3). The most important factors were a lack of the practice assistant's time (mentioned by 46%), room (30%) and funds (29%) (not asked in 1990). This seems to be an old problem: in 1990 the same drawbacks were mentioned. Factors that became far less important in the course of time are lack of expertise on the side of the practice assistant (decrease from 28% to 15%), the GP wanting to keep control (from 32% to 11%) and the acceptance of assistants by patients (from 31% to 11%).

Number of working hours

Considering the results so far, it could be expected that GPs work fewer hours when they have more assistance available. After all, they can save time by delegating activities. However, we have found that the more hours an assistant works, the more hours the GP works. The (unstandardised) regression coefficient (*b*) is 0.36, which means over 21 additional minutes GP working time per assistant-hour (these data were only available for 2001). Nevertheless, multi-

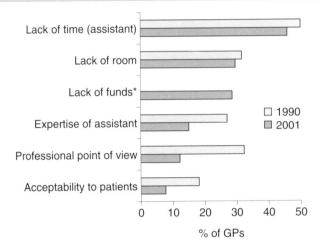

Figure 18.3 Factors that are seen by GPs to hamper task delegation in 1990 (*n* = 436) and 2001 (*n* = 185). *Not asked in 1990.

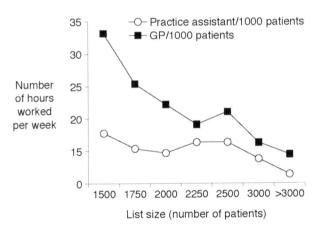

Figure 18.4 Number of hours worked by GPs and practice assistants per 1000 patients, per week by list size, 2001.

variate analyses showed that this relationship can be attributed to the list size. The number of hours worked per week by the GP (per 1000 patients) and the number of hours worked by the practice assistant (per 1000 patients) both decline with list size (*see* Figure 18.4). For the number of hours worked by the GP this relationship is the strongest.

There has been a slight increase from 0.84 full-time equivalent (fte) assistants per practice of 2350 patients in 1987 to 0.90 in 2001.

The practice nurse

One-quarter of the practices (25 out of 100) employed a practice nurse. Practice nurses worked approximately 0.20 fte (approximately one day a week) in a practice of 2350 patients. The practice nurse did not seem to thwart the activities of the assistants; the number of assistance hours did not differ between practices with a practice nurse and those without a practice nurse. Moreover, the number of hours worked by the GP does not differ either. So, it seems that in the practices with a practice nurse, some work is done that would otherwise have to wait before being done.

GPs are also very positive about task delegation to practice nurses: 73% of the GPs believe that a practice nurse reduces the workload of the GP, another 73% think it saves time and 78% think it improves the job satisfaction of the GP (not shown). However, the same hampering factors were mentioned as described above: a lack of time, room and funding. These aspects were mentioned by respectively 31%, 29% and 35% of the GPs (not shown)

What to think about it

In the course of time the job of practice assistants has developed. The role of the GP's wife assisting her husband has increasingly been taken over by a qualified assistant with a job contract, a separate working area and a clearly defined package of responsibilities.

A clear trend towards (medical) professionalisation among practice assistants is observed.

The results show a clear trend towards medical professionalisation among practice assistants. As the proportion of assistants with a vocational training is still growing, this trend will probably continue. In the near future, GPs will probably delegate more tasks. In healthcare policy, a trend towards delegation of more complex tasks to highly skilled support workers can be observed. This policy intends to solve problems of scarcity and workload. Our findings indicate that delegation of tasks to existing staff together with effective training gives promising results.

References

1 van den Berg MJ and de Bakker DH (2003) *Meta-analyse Introductie Praktijkondersteuning op HBO-niveau in de Huisartspraktijk in Nederland*. [Meta-analysis introduction practice support at vocational training level in GP practice in the Netherlands.] NIVEL, Utrecht.

2 Nijland A, de Haan J, van der Velden J and Meyboom-de Jong B (1990) De sociale en professionele kenmerken van de doktersassistente. [The social and professional characteristics of the practice assistant.] *Huisarts en wetenschap*. 33: 350–4, 363.

3 Nijland A, Pistor-Hendriks M, Groenier KH, Meyboom-de Jong B. and de Haan J (1991) Wil de huisarts taken delegeren aan de praktijkassistente? [Does the GP want to delegate tasks to the practice assistant?] In: Nijland A *De Praktijkassistente in de Huisartspraktijk, Progressie in Professionalisering*. [The practice assistant in GP practice, progression in professionalising.] NIVEL, Utrecht.

Chapter 19

Communication in general practice

Sandra van Dulmen and Jozien Bensing

What is this chapter about?

In this chapter, we explore the essence of the general practitioner (GP)–patient encounter by looking at what is actually being communicated in the consulting room. In terms of conversational input of GP and patient, the average GP–patient encounter appears quite equal. A more detailed analysis shows GPs taking the lead, by giving instructions and asking questions more often, and paying relatively little attention to psychosocial issues.

Patients' age, ethnicity and educational background influence the communication in the consulting room, in some respects favouring the younger, higher educated and native Dutch patient. GPs are found frequently being able to meet patients' preferences for support, information and advice. Compared to 1987, GPs give more information and allow patients more room in the decision-making process. The information exchange on possible other treatments and risks needs improvement.

Introduction

Various societal developments have taken place, which have contributed to a changing role of GPs and their patients. These developments include the epidemiological shift from acute to chronic illnesses; the change from illness-focused to patient-focused communication; the increased accessibility of information and a more equitable doctor–patient relationship. In addition, the position of patients in the Netherlands has been strengthened by the pro-patient legislation adopted by Parliament in the 1990s, e.g. the Medical Treatment Act (WGBO). The video-observation part of the second Dutch National Survey of General Practice (DNSGP-2) seeks to establish to what extent patients' needs and preferences are nowadays reflected in the communication between GPs and patients, and to what extent societal changes are reflected in the communication in the consulting room.

There is now ample evidence that communication should be considered as a powerful tool in medicine, not only in establishing a workable relationship with the patient, but also in both the diagnostic and therapeutic process.[1–5] It also works the other way around: good technical quality care, provided in an unsatisfactory environment and with unsatisfactory interactions, will not produce healthier patients, and negative expectancies increase the frequency of patients reporting all kind of symptoms.[4,6] Consciously or unconsciously, communication plays a crucial role in medicine. Sometimes this role is positive and leads to better understanding and coping, to better therapeutic decisions and more compliance; sometimes, however, the role of communication is negative and leads to misunderstanding, dissatisfaction, wrong decisions and sometimes even malpractice suits.[3,7] The success or lack of success can often be ascribed to communication processes, processes that will be unravelled in this chapter.

First, a general description of the communication in the consulting room is presented, followed by a description of the communication based on three sociodemographic characteristics: age, ethnicity and education of the patient (for the role of gender, *see* Chapter 20). Then, the preferences of patients for specific aspects of communication are described, together with the extent of GPs attending to these aspects during a consultation. Lastly, it is examined whether GPs encounter their patients differently after the introduction of the WGBO with respect to the provision of information and the level of patient centredness.

How was it done?

For a description of the methods of the first and second Dutch National Surveys of General Practice (DNSGP-1, 1987; DNSGP-2, 2001), *see* Chapter 2. Specific for the study described in this chapter is that data presented here are based on videotaped consultations with 142 GPs and 2094 patients, of whom 1787 were aged 18 years or older. A comparison was made with data from 210 videotaped consultations of the DNSGP-1 conducted in 1987.

Video observation

The verbal communication was rated using the Roter Interaction Analysis System.[8] This system distinguishes affect-oriented, task-oriented and process-oriented doctor–patient communication.

- *Affect-oriented communication* consists of social talk, agreements, expressions of concern or reassurance, paraphrases and differences of opinion.
- *Task-oriented communication* includes asking questions, giving information and giving advice (GP only) about medical/therapeutic matters, psychosocial problems, the patient's social situation and lifestyle.
- *Process-oriented communication* includes procedural utterances (giving instructions, asking whether the patient has understood).

The inter-observer reliability for the different communication categories was good (range of Pearson correlation coefficient $r = 0.72$–0.96).

Patient centredness

Patient centredness is the core concept in this study.

Patient-centred medicine in general practice means that GPs focus on 'being ill' instead of on the disease, that patients are well informed about possible diagnostic and therapeutic interventions and risks, and that GPs give their patients the room and encouragement to be involved in the decision about the treatment plan and to discuss preferences and concerns.

All these items were rated by observers on a five-point Likert scale.

Patient questionnaire

Before entering the consulting room of the GP, patients were asked to complete a questionnaire with questions about, for instance, their sociodemographic characteristics and their preferences and expectations of the visit, including information needs and role preference in decision making (WGBO aspects). Immediately after the visit, patients indicated, among other things, to what extent they perceived the GP as having performed the aspects they preferred.

What was found?

GP–patient communication: general findings

GP–patient communication is balanced in terms of their respective input. During the contacts, the contribution of GPs and patients in terms of the number of utterances is almost equal (*see* Table 19.1). Both the GPs and the patients communicate primarily in a task-oriented way; the GPs ask their patients on average 12 questions per visit and one in every four GP utterances concerns the provision of medical information. The patients, on the other hand, ask on average 3.5 questions, mostly on medical or therapeutic issues, and half of their utterances concern the provision of information. As expected, the GP takes the lead in the contact: one in every 10 GP utterances is rated as giving

Table 19.1 Mean frequencies of doctor and patient utterances in 2001
(n = 2094 consultations)

Type of talk	GP	Patient
All utterances	116.1	104.7
Task-oriented talk:		
biomedical questions	8.3	3.0
biomedical info	28.8	35.1
biomedical advice	5.1	–
psychosocial questions	3.8	0.5
psychosocial information	4.5	21.6
psychosocial advice	1.2	–
Affect-oriented talk:		
social talk	7.2	7.5
concern/optimism	1.3	1.5
encouragement	24.6	25.9
paraphrase/check	12.2	3.2
empathy	1.6	0.0
Process-oriented talk:		
instructions	10.7	0.8
seeking dialogue	1.5	0.4
disagreements	0.2	0.4
Other utterances	5.1	4.8

instructions to the patient, whereas the patients express only one structuring statement per contact. The GPs give five times more medical advice than advice on patients' lifestyle or psychosocial aspects. They show empathy 1.6 times per visit. Looking at patient centredness it appears that GPs behave generally in a quite patient-centred way; their average score is 3.8 (standard deviation (SD) 0.6) on a five-point scale. The extent of GPs encouraging patients to decide upon treatment appears somewhat lower than the room GPs allow for patients to express their opinion, but does seem to have increased compared to 14 years ago (mean score 3.1 in 1987 and 3.4 in 2001, $P \leq 0.01$).

Both GPs and patients communicate primarily in a task-oriented way.

The role of the patient's age

Older people talk more but receive less information and advice.

GPs are less inclined to encourage patients aged over 65 years, and they involve them less in decision making than younger patients. However, they are more affective towards patients in this age group than towards others. GPs express more concerns towards older patients and chat more with them than with younger adults. However, GPs ask older patients fewer questions and give less medical advice and information. The over 65s are less assertive than younger patients, although they are more likely to ask the GPs to repeat the information given.

The role of the patient's ethnicity

GPs are more task oriented in consultations with patients from non-western ethnic minorities.

The differences in communication are largely confined to a comparison between native Dutch and non-western immigrant groups. There is no difference with regard to the duration of a contact; however, non-western patients contribute less to the consultations. GPs are more patient centred in consultations with nationals by showing for instance more empathy and more understanding. Relatively speaking, GPs ask more medical questions in consultations with non-westerners but generally give less information. In these cases, however, both GPs and patients are more likely to check with one another that they have understood each other properly.

The role of the patient's education

Consultations with highly educated patients take longer than with those who are less well educated.

This difference is particularly marked during the decision-making phase of the consultation. Patients' assertiveness increases with their level of education. GPs are more likely to involve highly educated patients in decisions about their treatment than lower educated patients. There are relatively few differences in affective behaviour by GPs towards patients with different levels of education. GPs are more likely to ask patients with a low level of education whether they have understood what has been said. They ask highly educated patients fewer questions – particularly medical and therapy-related questions. By contrast, they give more information on these subjects to highly educated patients.

Patient preferences and GP performance

GPs meet almost all patient expectations.

The analysis of the questionnaire data showed that most patients (93%) want their GP to have time for them, to be pleasant (87%) and open (96%) to them, and to pay attention to what they are saying (96%) (affective behaviour). Almost all patients report that these expectations are met, even in cases where they had not attached much importance to these aspects prior to the consultation. Most instrumental aspects of a consultation are rated as important as well, such as getting clear information about the treatment (important to 94% of the patients) and getting to know how to cope with the complaints (94%). GPs are found to frequently give the desired information, explanations and advice, although in about 10% of the patients the doctor did not meet their preferences on getting to know what is wrong or receiving something from the doctor to relieve the complaints.

Patients' involvement in the decision-making process

Compared to 1987, GPs seem more patient centred.

The Medical Treatment Act served as an instrument to aid the research into the change in communication brought about by societal developments. Patients of 18 years and older consider it important to be informed about treatment and to decide for themselves or jointly with the GP on a course of treatment. However, this information is not as forthcoming as they would like, particularly where side-effects, risks and possible other treatments are concerned. Slightly over half of patients report involvement in the decision concerning treatment (see Figure 19.1). Compared to 1987, GPs seem more patient centred; they give more information (on average, 30 times per consultation in 1987 and 34 times in 2001; $P \leq 0.01$); they involve the patient more frequently in decisions, and they are more likely to request consent for a treatment (in 1.0% and 20.6% of the consultations, respectively; $P \leq 0.05$). This is reflected in the more democratic attitudes of GPs nowadays. However, GPs are less likely to involve the over 65s in decision making than younger adults.

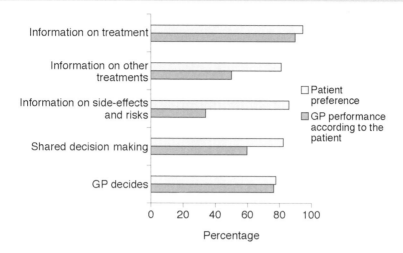

Figure 19.1 Percentage of patients indicating preference for the WGBO aspects and GPs performing these aspects (*n* = 1787).

What to think about it

The shift in morbidity to more chronic illnesses, combined with the increase in accessibility of knowledge and in the assertiveness of patients, was expected to lead to patients expressing clearer preferences with regard to what should take place during a consultation. However, changing structures in general practice may mean that GPs will be less able to deduce their patients' preferences than previously. These changing structures include the fact that GPs are increasingly working part-time and in group practices, as well as the introduction of GP co-operatives. This means that it can no longer be taken for granted that patients know their GP well. Nonetheless, the results of our research indicate that there is as yet no call for concern that GPs might not be able to meet their patients' expectations. In order to maintain a good quality of GP care, efforts must continue to be made to ensure a good balance in communication between doctor and patient.

When looking at patients' involvement in the decision-making process it appears that GPs gave less information during the consultation than patients had previously wanted. Yet, patients may have changed their mind about the relevance of specific aspects of communication and no longer needed the information. Another explanation for this may be that the consultation proceeded differently from what patients had originally expected.

In addition, the question arises as to whether GPs should in fact always be obliged to meet patients' requirement for information about treatment, possible associated risks and any other treatments. Not all patients want to make a decision or participate in the decision-making process, even if they are well informed. This concurs with the finding that highly educated patients value joint decision making about treatment more than less educated patients. Depending on the way the information is presented, less educated patients may have more difficulty understanding the information. This also concurs with the finding that many patients said the GP ultimately made the decision, although they did feel they had been included in the decision-making process.

Information about medical and therapeutic matters appears to contribute to the joint decision-making process, despite the influence of other factors on this process. Clearly, this makes sense, because the patient needs to know what is happening, in order to arrive at a well-considered decision, with possible implications for his or her health. The introduction of the WGBO legislation was a logical step towards increased involvement by patients in decision making, on the basis of informed consent. The more affective GPs appear to involve their patients more often in this process. This is a fairly obvious, but nonetheless important fact. Patients need both cure and care, if they are to get answers to their request for knowledge and understanding, and if they are to be known and understood and accordingly to be able to participate in the decision-making process. The change in communication behaviour is also reflected in the more democratic attitude of GPs towards patients. In this respect, the GP–patient relationship has progressed in tandem with societal developments. This is not only important, but also necessary to arrive at a patient-centred health service, based on joint decision making and informed consent.

References

1 White K (1988) *The Task of Medicine*. The Henry J Kaiser Family Foundation, Menlo Park, California.

2 Bensing JM (1991) *Doctor–patient Communication and the Quality of Care. An observational study into affective and instrumental behaviour*. NIVEL, Utrecht.

3 Roter DL and Hall JA (1992) *Doctors Talking with Patients; Patients talking with Doctors. Improving communication in medical visits*. Auburn House, Westport, Connecticut, London.

4 Crow R, Gage H, Hampson S, Hart J, Kimber A and Thomas H (1999) The role of expectancies in the placebo effect and their use in the delivery of health care: a systematic review. *Health Technol Assess*. **3**: 1–96.

5 Lipkin M, Putnam SM and Lazare A (1995) *The Medical Interview. Clinical care, education and research*. Springer Verlag, New York, Berlin Heidelberg.

6 Koehler WF, Fottler MD and Swan JE (1992) Physician–patient satisfaction: equity in the health services encounter. *Med Care Rev*. **49**: 455–84.

7 Levinson W, Roter DL, Mullooly JP, Dull V and Frankel RM (1997) The relationship with malpractice claims among primary care physicians and surgeons. *JAMA*. **277**: 553–9.

8 Roter DL (2001) *The Roter Method of Interaction Process Analysis*. The Johns Hopkins University, Baltimore.

Chapter 20

Have gender preferences and communication patterns changed?

Atie van den Brink-Muinen, Sandra van Dulmen and Jozien Bensing

What is this chapter about?

This chapter shows that despite their preferences, many patients do not have a female general practitioner (GP). Preferences for female GPs are not fulfilled for one-third of female and two-thirds of male patients. The reason is that the higher number of female medical students has not led to enough practising female GPs yet. Those patients that have a preference for a female GP are more often female and younger.

Furthermore, communication patterns have become more pragmatic. Nowadays, both male and female GPs talk less with their patients, express less empathy and concern, and talk less about biomedical and psychosocial issues than in 1987. Nevertheless, female GPs still talk more with patients than their male colleagues do. Compared with male GPs, they give more information, especially about biomedical issues. They also look more at their patients and are more affective. Communication patterns are not related to the patient's gender.

Introduction

Female GPs show more affective (socio-emotional) behaviour, such as empathy, partnership building, emotional support and reassurances.[1-5] They also have been found to encourage patients' input more through the use of concern and partnership statements.[6] Male GPs are likely to give more interpretations and paraphrases.[7] Concerning instrumental (task-focused) behaviour, information appears to be given more by female than male GPs.[5,8] Male GPs are likely to give more instructions, advice and suggestions for patient behaviour, and they appear to be more verbally dominant and imposing during the visit.[7,9] Female GPs seem more sensitive to patients' psychosocial problems, and give more psychosocial information to their patients than male GPs.[4,10,11] The non-verbal behaviour also differs according to the gender of the GP: female GPs look more often in the direction of the patient.[12]

Male and female GPs differ in their communication with patients.

Studies into differences in communication between cross-gender and same-gender-dyads have shown that in the female/female consultation the communication pattern differs from the other gender-dyads.[8] The female doctor gives more positive statements and looks more at the female patient. The atmosphere between female doctor and female patient is likely to be friendlier than between a female doctor and a male patient.[13,14] Female patients appear to find it easier to disclose information about themselves when the doctor is a woman, and they are likely to discuss psychosocial problems more often.[13] Because female doctors may be more inclined to look for psychosocial problems with women, there is probably a double effect. This assumption agrees with the higher amount of psychosocial problems diagnosed with female patients.[15] In the female/female dyad the contribution of doctor and patients is likely to be almost equal.[2]

Male patients are found to like psychosocial talk with male doctors but not with females, and, in general, to talk to female doctors as much as female patients do.[16] Female doctors are found to show more interest in male than female patients.[2]

Nowadays, around 65% of the students and 35% of the practising GPs are female. With the steady increase of the number of female GPs, the differences in communication between men and women are of increasing interest. One might expect that the growing number of female GPs has increased the possibility for choosing a female GP. More patients may want to see a female GP, and this gender preference is likely to be more often fulfilled nowadays.

Patients' main motives for preferring a female GP are that they feel more at ease during a physical examination, they talk more easily to a woman, and female GPs show more personal interest, have more experience with female health problems and a better understanding of their problems in general.[1,10] Some studies reported that highly educated and young patients and patients with specific female diseases more often prefer a female than a male doctor.[10,17] As recent societal development may have influenced communication, the question is raised whether GPs' communication patterns still differ between gender-dyads, i.e. M/M, M/F, F/M, F/F, GP and patient gender, respectively. Communication may have been influenced too by societal developments, such as a change to a more patient-centred communication and a more equal doctor–patient relationship, and by the increase of female GPs in general.[9]

The following questions will be addressed:

- have patients' preferences for GPs' gender changed over time, are their preferences fulfilled and which factors influence the patients' preferences?
- have male and female GPs' communication patterns with male and female patients changed over time?

How was it done?

Data sources

For the present study data from three databases were used:

- the first Dutch National Survey of General Practice (DNSGP-1, 1987): 16 GPs (12 male and 4 female) and 374 patients (both research questions)[18]

- the Dutch Health Care Consumer Panel: 961 people: a random sample of Dutch households (first research question)[19]
- the second Dutch National Survey of General Practice. (DNSGP-2, 2001): 142 GPs (108 male and 34 female) and 2784 patients (both research questions).[5,20]

Measurement instruments

For a description of the methods of the first and second Dutch National Surveys of General Practice (DNSGP-1, 1987 and DNSGP-2, 2001) *see* Chapter 2. Specific for the study described in this chapter is the following.

The participants of the Consumer Panel (1997) and those patients of the second National Survey (2001) whose contacts were videotaped, completed questionnaires about, among other things, sociodemographic variables (age, gender, educational level); health problem presented (International Classification of Primary Care (ICPC) coded);[21] and the preference for GP's gender (categories: male GP/female GP/no preference). Regarding the fulfilment of the patient's preference for GP's gender, in 2001 the patients were also asked whether they were registered with a male or a female GP.

To study the doctor–patient communication, in both national surveys consecutive general practice consultations were recorded on video on a randomly chosen day and approximately 15 GP–patient contacts were assessed.

The consultation length and duration of GPs' patient-directed gazes (as a percentage of the time the GP was on the screen and could look at the patient) were measured. Observers rated the verbal behaviour of GPs (frequencies of utterances) by means of Roters' Interaction Analysis System (RIAS).[22] The RIAS observation protocol assigns all verbal utterances to mutually exclusive categories, distinguishing between affective and instrumental communicative behaviour. Affective or socio-emotional communication (care-dimension) includes showing empathy, concerns, reassurance, encouragement, social talk and paraphrasing. Instrumental or task-focused behaviour (cure-dimension) consists of asking questions, giving information and counselling about biomedical or psychosocial issues, and structural utterances. The content of biomedical talk consists of medical and therapeutic issues. The content of psychosocial talk comprises psychosocial issues, feelings, social context (family, work) and lifestyle. The inter-rater reliabilities were satisfactory (Pearson's correlation coefficient between 0.72 and 0.95).

What was found?

Most patients still don't have a preference for their GP's gender

In 2001, 79.8% of the men and 68.6% of the women whose contact with the GP was videotaped had no gender preference (*see* Table 20.1). These percentages do not differ significantly from those in 1997. If patients do have a preference, both male and female patients have the highest preference for a GP of their own gender.

Table 20.1 Preference of patients (%) for a male or female GP in 1997 and 2001

	Male patients			Female patients		
	Male GPs	Female GPs	No preference	Male GPs	Female GPs	No preference
Consumer panel (1997)[a]	16.3	1.9	81.8	8.5	19.7	71.8
DNSGP-2 (2001)[b]	16.6	3.6	79.8	8.6	22.7	68.6

[a]478 male patients, 483 female patients.
[b]638 male patients, 972 female patients.

Factors determining patients' preferences

Both in 1987 and in 2001, the most common gender-dyad in general practice consultations was the male GP/female patient dyad, and next the male/male dyad (*see* Table 20.2). Female GPs see for the greater part female patients. The female/male dyad occurs relatively rarely, but has increased over time.

Younger patients and female patients prefer a female GP more often than older patients and male patients do (*see* Table 20.3). The chance that a female patient prefers a female GP is 7.5 times higher than for a male patient. Likewise, for every year increase in age, the chance that he/she will prefer a female GP is 0.98 higher, i.e. the chance becomes smaller. The patient's educational level does not influence this preference, neither does the presentation of typical female or male health problems.

Are patients' preferences met?

From the DNSGP-2 study (2001) it appears that nearly all male and female patients who prefer to be registered with a male GP do indeed have a male GP (98.9% and 98.6%). However, more than half of the male patients (60.0%, $n = 14$) and one-third of the female patients (33.0%, $n = 28$) who prefer a female GP do not have one.

Table 20.2 GPs' gender by patients' gender (gender-dyads) of videotaped consultations in 1987 and 2001

	Male GPs				Female GPs			
	Male patients		Female patients		Male patients		Female patients	
	n	%	*n*	%	*n*	%	*n*	%
1987	114	30.5	185	49.5	7	4.5[a]	58	15.5
2001	671	32.0	926	44.2	161	7.7	337	16.1

[a]$p \leq 0.01$ between 1987 and 2001.

Table 20.3 Odds ratios of preferring a female GP compared to 'no gender preference' (2001) (*n* = 1005)

Patient characteristics	OR	95% CI
Patient's age (years)	0.98	0.97– 0.99
Patient's gender (1 = female)	7.50	4.12–13.65
Patient's educational level (1 = low, 2 = average, 3 = high)	1.09	0.81– 1.47
Women's health problem (1 = yes)	1.23	0.78– 2.06
Men's health problem (1 = yes)	1.06	0.12– 9.49

OR: odds ratio; CI: confidence interval.

Consultation length is equal for all gender-dyads in 2001

In 1987, the consultations of male GPs with their male patients were the shortest. In 2001, these had lengthened and are now of the same duration as the consultation lengths of the other gender-dyads (*see* Table 20.4).

Looking patients in the eye is a characteristic of female GPs

In 1987, female patients were more looked at by female GPs than by male GPs. In 2001, the percentage of patient-directed gazing seems to be a characteristic of GPs' gender and unrelated to patients' gender. Female GPs look longer in the direction of their patients than male GPs.

Female GPs (still) are more affective ...

In 2001, female GPs communicated still more affectively than male GPs, although female GPs are less affective towards their female patients compared with 1987 ($P < 0.01$). The differences between opposite-gender dyads (M/F and F/M dyad), apparent in 2001, did not exist in 1987. Nowadays, male GPs are less affective towards female patients than female GPs are towards male patients.

... and they give more information

Female GPs give more information to the patients than male GPs. This was the case in 1987 and is still so in 2001. But the relative amount of instrumental talk (giving information and advice, asking questions, structuring) during consultations has changed. Both male and female GPs' instrumental talk with their female and male patients has decreased since 1987 ($P < 0.01$). The changes regarding instrumental talk between the gender-dyads are comparable to the changes regarding affective talk: the differences between opposite-gender-dyads (M/F and F/M dyad), apparent in 2001, also did not exist in 1987.

GPs' communicative behaviour: biomedical and psychosocial talk

Female GPs talk more about biomedical issues, i.e. questions, information and advice about medical and therapeutic issues, during consultations than their male colleagues. This was the case in 2001, as well as in 1987, except for female GPs who talked in 1987 with male patients as much as male GPs and their male and female patients. The amount of biomedical talk of female GPs with their female patients decreased between 1987 and 2001 ($P < 0.01$), while the biomedical communication pattern of the other gender-dyads has not changed over time (*see* Table 20.4).

In 2001, male and female GPs talk less about psychosocial issues with their male and female patients than in 1987 ($P \leq 0.05$). There are no differences between the four gender-dyads in psychosocial talk.

What to think about it

Preferences for GPs' gender did not change

The preference to be registered with a male or female GP has not changed over time. Still, 70% to 80% of the patients do not have a preference at all. If patients do have a preference, they mostly want a GP of their own gender. Whether these gender preferences are based on the same motives as in 1993 is not known. However, feeling more at ease and understood, and talking more easily with a female GP are motives that may be rather stable.

The higher number of practising female GPs probably explains the higher percentage of male patients visiting a female GP in 2001 compared to 1987. However, still more men prefer a female GP, as becomes clear from the finding that more than half of the male patients do not visit a female GP contrary to their wish. However, this concerns only 14 male and 28 female patients, so these results should be interpreted carefully. The preference for a female GP is also not fulfilled for one-third of the female patients. Patients preferring a male GP, on the contrary, nearly always have a male GP. This is understandable, because there are (still) more male than female GPs.

To fulfil patients' preferences, more female GPs are needed in the future, the more so because young patients prefer a female GP more often than older patients do. The proportion of female medical students has already been higher for years, and the proportion of female GPs is also steadily increasing. So, patients' preferences for a female GP may be more often fulfilled in the future. However, women are more likely to quit working as a GP.[23] Better working conditions, the possibility of working part-time and regulations for maternity and parental leave are likely to contribute to a higher participation of women in the GP profession. The new professions of physician assistant and nurse practitioner may take over some of GPs' workload and, therefore, will raise the willingness of female students to become a GP. As a consequence, the availability of female GPs may further increase in the near future.

Table 20.4 Communication characteristics and GPs' communicative behaviour in 1987 and 2001

	Male GPs		Female GPs	
	Male patients	Female patients	Male patients	Female patients
Consultation length (min) mean (SD)				
1987	8.2 (4.3)^{b,d}	10.0 (5.6)^a	11.1 (4.8)	11.3 (9.7)^a
2001	9.4 (4.6)	9.6 (4.6)	9.8 (5.0)	10.2 (4.5)
Patient-directed gaze (%) mean (SD)				
1987	54.6 (23.5)	47.7 (18.9)^d	53.4 (16.8)	68.8 (57.0)^b
2001	54.6 (21.4)^{c,d}	55.3 (20.5)^{c,d}	61.6 (18.9)^{a,b}	61.6 (18.8)^{a,b}
Affective talk (mean number of utterances (SD))				
1987	38.4 (29.7)^{c,d}	48.0 (33.0)^d	62.7 (35.1)^a	67.1 (29.3)^{a,b}
2001	43.5 (27.2)^{c,d}	44.9 (26.3)^{c,d}	55.8 (32.8)^{a,b}	55.7 (28.9)^{a,b}
Instrumental talk (mean number of utterances (SD))				
1987	68.3 (36.9)^{c,d}	80.9 (42.0)^d	105.4 (53.0)^a	111.1 (51.9)^{a,b}
2001	64.9 (32.4)^{c,d}	67.8 (32.8)^{c,d}	78.4 (41.7)^{a,b}	76.7 (35.8)^{a,b}
Biomedical talk (mean number of utterances (SD))				
1987	35.7 (24.8)^d	39.6 (24.5)^d	50.9 (29.9)	61.0 (31.1)^{a,b}
2001	39.1 (22.2)^{c,d}	41.3 (23.7)^{c,d}	48.1 (30.1)^{a,b}	48.0 (26.0)^{a,b}
Psychosocial talk (mean number of utterances (SD))				
1987	6.2 (11.8)	7.7 (14.1)	14.8 (18.9)	11.4 (20.3)
2001	3.5 (8.2)	4.2 (8.2)	3.8 (5.6)	4.4 (8.1)

SD: standard deviation.
Score differs significantly from the score of:
^{a}male GP/male patient consultations (1987: n = 114; 2001: n = 671)
^{b}male GP/female patient consultations (1987: n = 185; 2001: n = 926)
^{c}female GP/male patient consultations (1987: n = 17; 2001: n = 161)
^{d}female GP/female patient consultations (1987: n = 58; 2001: n = 337).

GPs' communication patterns with their patients changed

The communication of male and female GPs with their male and female patients (the four gender-dyads) has changed since the late 1980s. The consultation length and GPs' patient-directed gaze have remained unchanged, except for the male/male consultations, which have become somewhat longer. Nowadays, the consultation length of the four gender-dyads has become about equal.

Overall, GPs talk less with their patients than in 1987. This is more apparent in their task-focused than socio-emotional (affective) communication, and more in information giving and question asking about psychosocial than biomedical issues. Female GPs' communication with female patients has changed over time in all respects. In 2001, they showed less empathy, concern and reassurance to their female patients, they gave less information and they also talked less often about biomedical and psychosocial issues compared to 1987. This does not mean that female GPs talk less than their male colleagues nowadays, but less than they did in 1987.

Doctor–patient communication has become more pragmatic.

The overall decrease in communication, including psychosocial communication, was not expected in view of the more patient-centred behaviour and more equal doctor–patient relationship nowadays. The decrease may be a sign of the more business-like communication in medical consultations and the consumerist behaviour of patients. An additional explanation may be that all GPs have a computer on their desk nowadays. They need to register the information of the patients and the diagnoses, which takes time during which GPs mostly do not talk with their patients. It was demonstrated in an earlier study that there are more silences during the consultations nowadays than in the 1980s, when GPs did not have computers at all.[5] Specific attention should be given to the decrease of showing empathy and concern and talking about psychosocial issues. GPs should not neglect that this kind of communication is important for a good doctor–patient relationship and a good quality of care.

The differences in communication between the four gender-dyads have remained about equal over time. Male GPs talk in the same way with male and female patients, and this is also true for female GPs. However, there are still differences between male and female GPs. Female GPs look more often at their patients than male GPs. This may be interpreted as showing interest in the patients and may encourage the patients to disclose their – sometimes embarrassing – problems.[24]

Female GPs are still more affect-oriented, they show more empathy, concern, reassurance and encouragement, and they give more information to their patients and ask more questions than male GPs do. These gender differences are rather stable over time. It is remarkable that female GPs' communication with female patients has diminished over time in all respects. Possibly, they have adapted their communication pattern because of a higher workload than before.

In medical training it should be emphasised that communication is an essential part of the medical consultation. In spite of the trend to a more business-like communication, GPs have to show empathy and concern when necessary, and they have to talk with their patients about all relevant issues.

References

1 Bensing JM, van den Brink-Muinen A and de Bakker D (1993) Gender differences in practice style: a Dutch study of general practitioners. *Med Care*. **31**: 219–29.
2 Hall JA, Irish JT, Roter DL, Ehrlich CM and Miller LH (1994) Gender in medical

encounters: an analysis of physician and patient communication in a primary care setting. *Health Psychol.* **13**: 384–92.

3 van den Brink-Muinen A (1996) Women's health care: for whom and why? *Soc Sci Med.* **44**: 1541–51.

4 Roter DL and Hall JA (2001) How physician gender shapes the communication and evaluation of medical care. *Mayo Clin Proc.* **76**: 673–6.

5 van den Brink-Muinen A, van Dulmen AM, Schellevis FG and Bensing JM (eds) (2004) *Tweede Nationale Studie naar Ziekten en Verrichtingen in de Huisartspraktijk. Oog voor communicatie: huisarts-patiënt communicatie in Nederland.* [Second Dutch National Survey of General Practice. Focus on communication: doctor–patient communication in the Netherlands.] NIVEL, Utrecht. *See also* www.NIVEL.nl/nationalestudie

6 Lorber J (2000) What impact have women physicians had on women's health? *J Am Med Women's Assoc.* **55**: 13–15.

7 Roter DL and Hall JA (1998) Why physician gender matters in shaping the physician–patient relationship. *J Women's Health.* **7**: 1093–7.

8 van den Brink-Muinen A, van Dulmen AM, Messerli-Rohrbach V and Bensing JM (2002) Do gender-dyads have different communication patterns? A comparative study in Western-European general practices. *Patient Educ Couns.* **48**: 253–64.

9 Bensing JM and Verhaak PFM (2004) Communication in medical encounters. In: Kaptein A and Weinman J (eds) *Introduction to Health Psychology.* Oxford: Blackwell Publishers, Oxford, pp. 261–87.

10 van den Brink-Muinen A, de Bakker DH and Bensing JM (1994) Consultations for women's health problems: factors influencing women's choice of sex of general practitioner. *Br J Gen Pract.* **44**: 205–10.

11 van den Brink-Muinen A, Bensing JM and Kerssens JJ (1998) Gender and communication style in general practice: differences between women's health care and regular health care. *Med Care.* **36**: 100–6.

12 Hall JA (1999). How big are nonverbal sex differences? The case of smiling and sensitivity to nonverbal cues. In: Canary DJ and Dindia K (eds) *Sex Differences and Similarities in Communication: critical essays and empirical investigations of sex and gender in interaction.* Erlbaum, Mahwah NJ, pp. 155–77.

13 Roter DL, Lipkin S and Korsgaard A (1991) Sex differences in patients' and physicians' communication during primary care visits. *Med Care.* **29**: 1083–93.

14 Hall JA, Epstein AM, De Ciantis MC and McNeil BJ (1993) Physicians' liking for their patients: more evidence for the role of affect in medical care. *Health Psychol.* **12**: 140–6.

15 Roter DL, Stewart DM, Putnam SM, Stiles W and Inui TS (1997) Communication patterns of primary care physicians. *JAMA.* **277**: 350–6.

16 Hall JA, Irish JT, Roter DL, Ehrlich CM and Miller LH (1994) Satisfaction, gender, and communication in medical visits. *Med Care.* **32**: 1216–31.

17 Roter L (1991) The influence of patient characteristics on communication between the doctor and the patient. *Huisarts en Wetenschap.* **34**: 295–301.

18 Bensing JM, Foets M, van der Velden J, van der Zee J (1991) *De Nationale Studie van Ziekten en Verrichtingen in de Huisartspraktijk Achtergronden en Methoden* [Second Dutch National Survey of General Practice. Background and methods.] *Huisarts en Wetenschap.* **34**: 51–61.

19 Kerssens JJ, Bensing JM and Andela MG (1997) Patients' preferences for health professionals' gender. *Soc Sci Med.* **44**: 1531–40.

20 Schellevis FG, Westert GP, de Bakker DH *et al.* (2003) De Tweede Nationale Studie naar ziekten en verrichtingen in de huisartsenpraktijk: aanleiding en methoden [Second Dutch National Survey of General Practice.] *Huisarts en Wetenschap.* **46**: 7–12.

21 Lamberts H and Woods M (1987) *International Classification of Primary Care (ICPC).* Oxford University Press, Oxford.

22 Roter DL (2001) *The Roter Method of Interaction Process Analysis*. The Johns Hopkins University, Baltimore.

23 Kenens R and Hingstman L (2003) Cijfers uit de Registratie van Huisartsen, Peiling 2003 [Figures from the registration of general practitioners in 2003.] NIVEL, Utrecht.

24 Bensing JM, Kerssens JJ and van der Pasch M (1995) Patient-directed gaze as a tool for discovering and handling psychosocial problems in general practice. *J Nonverbal Behav*. **19**: 223–42.

Part 5

Quality

Chapter 21

Quality of primary care

Roger Jones

What is this chapter about?

Nowadays 'quality of healthcare' receives much attention. This chapter compares the process of quality measurement and quality assurance in primary care between the Netherlands and the UK.

In the DNSGP-2 several quality indicators explicitly developed for general practice were studied: adherence to guidelines, quality of practice management and views of the patient on the quality of services provided. The study shows that quality standards in Dutch general practice are high. However, there is no formal quality cycle in which guidelines are set, outcomes measured and re-evaluated: compliance depends on professional attitudes and commitment. This contrasts with the UK where a more formal cycle of quality of care is in place with contractual financial incentives for achieving quality targets: the Quality and Outcomes Framework.

Introduction

It is, perhaps, self-evident that we should strive for the highest possible quality in the provision of healthcare, but it is also worth considering why we should be particularly interested in the quality of the provision of primary care.

Primary care is, as Starfield has repeatedly argued, an essential component of any cost-effective healthcare system.[1] Its central activities – first contact, personal care, continuity, comprehensiveness and co-ordination – need to be added to the key gatekeeper role which strong primary care systems play in many countries. The use of appropriate technology, with investigations and management being conducted parsimoniously, against a background knowledge of patients' personal, family and psychosocial milieux, is a further hallmark of sophisticated primary care.

However, the identification of quality standards and outcomes depends on the establishment of a firm evidence base, derived from research conducted in primary care. We cannot simply transfer evidence collected in secondary and tertiary settings to inform quality standard-setting in primary care. This process must, additionally, encompass the demands and perspectives of patients, policy makers and funders, as well as the healthcare professionals delivering services.

Evidence collected in other healthcare settings cannot simply be applied in primary care.

It is important to continue to re-iterate these truths, widely accepted in the primary care community but easily forgotten in policy and administrative circles, where organisational memories are often short and decision makers are easily dazzled by high technology and life-or-death struggles in tertiary referral settings. How often have we heard health ministers measuring the scale of political investment in healthcare by the number of new hospitals that have been built?

Any discussion of quality of care needs to pay attention to quality measurement, quality assurance and quality development. Richard Grol, in the Netherlands, has led much of our thinking in this area, and has identified a quality cycle, analogous to an audit cycle, in which standards are set, mechanisms put in place to achieve them, outcomes measured and mechanisms re-evaluated, in the constant effort to meet predetermined quality standards.[2] This theme has informed much of the work of the National Primary Care Research and Development Centre in Manchester, UK, where Roland and Marshall have pioneered many quality assurance initiatives in the UK, and have laid the basis for the Quality and Outcomes Framework in the NHS.[3]

Quality indicators in the Netherlands: second Dutch National Survey of General Practice

In the second Dutch Survey of General Practice (DNSGP-2) quality indicators are located within three main themes. These are (1) adherence to clinical practice guidelines; (2) practice management criteria; and (3) patients' views of services. The survey methodology is described elsewhere in this book and information was collected from the sampling frame of general practitioners (GPs) and their practices to determine the extent to which performance measured up against quality criteria within each of these three domains.

Quality indicators: adherence to guidelines

Adherence to guidelines was examined in DNSGP-2 under the four main headings of diagnosis, prescribing, referral and prevention. Within each of these significant and gratifying improvements between the two surveys have taken place, with an overall increase in adherence rates to guidelines provided by the Dutch College of General Practice from 53% to 74%, with a wide range within and between guidelines. Adherence to prescribing guidelines is still somewhat low at 68%, but 89% of specialist referrals conform to clinical practice guidelines. Prevention targets in the Netherlands are similar to those of the UK, and 75% of high-risk patients had been vaccinated for influenza according to the second survey, with a cervical cytology coverage overall of 66%, which was, interestingly, substantially increased when GPs issued personal invitations to patients to attend for this procedure.

Guideline development and implementation has become something of a science in itself, and much has been written about the benefits and disadvantages of top-down versus bottom-up guidelines, the need for local modification of nationally-generated guidelines to create local ownership, the role of incentives and rewards, of IT decision support, of feedback to individual GPs and of the integration of guideline dissemination into continuing medical education and continuing professional development.[4]

The results of DNSGP-2 offer an interesting research opportunity to examine barriers and facilitating factors involved in guideline implementation amongst individuals and practices characterised by high and low rates of uptake and adherence.

Quality indicators: practice management

Three themes were examined under this quality criterion, including working patterns of GPs, and in particular the burden placed on them by their clinical work, the extent to which clinical tasks were appropriately delegated to other members of the primary care team and a number of detailed criteria related to practice management and administration systems; these include the way that practice equipment was held and maintained, the extent of delegation and co-operation within the primary care team, the way that services, including accessibility to patients, were organised, the quality of record keeping and also the quality of routine activities such as referral and prescribing.

This package of quality indicators relating to practice management provides a comprehensive overview of the way in which practices are run in the Netherlands, with the results of the DNSGP-2 demonstrating high standards and a commitment to quality.

Quality indicators: patients' views

Finally, patients' views have been incorporated substantially into the quality framework of DNSGP-2. Key aspects of patients' and users' views included the use of satisfaction surveys, feedback on GPs' diagnostic style, including the balance of their attention to physical and psychological issues in the consultation, privacy, accessibility and availability for house calls, practice organisation and, most interestingly perhaps, patients' views about GPs' health, their level of interest in individual patients and, conversely, their apparent level of burnout. This, once again, provides a comprehensive approach to the assessment of users' views in primary care, and information collected by individual practices can form a firm basis for practice quality improvement and development.

These results show that patients being cared for in Dutch general practice, while informed and critical, are highly appreciative of many organisational and professional aspects of the services that they have encountered.

Although these results are highly encouraging, they do not form part of a formal quality cycle, and the Dutch system does not, at present, incorporate methods of incentivising improvements in organisation and service delivery in primary care. However, in the UK a more structured approach has been developed, in which financial incentives are used to promote 'quality of care'.

Quality indicators in the United Kingdom: the Quality and Outcomes Framework

A new National Health Service (NHS) contract for GPs has recently been created in the United Kingdom (UK) in which core practice funding is supplemented by financial rewards related to the Quality and Outcomes Framework (QOF). Very similarly to the DNSGP-2 criteria, the QOF has four domains – clinical services, organisational aspects, the provision of additional services (such as cervical cytology, maternity care and child surveillance) and the patient/user experience.

The QOF itself, which provides practices with the opportunity to substantially increase their income by accumulating points awarded for reaching a range of targets, effectively embeds guidelines into the contractual arrangements for GPs. In the UK, guidelines have been big business for many years, and arrive on GPs' desks from many destinations – Royal Colleges, specialist societies, pharmaceutical companies, local primary care organisations, the National Institute for Clinical Excellence (NICE) and, via computers, in decision support and reminder systems provided by primary care software suppliers. However, sustained implementation has always been a significant problem, and the 'implementation corner' has been cut in the new contract by the provision of financial incentives related to the QOF.

Compliance to quality targets in the UK is stimulated by financial incentives.

Two examples of targets taken from the QOF are shown in Tables 21.1 and 21.2, relating to the management of stroke and of long-term mental illness (LTMI). Highly specified targets are provided for a range of measures related to the treatment and prevention of stroke, and similar high-specified criteria are applied to the management of LTMI. While recognising that this is the first iteration of the QOF, it is notable that, in relation to mental health for example, nothing appears about the detection of depression, benzodiazepine and antidepressant prescribing or attempted suicide. Some chronic and acute disease areas, notably gastrointestinal and musculoskeletal disorders, are absent altogether from the framework.

Practice management criteria within the QOF include targets relating to records – patient information materials, patient communication by telephone, electronic and paper media, staff education and training, practice and staff management and medicines management. There is less in the QOF about quality cycles, although these are, perhaps, implicit in the clinical management targets. Individual practices have the responsibility for reviewing their performance in relation to QOF targets and, through developing their own audit and quality cycles, putting in place the necessary improvements to meet them.

Finally, patients' experiences are assessed through measurement of consultation length, using consultation length as a proxy for quality, as described by Howie and colleagues, and also by the conduct of patient surveys, including the General Practice Assessment Survey (GPAS) questionnaire and the Improving Practice Questionnaire. [6–8]

Table 21.1 Indicators used in the Quality and Outcomes Framework for Stroke Management and the percentage of GPs reaching the target[5]

Topic	Target (%)
Stroke/TIA register	–
Δ by computed tomography or MRI	80
Smoking status	90
Smoking cessation	70
BP measured	90
BP ≤150/90 mmHg	70
Cholesterol	90
Total cholesterol ≤5 mmol/l	60
Antithrombotic	90
Influenza vaccine	85

BP: blood pressure; MRI: magnetic resonance imaging; TIA: transient ischaemic attack.
Δ: diagnosis

Table 21.2 Indicators used in the Quality and Outcomes Framework for Mental Health and the percentage of GPs reaching the target[5]

Topic	Target (%)
Long-term mental illness register (LTMI)	–
LTMI review within 15 months	90
Lithium measurement within 6 months	90
Lithium: creatinine and thyroid function tests within 15 months	90
Lithium in therapeutic range within 6 months	70

Conclusions

From a UK perspective the striking feature of the Dutch quality assurance programmes is their similarity, in the choice of themes and in much detail, to the quality criteria selected in the UK. The combination of clinical management guidelines, practice management and patients' views provides a widely applicable framework for judging the quality of primary care delivered by individuals and their teams.

Perhaps the most striking dissimilarity is the way in which the QOF in the UK has been linked to explicit contractual and financial quality targets, providing substantial financial incentives for achieving them. This contrasts with the methods used for dissemination and implementation of guidelines in the Netherlands, which depend more on professional attitudes and commitment.

Nonetheless, it is important to recognise that in any quality assurance system it is only possible to 'measure the measurable' and this can result in an undue emphasis on the more traditional chronic disorders, to the exclusion of other important clinical areas. Further, more subtle constituents of high-quality primary care may, because they are difficult to measure, not appear as quality targets, although the Dutch approach to using patient-reported assessments of physicians' engagement with their patients, and in particular their psychosocial problems, is innovative and apparently effective.

The trap for every quality measurement system is its focus on what is easy to measure. But that might not be the most important!

Additionally, any quality framework needs to be sensitive to the practice context, and potentially confounding variables in the population denominator, such as unusual demographic or case-mix features and large concentrations of ethnically distinct or refugee populations.

In future it will become increasingly important to measure primary care professionals' impact on health promotion and disease prevention, and the extent to which, in the context of an increasingly prominent public health agenda, ingredients such as motivational interviewing and reduction of risky behaviours, obesity and alcohol and tobacco abuse are effectively performed in primary care.

The continued evolution of quality frameworks for primary care requires continuing patient and professional input and also depends critically on two other key factors. The first of these is well-conducted research based in primary care, essential in generating the evidence base to support a focus on quality outcomes. The second relates to the curricular content of undergraduate medical training, with the need to increase the emphasis on disease prevention and health promotion and, perhaps, reduce the impact of the 'cure' paradigm in medical school teaching.

References

1 Starfield B (1994) Is primary care essential? *Lancet*. **344**: 1129–33.

2 Marwick J, Grol R and Borgiel A (1992) *Quality Assurance for Family Doctors*. Report of the Quality Assurance Working Party of the World Organisation of Family Doctors. WONCA, Jolimont.

3 Marshall M, Campbell S, Roland M and Hacker J (2001) *Quality Indicators for Common General Practice Problems*. Royal Society of Medicine Press, London.

4 Michie S and Johnston M (2004) Changing clinical behaviour by making guidelines specific. *BMJ*. **328**: 343–5.

5 www.bma.org/ap.nsf/Content/NewGMSContract (accessed 19 September 2005).

6 Howie JGR, Heaney DJ, Maxwell M *et al.* (1999) Quality at general practice consultations: cross-sectional survey. *BMJ*. **319**: 738–43.

7 Ramsay J, Campbell JL, Schroter S, Green J and Roland M (2000) The General Practice Assessment Survey (GPAS): tests of data quality and measurement properties. *Fam Pract*. **17**: 372–9.

8 Greco M, Powell R and Sweeney K (2003) The Improving Practice Questionnaire (IPQ): a practical tool for general practices seeking patients' views. *Educ Primary Care*. **14**: 440–8.

Chapter 22

Assessment of primary care by clinical quality indicators

Jozé Braspenning, François Schellevis and Richard Grol

What is this chapter about?

This chapter describes to what extent the care delivered in general practices is in agreement with clinical guidelines. Recommendations for good practice have been summarised in 139 indicators from 70 national guidelines. In this study, data on contacts, prescriptions, and referrals for a wide range of medical conditions were available for 106 quality indicators. Indicators on prevalence showed that detection rates could be improved for hypertension, hypercholesterolaemia, heart failure, alcohol abuse, dementia, anxiety, asthma in children, urine incontinence, hearing problems, and osteoporosis. Diagnostic imaging was requested according to the guidelines (76%), but this was less the case for laboratory tests (53%). Prescription-related indicators showed that the guidelines were more often followed when they related to not prescribing certain drugs (78%), rather than when they advised specific drugs (62%). Adherence was particularly high for referrals (89%). The indicators for preventative activities showed a high level of adherence (75%) but here too some improvement is possible. The indicators provide reference figures for current performance in general practice in the Netherlands. The adherence rates tell us about the quality of care delivered; the variance between practices provides further information on possible quality improvement.

Introduction

Since 1989, the Dutch College of General Practitioners has developed clinical guidelines for general practitioners (GPs). About 80% of the general practitioners appreciate these guidelines.[1] However, we know less about the adherence to these guidelines in general practices. A Dutch review study showed that in five years (1997–2003), only 22 studies evaluated the performance in general practices, of which 13 determined the adherence to a specific clinical guideline.[2] This type of information is much needed. Transparency of performance is for professionals an instrument to improve the quality of care provided.

Previous Dutch studies on adherence to guidelines focus on specific conditions such as asthma and chronic obstructive pulmonary disease (COPD), (threatening) miscarriage, low back pain or hypertension.[3–6] Two studies are available measuring the performance in general practice based on several different guidelines.[7,8] These two studies made use of registration forms that had to be filled in by the GP after the consultation. This type of data collection is very time consuming, especially when the number of guidelines is increasing. Data from routine collection in general practices, e.g. electronic medical records (EMR), seems a welcome solution.

To measure the performance we have developed in an earlier study 139 quality indicators based on the Dutch clinical guidelines.[9,10]

A quality indicator is a measurable element of practice performance for which there is evidence or consensus that it can be used to assess the quality, and hence change the quality, of care provided.[11]

Following Donabedian's description of different aspects of quality of care, three types of quality indicators can be distinguished: structure, process and outcome indicators.[12] Applied to diabetic care, having specific clinic hours for diabetics is a structure indicator, performing feet examination is a process indicator and the haemoglobin A_{1c} (HbA_{1c}) value is an outcome indicator (a proxy for possible complications in the future). These indicators have been used in the second Dutch National Survey of General Practice (DNSGP-2) to describe the quality of primary care.[13,14]

In this chapter, we focus on the extent of agreement between the care delivered in Dutch general practices and clinical guidelines.

How was it done?

For a description of the methods of the (first and) second Dutch National Surveys of General Practice (DNSGP-1, 1987 and DNSGP-2, 2001), *see* Chapter 2. The following is specific for the study described in this chapter.

Quality indicators

The Dutch College of General Practitioners developed 70 partly evidence-based and partly consensus-based guidelines.[9,10] These guidelines represent for the most part medical decisions in general practice and they are regularly being revised according to new or better evidence. The subjects addressed vary from acute otitis media to low back pain, from diabetes mellitus to asthma and from screening on cervical cancer to osteoporosis. Indicators were extracted from these guidelines using an iterative rating consensus procedure.[14] In five consensus rounds, indicators were identified that expressed quality of care in terms of expected health benefits and reducing harm or costs. The indicators were formulated using diagnostic and medication codes, e.g. International Classification of Primary Care (ICPC) and Anatomical Therapeutic Chemical Drug Classification (ATC).[15,16] Furthermore, the data from a national health information network for general practices (LINH, *see also* Chapter 30) were explored in order to get information on the number of indicators that could become available from routinely collected data. This procedure resulted in 139 indicators from 61 guidelines. For these indicators, specific information was available in the electronic medical records and this could be extracted in a uniform and structured manner. For 13 of these indicators we used additional electronic questionnaires (*see* Table 22.1 for an overview).

Most of the indicators are process indicators ($n = 124$) that have been categorised in indicators on diagnostics ($n = 13$ on the prevalence and $n = 21$ about testing); on medication ($n = 52$); on referrals to primary and secondary care ($n = 28$); on prevention ($n = 9$); and on health education ($n = 1$). Furthermore, 10 structure indicators and 5 outcome indicators were involved in the study.

Table 22.1 The 61 Dutch guidelines from which 139 quality indicators were derived

Guideline	Number of indicators	Guideline	Number of indicators
Hypertension	8	Eye diagnostics	1
Hypercholesterolaemia	4	Red eye	1
Peripheral artery disease	1	Acute otitis media	2
Angina pectoris	1	Otitis media with effusion in children	1
Transient ischaemic attack (TIA)	2	Otitis externa	2
Heart failure	4	Hearing complaints	3
Diabetes mellitus, type 2	10	Atopic dermatitis, eczema	2
Asthma in children	3	Acne	3
Asthma and COPD in adults: diagnostics	1	Venous ulcer of the leg	2
Asthma among adults: treatment	2	Psoriasis	2
COPD: treatment	3	Dermatophytosis	1
Depression	4	Bacterial skin diseases	3
Anxiety	2	Pressure sores	1
Dementia	1	Vaginal discharge	1
Disturbance of sleep	1	(Threatening) miscarriage	1
Problematic alcohol use	1	Subfertility	1
Stomach ache, pain	5	Vaginal bleeding	1
Acute diarrhoea	2	Pregnancy and puerperium	1
Ankle sprains	3	Intra-uterine device	1
Shoulder complaints	2	Amenorrhea	1
Low back pain	2	Pelvic inflammatory disease	1
Lumbar radiation	2	Genital herpes	1
Tennis elbow	2	Urethritis in men	2
Non-traumatic knee disorders in children and adolescents	1	Lower urinary tract symptoms	3
Sprains and strains of knee	1	Nephrolithiasis	2
Non-traumatic knee disorders	1	Urinary tract infection	2
Osteoporosis	5	Urine incontinence	2
Migraine	2	Enuresis	2
Influenza and influenza vaccination	6	Acute sore throat	3
Screening for cervical cancer	2	Sinusitis	4
		Fever in children	2

Data collection

For some indicators extra information was necessary. For instance, to calculate an indicator score on referral in cases of low back pain it was necessary to know whether the low back pain complaints were acute or not. For this information, an electronic questionnaire was developed that was triggered by the diagnostic ICPC code and was to be answered by the GP. This additional questionnaire was activated in the software system in the practices for three months.

Participating practices

In 101 out of 104 practices, data for the prevalence indicators could be collected; for referral and prescription indicators these numbers were respectively 99 and 97 practices. For some indicators, lower numbers of practices participated, as can be seen in the tables. Availability of extraction software in specific practices and additional questioning were the main reasons for getting less response.

Analyses

Except for the prevalence indicators, the indicators were formulated in such a way that a higher percentage represents closer adherence to the guidelines. Prevalence indicators were expressed in a number per 1000 patients. The percentage is an overall mean for all practices and is accompanied by a standard deviation to show the variation among practices. The unit of analysis is not the same for all indicators. Units of analysis could be the GP, the patient or the disease episode. For most structure indicators, the unit of analysis was the GP. For the prevalence figures and the prevention indicators, the unit of analysis was the patient, and for all other indicators it was the disease episode.

What was found?

Adherence to guidelines

Diagnostics

There is variation in the rate of (early) detection of chronic conditions. The indicators studied included the prevalence of diabetes mellitus, hypertension, hypercholesterolaemia, heart failure, problematic alcohol use, dementia, depression, anxiety disorders, urine incontinence, hearing impairment, asthma in children and osteoporosis (see Table 22.2). There was considerable divergence for the prevalence of hypertension (mean annual prevalence of 57.1 per 1000 patients), but also for instance for osteoporosis (mean annual prevalence of 4.2 per 1000 patients).

Requests for imaging diagnostics are largely conducted according to guidelines (76%). Guidelines about laboratory testing are adhered to in 53% of cases. Guidelines indicating when a certain test should be carried out are better adhered to than guidelines indicating there is no need for testing. Altogether, the rate of adherence to guidelines for diagnostics is 65% (see Table 22.3). Some examples are given in Table 22.4.

Table 22.2 Quality indicators on prevalence in Dutch general practice

Condition	Prevalence rates per 1000 patients in general practice				
	Age (years)	Total	95% CI	Men	Women
Diabetes mellitus	All	26.3	24.4–28.2	24.5	28.0
Hypertension	All	57.1	52.0–62.2	43.6	70.4
Hypercholesterolaemia	All	17.8	15.0–20.6	19.5	16.0
Heart failure	All	7.4	6.7–8.1		
	45–64			3.9	2.0
	65–74			25.9	17.8
	≥75			95.2	87.4
Asthma in children	<1			139.7	81.7
	1–4			66.4	43.5
	5–14			44.3	33.1
Depression	All	21.2	19.1–23.3	13.7	28.6
Anxiety disorders	All	7.1	6.0–8.2	4.5	9.6
Senile dementia	65–74	1.7	1.5–1.9	3.3	2.8
	≥75			22.0	28.3
Problematic alcohol use	All	1.7	1.4–2.0	2.6	0.9
Urine incontinence	All	6.0	4.8–7.2	2.1	9.9
Hearing impairment (presbyacusis)	All	2.3	2.0–2.6	2.6	2.1
Osteoporosis	45–64	4.2	3.4–5.0	1.1	8.5
	65–74			3.9	28.1
	≥75			8.6	42.3

Source: Van der Linden *et al.* (2004)[17]

Table 22.3 Adherence to Dutch guidelines: practice means in % and range between indicators

	% Adherence	Range between indicators (%)
Diagnostics, 11 indicators	65	13–96
imaging techniques	76	13–96
laboratory testing	53	32–78
Medication, 44 indicators	68	10–99
don'ts	78	33–99
dos	62	10–99
Referral primary and secondary care, 25 indicators	89	41–100
Total	74	10–100

Medication

Guidelines are reasonably well adhered to when they indicate that a certain drug is not needed or should not be administered ('don'ts': 78%). Guidelines suggesting the prescription of a specific drug are less well followed ('dos': 62%). Altogether, the rate of adherence to prescription guidelines is 68% (*see* Table 22.3). An example is shown in Box 22.1.

Table 22.4 Example of quality indicators

	% Adherence	Standard deviation
Diagnostics		
Percentage of episodes of low back pain in which no X-ray was requested (n = 2244 episodes in 57 practices)	90	9.1
Percentage of episodes of acute diarrhoea in which the faeces were not tested (n = 641 episodes in 67 practices)	34	28.1
Medication		
Percentage of episodes of lower urinary tract symptoms in which no finasteride has been prescribed (n = 2023 episodes in 97 practices)	94	9.3
Percentage of episodes of urinary tract infection in which nitrofurantoin or trimethoprim has been prescribed (n = 14 155 episodes in 97 practices)	68	15.7
Referrals		
Percentage of episodes of ankle sprain that was not referred to a physiotherapist (n = 3032 episodes in 99 practices)	89	13.1
Percentage of episodes of non-traumatic knee disorders in patients aged up to 22 years that was not referred to an orthopaedic specialist (n = 6512 episodes in 99 practices)	100	1.4

Box 22.1 An example on antibiotic policy

In the Netherlands, some 80% of all antibiotics are prescribed in general practice. The guidelines recommend restrictive prescribing of antibiotics, on account of preventing antibiotic resistance; and when antibiotics are needed, a first-choice drug is proposed. Nine guidelines concern prescribing of antibiotics, on which 13 indicators are based. There is a 62% adherence rate for prescribing antibiotics. A recommendation not to prescribe an antibiotic is better adhered to than recommendations for a first-choice antibiotic. The rate of compliance with guidelines varies considerably per indicator and also varies between the different indicators. The variation is greater when the guideline recommends a specific antibiotic than when an antibiotic is not recommended. Two-thirds of the patients with sinusitis get antibiotics (67% of episodes); there is a very high rate of compliance with the guideline on prescribing antibiotics for asthma in children. Antibiotics are prescribed in only 6% of cases. A high rate of compliance with the recommendations on antibiotic prescriptions does not mean that the recommendations on first-choice antibiotics are adhered to as well. In the same general practices under-prescribing as well as over-prescribing can occur. In Table 22.4 we show some examples.

Referrals

Of all referral indicators, 89% are according to the guidelines (*see* Tables 22.3 and 22.4). For referrals to physiotherapy, this is 83% when we exclude the very low number of referrals to the physiotherapist in case of urine incontinence in women (19.4%). The other referrals to secondary care have a mean number of guideline adherences of 93%. Differences between general practices are small, and even smaller as the rate of adherence approaches 100%.

Prevention

Of all patients in high-risk groups, 75% are vaccinated against influenza. The vaccination rate is particularly high among patients with cardiovascular diseases and diabetics. The vaccination rate among lung patients and of elderly patients (over 65 years) without a medical indication could be higher.

The average net uptake rate for population screening for cervical cancer is 74%. The uptake rate is considerably higher, i.e. 10–15%, when the practice is actively involved in inviting the eligible women.

Number of quality indicators

We have started off with 139 indicators but we could collect data for only 106 indicators. Although we already knew our dataset, we were too optimistic about collecting reliable data for clinical parameters, such as blood pressure and blood glucose. We were not able to decide if the measurements had taken place (process indicators), and we stayed unaware of the actual outcomes (outcome indicators).

What to think about it

Measuring the quality of care is not an easy task. It has become clear that it is possible to measure the quality of care on the basis of these indicators. The information about medical performance has mainly been derived from the electronic patient record systems, supplemented with a brief electronic questionnaire. A new challenge emerges once the data have been collected. How can the results be presented in a way that does justice to the data and delivers a clear message? According to O'Leary (1995), chairman of the Joint Commission on Accreditation of Healthcare Organizations:[18]

> ... *the problem with measurement is that it can be a loaded gun – dangerous if misused and at least threatening if pointed in the wrong position.*

We can calculate a total score, which indicates to what extent the actual performance in general practice agrees with the guidelines. For general practice performance, this score is 74%. Literature review shows that this figure was 55% in the period prior to 2001.[2] Although the tasks performed are not entirely comparable, these statistics clearly indicate an increase. The figure of 74% may also be regarded as high in international context.[19–21] However, there was considerable divergence in scores between the different indicators and between practices. Categorising the indicators according to different aspects of performance draws a clearer picture. Describing all the separate indicators is not an easy task. Clearly, it would help to divide them into categories, but further study is needed on the possibility of categorising groups of indicators. Which indicators can be summed up in categories on the basis of strong links, and which cannot? If some groups can be put together because they more or less cover the same area, would we need fewer indicators in future? This would make the task of determining the quality of performance easier.

We can establish where there is room for improvement by examining the scores for the different indicators. With regard to referrals, the figures show that there is a high adherence rate to the guidelines. However, a relatively large number of unnecessary referrals to physiotherapy have been made (one in five). With regard to prescribing drugs, there was a clear distinction between the 'dos' and 'don'ts'. Evidently, Dutch GPs are more likely to refrain from prescribing, than to prescribe first-choice medication.

The indicators had a maximum score of 100% and a minimum score of 0%. An adherence rate of 100% was not expected, because situations will always arise where a doctor's judgement regarding a specific patient will indicate a deviation from the guideline. For some indicators, an adherence rate of 100% is almost attainable, whereas for other indicators the expected rate is much lower. This difference is partly linked to the guidelines themselves, since some guidelines contain more strict recommendations than others.

For a number of indicators there were problems in gathering valid and reliable information on the basis of the routine data registered in the electronic patient record system. The problems concerned data on giving information and advice, and data about certain measurements taken and the results, such as blood pressure, cholesterol level and glucose levels. The current electronic patient record systems do not facilitate registration of these data in a uniform and accessible way. We recommend that electronic patient record systems should be equipped with suitable software capable of supporting disease management in the area of diabetes mellitus, asthma and COPD, as well as risk factors for cardiovascular disease.

The quality of GP care in the Netherlands measured by adherence to guidelines is rather good.

It can be concluded that the quality of GP care in the Netherlands measured by adherence to guidelines is rather good; however, specific fields for quality improvement for certain practices also became clear. To get a broader view on the quality in practice, other aspects should be measured as well, such as practice management and patients' experience.[22,23] For the latter, *see also* Chapters 23 and 24.

References

1 Geijer RMM and Meulenberg F (1999) Dertig standaarden geactualiseerd: waakzaam afwachten en/of gestructureerde zorg? [Thirty standards made up to date: waiting and being on guard and/or structured care?] In: Geijer RMM, Burgers JS, Van der Laan JR *et al.* (eds) *NHG-Standaarden voor de Huisarts I.* [NHG-standards for GPs I.] Elsevier/Bunge, Maarssen, pp. 1–10.

2 Braspenning J, Schiere AM, van Roosmalen M, Mokkink H and Grol R (2004) Kwaliteit van Huisartsgeneeskundig Handelen Moeilijk te Meten. Een literatuur-overzicht over 1997–2003. [Quality of interventions in general practice hard to measure. A literature survey of 1997–2003.] *Huisarts en Wetenschap.* **47**: 184–7.

3 Smeele IJ, Grol RP, van Schayck CP *et al.* (1999) Can small group education and peer review improve care for patients with asthma/chronic obstructive pulmonary disease? *Qual Health Care.* **8**: 92–8.

4 Fleuren M, Van der Meulen M and Wijkel D (2000) Do patients matter? Contribution and care provider characteristics to the adherence of general practitioners and midwives to the Dutch national guidelines on imminent miscarriage. *Qual Health Care.* **9**: 106–10.

5 Schers H, Braspenning J, Drijver R, Wensing M and Grol R (2000) Low back pain in general practice: reported management and reasons for not adhering to the guidelines in the Netherlands. *Br J Gen Pract.* **50**: 640–4.

6 Frijling BD, Spies TH, Lobo CM *et al.* (2000) Blood pressure control in treated hypertensive patients: clinical performance of general practitioners. *Br J Gen Pract.* **51**: 9–14.

7 Grol R, Dalhuijsen J, Thomas S *et al.* (1998) Attributes of clinical guidelines that influence use of guidelines in general practice: observational study. *BMJ.* **317**: 858–61.

8 Spies TH and Mokkink HGA (1999) Toetsen aan standaarden. [*Using Guidelines in Clinical Practice.*] Centre for Quality of Care Research/Dutch College of General Practitioners, Nijmegen/Utrecht.

9 Geijer RMM, Burgers JS, van der Laan JR *et al.* (eds) (1999) *NHG-Standaarden voor de Huisarts I.* [NHG-standards for GPs I.] Bunge, Utrecht.

10 Thomas S, Geijer RMM, van der Laan JR and Wiersma TJ (1996) *NHG-Standaarden voor de Huisarts II.* [NHG-standards for GPs II.]. Bunge, Utrecht.

11 Lawrence M and Olesen F(1997) Indicators of quality in health care. *Eur J Gen Pract.* **3**: 103–8.

12 Donabedian A (1980) *Explorations in Quality Assessment and Monitoring (vol 1): the definition of quality approaches to its assessment.* Health Administration Press, Michigan, Ann Arbor.

13 Braspenning JCC, Drijver R and Schiere AM (2003) *Kwaliteits- en Doelmatigheidsindicatoren voor het Handelen in de Huisartspraktijk. Handboek Kwaliteit van Zorg.* [Quality and efficiency indicators for GPs' interventions. Manual of Quality of Care.] Maarssen: Elsevier, Maarssen, C4.4: 1–30.

14 Campbell SM, Braspenning J, Hutchinson A and Marshall M (2002) Research methods used in developing and applying quality indicators in primary care. *Qual Saf Health Care.* **11**: 358–64.

15 Lamberts H and Wood M (1987) *ICPC: International Classification of Primary Care.* Oxford University Press, Oxford.

16 *Diagnostisch Kompas 1999/2000.* [Diagnostic Compass 1999/2000.] College voor zorgverzekeringen, Amstelveen.

17 van der Linden M, Westert GP, de Bakker DH and Schellevis FG (2004) *Tweede Nationale Studie naar Ziekten en Verrichtingen in de Huisartspraktijk. Klachten en aandoeningen in de bevolking en in de huisartspraktijk.* [Second Dutch National Survey of General Practice. Complaints and illnesses in general practice.] NIVEL/RIVM, Utrecht/Bilthoven. *See also* www.NIVEL.nl/nationalestudie

18 O'Leary DS, Nadzam DM, Loeb JM and Jessee WF (1995) Framework for performance measurement of health care networks and health plans. *Manag Care Q.* **3**: 48–53.

19 Schuster M, McGlynn E and Brook R (1998) How good is the quality of health care in the United States? *Milbank Q.* **76**: 517–63.

20 Seddon ME, Marshall MN, Campbell SM and Roland MO (2001) Systematic review of studies of quality of clinical care in general practice in the UK, Australia and New Zealand. *Qual Health Care.* **10**: 152–8.

21 McGlynn EA, Ash SM, Adams J *et al.* (2003) The quality of health care delivered to adults in the United States. *N Engl J Med.* **348**: 2635–45.

22 Van den Hombergh P (1998) *Practice Visits. Assessing and improving management in general practice.* [dissertation] KUN, Nijmegen.

23 Grol R, Wensing M, Mainz J *et al.* (2000) Patients in Europe evaluate general practice care: an international comparison. *Br J Gen Pract.* **50**: 882–7.

Chapter 23

Practice visits in the Dutch National Survey of General Practice: a useful research instrument for data on practice management

Pieter van den Hombergh, Yvonne Engels and Richard Grol

What is this chapter about?

Data on practice management and the practice setting are collected in order to provide feedback for 'individual' practices and benchmarks for quality improvement of practice management. In the second Dutch National Survey of General Practice (DNSGP-2), data were collected using the visit instrument to assess practice management (VIP method). In this chapter we will outline the scope of the VIP method, the data it provided for the DNSGP-2; finally, examples of variation in practice management are presented.

The practice visit method consists of 303 indicators describing 56 dimensions of practice management. The dimensions make up four major areas of practice management (infrastructure, team, communication and quality and safety). Instruments are questionnaires for patients (practice and general practitioner (GP) level), questionnaires for practices and individual GPs, practice assistants and a direct observer in the practice. The visit takes half a day. The practice received feedback and the data were used for analysis in the DNSGP-2.

Variation in practice management was demonstrated in the sample of 181 GPs of 98 practices. Variations in the four major aspects are demonstrated, its use for feedback to the GP and the practice as well as its use for benchmarking. The VIP provided valuable data for monitoring future trends.

Introduction

The practice setting is not only determined by the qualities of its staff (GP and auxiliary staff), but is also a major determinant of the quality of care. Data on practice management and setting provide feedback for each practice and benchmarks for quality assurance (QA). In the Netherlands, data on practice management are almost exclusively collected using the visit instrument to assess practice management (VIP method). The VIP was developed in the 1990s.[1] The method provides data for feedback at local, regional and national level, making it a useful research tool for analysis and the monitoring of future trends of practice management.[2,3] The second Dutch National Survey of

General Practice (DNSGP-2) added the VIP method to its set of instruments to measure practice management quality at national level. In this chapter we will give a short outline of the VIP method and some of its data on variation in the DNSGP-2.

The visit instrument to assess practice management (VIP)

Structure of the VIP instrument

In 1997, the Centre for Quality of Care Research (WOK) developed the VIP; a valid, reliable, and feasible method to assess practice management.[4] The Dutch College of General Practitioners decided to support practice visits using the VIP. Since 1998, it has been used by more than 2500 GPs in about 1300 practices. The VIP consists of 303 indicators describing 56 dimensions of practice management. The dimensions make up four major areas or chapters of practice management:

1 infrastructure, e.g. premises, equipment, service and organisation
2 team, e.g. task division, workload and job stress of the GPs
3 communication, e.g. with colleagues/care providers, time spent on meetings, patient information, computerised patient records, ICT
4 QA and safety, e.g. continuous medical education, audit, QA-activities.

Procedure

Questionnaires cover both the practice organisation and the management of the GP. Questionnaires are completed by each GP working in the practice, a practice assistant, 30 patients per practice and 30 per GP. An observer prepares a preliminary report with these data and completes the feedback report with a practice observation. This visit takes half a day. The GP invests one hour in answering the questionnaire and works normally during the visit. The time required to discuss the results is one hour or more. Practice visits by a non-physician observer instead of a colleague were found to be more feasible and better accepted.[5]

Feedback and benchmarking

Individual feedback and benchmark exemplified in a dimension

Table 23.1 gives an impression of the results on the dimension: 'Delegation of medical technical tasks' showing both the feedback to the practice and variation in general practice management.

Benchmarking was visualised by information on the variation in score on dimension. One's score can be compared to the score of colleagues and other practices in a histogram (see Figure 23.1). Histograms not only show the average score of GPs or practices, but also 'best practice'. 'Best practice' is the score at the right tail of the histogram and 'bad practice' the score at the left tail. Thus, feedback in a histogram provides more than one reference point for the GP and

Table 23.1 Example of the feedback on the aspect 'Delegation of medical technical tasks' of the dimension 'Team' in the VIP

Medical tasks delegated to the practice assistant	Yes (Θ) or No (N)	Reference[a] (%)
1 Removal of sutures (=an indicator)	N	82
2 Blood sampling (venapuncture)	N	39
3 Ear syringing	Θ	71
4 Liquid nitrogen application to warts	Θ	73
5 Removal of splinters	N	37
6 Treatment of small (cut-) wounds with glue	N	33
7 Audiometry	Θ	26
8 Recording an ECG[b]	N	18
9 Intracutaneous allergy test	N	24
10 Taping of a sprained ankle	N	34
11 Giving injections	N	93
12 Removal of a foreign body from the eye	N	9
13 Pressure gradient bandage for leg ulcer	N	24
Add up your 'yes' scores and compare. Plot your score in the histogram (*see* Figure 23.1)	Total: 3	Average: 5.9

[a]Percentage of practices answering 'yes'.
[b]ECG: electrocardiogram.

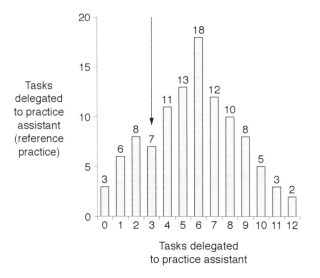

Figure 23.1 Medical tasks delegated to the practice assistant (compared with 106 reference practices).

the practice. This holds true, while a positive score on an indicator is in line with the Dutch College guidelines and recommendations for the profession. The effects of quality improvement (QI) can thus be simply demonstrated as movement to the right on the Gaussian curve.

Variation in practice management: the DNSGP-2

The DNSGP-2 used the VIP method to collect data on practice management at national level. The sample of 181 GPs of the 98 practices showed interesting variation in practice management.[6] The data could be compared to the larger database of VIP of 1874 GPs in 1055 practices and confirmed the reliability of the data.

Remarkable variation was found on the 56 dimensions and 303 indicators. A few examples of dimensions and indicators (bulleted points in) are shown in Tables 23.1 and 23.2. Some more instructive results in the table will be described here.

Infrastructure

As an example, only 73% of the practice assistants have their own room to address patients, hampering delegation of tasks. Some 45% of the patients reported that the emergency service of the practice could improve.

Team

Only half of the medical technical and diagnostic tasks were delegated to the practice assistant. An even lower fraction of preventive tasks, like cardiovascular risk profiling, routine in only 16% of the practices, was delegated.

Workload and job stress

GPs varied in reported workload (49 ± 11 h worked per week) and this was on average 6 h more than they would prefer to work. GPs over 45 years of age worked even longer hours (53 h). For single-handed GPs (working 53 h) and female GPs (working 43 h), the discrepancy between actual workload and preferred workload was even more than 6 h (8 and 9 h respectively).[7]

Communication

Background information on the patient history and a problem list was available in half of the records.

Quality assurance and patient safety

Pharmacotherapy was audited in groups with a pharmacist by 68% of the GPs.

Use of 'College-approved' patient leaflets scored 95%, showing tremendous speed of implementation since the leaflets were introduced in the late 1990s. An annual report and policy plan was reported by 22% of the practices, up from practically zero in the 1990s.

The examples show the considerable variation leaving room for improvement. It is for the profession to provide guidelines on benchmarks for dimensions and indicators. Extensive information on the 306 indicators and scores on the 56 dimensions can be found in the final report of the DNSGP-2.[8]

Table 23.2 **Examples of variation in score on 56 dimensions and 303 indi-cators in the DNSGP-2 (*n* = 98 practices)**

Chapter/*Dimension*/• indicator	*Mean ± SD*
I Infrastructure	
Practice size/surface (m²)	*87.5 (±31.7)*
• practice assistant has her own room (%)	73
Presence of medical instruments (out of 12 items)	*6.7 (±2.2)*
Presence of vials in the doctor's bag (out of 18 vials)	*13.2 (±2.5)*
Service and accessibility (30 patient questionnaires per practice)	
• time needed to contact the practice by phone (min)	5.4 (±3.6)
• waiting time before the consultation (min)	11.3 (±3.8)
Accessibility of the practice (5 items, score: –200% to +300%) (%)	*232 (±36)*
• when phoning the practice, the patient got > one answering device (%)	25
• practice can be reached easily in an emergency (%)	81
• emergency service of practice could improve (%)	45
Service/organisation of the surgery hours (5 items, score –200% to +300%) (%)	*154 (±56)*
• it is easy to contact the GP by phone (%)	73
II Team (delegation and collaboration)	
Preventive tasks delegated (out of 4 items)	*1.6 (±1.2)*
• cardiovascular risk profiling (%)	16
• PAP smear (%)	42
Medical technical and diagnostic tasks delegated (5 items)	*2.4 (±1.5)*
• ear syringing	*71%*
Medical technical and diagnostic tasks delegated (13 items)	*7.1 (±2.7)*
Collaboration with colleagues (8 items)	*6.7 (±1.4)*
Collaboration with other care providers (out of 13)	*5.4 (±2.5)*
Workload of GP (scored on 7 activities)	
• number of hours worked by full time GPs (hours a week)	49 (±11)
Job stress of GP (5 scales)	
III Communication (information and patient records)	
Patient score of information provided by GP and practice (% out of 300%)	*166% (±34)*
Background information of patient recorded (4 items)	*2.0 (±0.60)*
IV Quality assurance and patient safety	
Assessment in the GP group on quality assurance (7 items)	*3.2 (±1.8)*
• policy for patient with chronic disease	*46%*
Data-supported assessment of GP care (5 items)	*1.6 (±1.2)*
• GP assesses his prescription in a GP group (%)	68
• video of consultation for assessment (%)	32
Items demonstrating QI in the practice (no dimension)	–
• maintenance and calibration of equipment (%)	74
• use of 'College-approved' patient leaflets (%)	95
• protocols for treatment procedures (%)	32
• annual report and policy plan (%)	22
• patient knows how to file a complaint (%)	55

SD: standard deviation.

What to think about it

The VIP was successfully introduced in the set of instruments of the DNSGP-2, providing valuable data on present variation in practice management and data for monitoring future trends.

It provided benchmarks for practice accreditation as projected by the Dutch College.

The data in the VIP are the property of the GP and help the practice to account for transparency of their quality of care to government, health insurers and patients. This is in line with the new insights into evidence-based implementation.[9]

Collecting data in practice visits is a step forward towards blending research, individual feedback and benchmarking to the benefit of all stakeholders, without putting too great a burden on the practice. It allows quality management and unprecedented transparency.

References

1 van den Hombergh P, Grol R, van den Hoogen HJM and van den Bosch WJHM (1999) Practice visits as a tool in quality improvement: acceptance and feasibility. *J Qual Health Care*. **8**: 167–71.

2 Grol R (1994) Quality improvement by peer review in primary care: a practical guide. *J Qual Health Care*. **3**: 147–52.

3 van den Hombergh P. *Practice Visits. Assessing and improving management in general practice.* http://webdoc.ubn.kun.nl/mono/h/hombergh_p_van_den/pracvi.pdf (accessed 19 September 2005).

4 van den Hombergh P, Grol R, van den Bosch WJ and van den Hoogen HJ (1998) Assessment of management in general practice: validation of a practice visit method. *Br J Gen Pract*. **48**:1743–50.

5 van den Hombergh P, Grol R, van den Hoogen HJ and van den Bosch WJ (1999) Practice visits as a tool in quality improvement: mutual visits and feedback by peers compared with visits and feedback by non-physician observers. *J Qual Health Care*. **8**: 161–6.

6 Roosmalen M, Engels Y, Braspenning J *et al.* (2004) De praktijkvoering (VIP) [Practice management according to the visit instrument practice management.] In: Braspenning JCC, Schellevis FG, Grol RPTM (eds) *Tweede Nationale Studie naar Ziekten en Verrichtingen in de Huisartspraktijk. Kwaliteit huisartsenzorg belicht.* [Second Dutch National Survey of General Practice. Focus on Quality of General Practice Care.] NIVEL/WOK, Utrecht/Nijmegen. pp 74–83. *See also* www.NIVEL.nl/nationalestudie (accessed 2 January 2006).

7 Engels Y, Mokking H, van den Hombergh P *et al.* (2004) Praktijkvoering: werkbelasting en delegeren [Practice management: workload and delegation] In: Braspenning JCC, Schellevis FG, Grol RPTM (eds) *Tweede Nationale Studie naar Ziekten en Verrichtingen in de Huisartspraktijk. Kwaliteit huisartsenzorg belicht.* [Second Dutch National Survey of General Practice. Focus on Quality of General Practice Care.] NIVEL/WOK, Utrecht/Nijmegen. pp 38–47. *See also* www.NIVEL.nl/nationalestudie (accessed 2 January 2006).

8 Braspenning JCC, Schellevis FG, Grol RPTM (eds) *Tweede Nationale Studie naar Ziekten en Verrichtingen in de Huisartspraktijk. Kwaliteit huisartsenzorg belicht.* [Second Dutch National Survey of General Practice. Focus on Quality of General Practice Care.] NIVEL/WOK, Utrecht/Nijmegen. *See also* www.NIVEL.nl/nationalestudie (accessed 2 January 2006).

9 Grol R and Grimshaw J (1999) Evidence-based implementation of evidence-based medicine. *J Qual Improv*. **25**: 503–13.

Chapter 24

Quality of general practitioner care from the patients' perspective: facts, trends and differences

Herman Sixma and Peter Spreeuwenberg

What is this chapter about?

The aim of this chapter is to assess the quality of general practitioner (GP) care in the Netherlands from the patients' point of view and to look at the changes in quality of GP care between 1987 and 2001. Finally, we explore the differences in quality of care between practices.

   We conclude that, although Dutch patients are usually very satisfied with their GPs, results show that quality improvement on items that refer to organisational quality is possible.

Introduction

Patient views on quality of care are of paramount importance with respect to the implementation of quality assurance (QA) and quality improvement (QI) programmes.[1,2] Also, patient views on quality of care play an important role in mutual relationships between patients and healthcare providers, compliance with medical regimes and continued use of medical services.[3–5] However, the relevance of studies in which patient views are measured in terms of patient satisfaction is often questioned because of conceptual and operational problems. These problems refer to the reliability and validity of patient satisfaction ratings, the determinants associated with patient satisfaction and the ambiguity of the concept.[6,7] In general, patients are not involved in the development of survey instruments and, thus, the instruments tend to reflect the perspective of professionals rather than the distinct view of the patients.[8] Secondly, results from such studies show that patient satisfaction ratings are usually high and almost unrelated to outcome variables such as clinical outcome and levels of adherence,[9] and therefore not very suitable for application in quality improvement studies. Finally, the theoretical foundation for patient satisfaction studies can often be characterised as insufficient.[6,10]

Patient views are important but problematic to assess.

New developments

To deal with these problems, initiatives developed on both sides of the Atlantic over the last 15 years resulted in a new approach of the concept and in a new series of instruments measuring patient views on quality of care.[11–14] Quality of care from the perspective of the users of health and social care services is usually seen as a multidimensional concept.[15–17] There are also new elements. These include the way patients are involved in both development and assessment studies, often on the basis of shared decision making with researchers. They also include the combination of qualitative and quantitative research strategies as a basis for instrument development. Within the instruments the general focus is on questions asking for 'reports' rather than ratings of satisfaction or excellence. In this approach questions like 'Does the GP clearly explain the side-effects of prescribed medicines during the consultation?' (answering categories: 'always', most of the time', 'sometimes', 'never') are preferred above questions like 'How satisfied are you with the information you receive from your GP about the side-effects of prescribed medicines?' (answering categories: 'very satisfied' to 'very dissatisfied'). Within the field of quality of care research, there is a general agreement that questions asking for 'reports' tend to reflect better the quality of care and are more interpretable and actionable for quality improvement purposes than ratings of satisfaction or excellence.[18] In line with these developments, two of these second generation instruments measuring quality of care from the perspective of GP patients were applied in the second Dutch National Survey of General Practice (DNSGP-2).

The aim of this chapter is threefold. First, we will explore the weak and strong points of GP care in the Netherlands, looking through the eyes of the patients. Second, we will look at the changes in quality of care ratings over time, by comparing results from the first and second Dutch National Surveys of General Practice (DNSGP-1 and DNSGP-2). Finally, we will explore the differences between GPs and/or GP practices in overall quality of care ratings and look at the relationship between patient characteristics, GP characteristics and overall quality of care ratings by means of multilevel analysis.

How was it done?

Patients

From all 12 699 Dutch speaking patients who completed a health interview (*see* Chapter 2), a subsample of approximately 10 000 respondents aged 12 years or older answered questions about their perceived quality of GP care. Apart from age, the distribution of the respondents according to sex and place of residence is comparable with the sample population.

Questionnaires

Quality of GP care is measured by two instruments:

- *Clients Evaluate Practice locations (CEP) questionnaire*:[19,20] the 12 items included in the shortened version of the CEP instrument ($\alpha = 0.93$) refer to process quality (α = 0.89) and organisational quality (α = 0.84). CEP items have 6–point answering categories, ranging from 1 'inadequate' to 6 'excellent'

- *QUOTE (QUality Of care Through the Eyes of) GP patients questionnaire:*[21] the questionnaire consists of 22 items, with quality of GP care aspects being formulated as importance and performance statements. Items also refer to organisational aspects as well as aspects related to the actual care-giving process. These can be grouped together in (sub)scales that refer to overall quality (α = 0.89), process quality (α = 0.86) and organisational quality (α = 0.73). Importance and performance ratings are measured by 4–point response categories.

Scale scores derived from the CEP questionnaire and the QUOTE-GP patients' questionnaire correlate between 0.52 and 0.65, indicating that both instruments are roughly measuring the same underlying concept, but different aspects.

For part of the analyses, quality of care (QoC) ratings based on the QUOTE-GP patients and CEP questionnaires were dichotomised into 'positive' and 'negative' judgements. Included in the health interviews were four separate items on the perceived quality of GP care outside office hours. Other variables included in the analysis refer to sociodemographic characteristics of patients and GP and practice characteristics (e.g. GP job satisfaction, GP sex, GP age, number of days working in general practice, practice location). Variables at the GP and/or practice level were derived from questionnaires completed by all GPs who participated in DNSGP-2.

Analyses

The hierarchical database structure reflects the multistage sampling design of the study, with patients being linked to GPs, and GPs – when not working solo – being nested within general practices. This unique database structure offers possibilities to distinguish between differences in QoC ratings at patient level and differences at GP and/or practice level. It also offers possibilities to (1) aggregate scores on the level of individual GPs and/or practices; and (2) combine data from the interviews with characteristics of the participating GPs and practice staff members as well as other practice characteristics. For the part of our analyses in which we look at differences between GPs and/or practices, patient data were grouped together on the level of 126 GPs and analysed in a two-level regression model.[22–24] Approximately 60 patients per GP were included in these analyses. Patients that could not be linked to a specific GP were excluded from these analyses. Finally, trends in quality of care ratings on specific items were analysed by comparing DNSGP-2 data with the results of health interview data collected in 1987 as part of the DNSGP-1 study.

What was found?

Patients are satisfied with their GP

In general, patients are positive in their QoC ratings of Dutch GPs and the way GP practices are organised and functioning. The average percentage of negative ratings based on all 22 QUOTE GP patients items is 16.8%. For the 12 CEP items, an average of 7% of the respondents report negative ratings, 31% consider QoC 'sufficient' or 'amply sufficient', and 62% rate the quality of GP care as 'good' or 'excellent'. On average, QoC ratings derived from items that refer to process quality are somewhat more positive than ratings that refer to the way GP practices are organised and functioning.

Looking at the QoC ratings on the level of the individual items, Figure 24.1 shows that the average percentage of positive ratings for items that refer to process quality varies between 77% ('patients' complaints are labelled as psychosocial') and 96% ('GP explains about treatment'). For six out of the 22 aspects that refer to process quality, percentages of patients with positive ratings

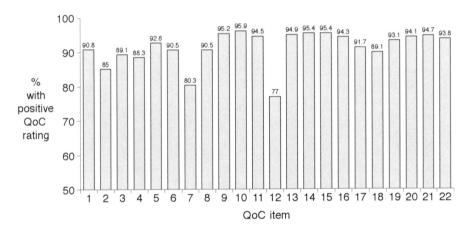

Figure 24.1 Quality of GP care (process aspects) from the patients' perspective, based on the QUOTE-GP patients and CEP instruments in 2001; percentages of respondents with positive QoC ratings. The QOC items are as follows:

1 patients are taken seriously (QUOTE-GP)
2 possibility to discuss all problems (QUOTE-GP)
3 enough time during consultations (QUOTE-GP)
4 willingness to discuss mistakes/shortcomings (QUOTE-GP)
5 shared decision making (QUOTE-GP)
6 access to patient files (QUOTE-GP)
7 referral according to patients' ideas (QUOTE-GP)
8 explanation about prescribed medicines (QUOTE -GP)
9 explanation about treatment (QUOTE-GP)
10 explanation about treatment (CEP)

11 explanation about complaint (QUOTE-GP)
12 complaints are related to psychosocial factors (QUOTE-GP)
13 adequate information on results examination (QUOTE-GP)
14 staff personnel with the right attitude (CEP)
15 patients' complaints are treated well (CEP)
16 effective treatment (CEP)
17 makes me feel better (CEP)
18 personal interest (CEP)
19 understands my problems (CEP)
20 treatment possibilities are discussed (CEP)
21 information about treatment (CEP)
22 treatment advices are emphasised (CEP).

fall below 90%. Quality aspects that refer to the way GP practices are organised (*see* Figure 24.2) show considerable differences in the percentages of positive ratings, varying between 47% ('conversations with the GP and staff cannot be overheard by people in the waiting room') and 94% ('GPs keep their appointments strictly'). For 10 out of 12 aspects, average percentages of positive ratings drop below 90%, indicating possibilities for quality improvement.

For patients, not all quality aspects are of equal importance. Results from the importance part of the QUOTE-GP patients questionnaire show that on a scale ranging from '1' (not important) to '4' (extremely important), average scores vary between 3.47 ('GPs should always take me seriously') and 2.08 ('time spent in the waiting room should not exceed 15 minutes'). Other QoC aspects with relatively high importance ratings refer to information that patients expect from their GP (explanation about their complaints, information about the results from examinations or diagnostic tests, information on prescriptions and (side-) effects of medicines), the accessibility of general practice by telephone and privacy aspects ('my conversation with the GP or staff personnel should not be overheard by people in the waiting room'). Over 30% of the patients rate these aspects as 'extremely important'. Apart from the accessibility by telephone, QoC aspects with relatively low importance scores refer to the costs associated with prescribed medicines, always seeing the same GP and the referral policy of the GP.

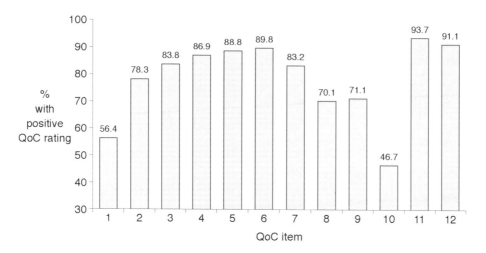

Figure 24.2 Quality of GP care (organisational aspects) from the patients' perspective, based on the QUOTE-GP patients and CEP instruments in 2001; percentages of respondents with positive ratings. The QOC items are as follows:

1 waiting time <15 min (QUOTE-GP)
2 accessibility by telephone (QUOTE-GP)
3 willingness to do house calls (QUOTE-GP)
4 consultation within 24 h (QUOTE-GP)
5 consultation as soon as possible (CEP)
6 consultation at convenient hours (CEP)
7 prescribed medicines without additional costs (QUOTE-GP)

8 consultation about referrals (QUOTE-GP)
9 always seeing the same GP (QUOTE-GP)
10 privacy within practice facility (QUOTE-GP)
11 GP keeps his/her appointments strictly (QUOTE-GP)
12 information about practice organisation (QUOTE-GP).

Changes in satisfaction over time

Trends in QoC ratings for Dutch GPs are difficult to establish, because instruments used in DNSGP-2 differ from the way this concept was measured in DNSGP-1. Four specific items that deal with the accessibility of the GP outside office hours are similar. For another five QUOTE-GP items the wording of the aspects and answering categories is slightly different but allows comparison (*see* Table 24.1).

Since 1987, patients report higher QoC ratings on 'process quality' items such as 'being taken seriously', 'explanation about complaints' and 'willingness to also discuss non-medical problems'. Aspects that refer to the organisational QoC (e.g. willingness to do home visits, enough time, accessibility during the weekends, nights and in the holiday season) show somewhat lower ratings and higher percentages of patients who are worried about the accessibility of GP care outside the office hours.

Although QoC ratings for the Dutch GPs are generally high, there are differences between GPs and/or practices. Based on the overall QoC ratings, derived from the QUOTE-GP patients' instrument, average ratings for GPs vary between 3.04 and 3.59 on a 1–4 scale (average: 3.31). Broken down in 'process' and 'structure' subdimensions, the variation in QoC ratings between GPs is somewhat larger and varies between 0.3 and 0.4 points around the mean score. Based on the overall QoC ratings derived from the CEP instrument (12–item version) the average QoC rating is 4.51 on a 1–6 scale. According to this scale, the GP with the highest 'improvement potential' rates 3.67, and the GP that can be characterised as 'best practice' scores a 5.02 rating. Differences between GPs and practices remain significant if we control for case mix and patient mix variables.

Explanation of differences in satisfaction

When variance in patients' overall QoC ratings is broken down in a component at patient level and a component at GP/practice level, the results show that

Table 24.1 Patients' ratings on quality of GP care, comparison between 1987 (DNSGP-1, n = 7679–10 112) and 2001 (DNSGP-2, n = 8007–9256); percentages 'yes'

	% saying yes	
Quality aspects	1987	2001
Patients are always taken seriously	82.7	90.8
Adequate explanation about complaints	82.8	94.5
Willingness to discuss all kind of problems	84.1	85.0
Willingness to do house calls	92.7	83.8
Enough time during consultation	90.8	89.1
Good accessibility during weekends/holidays	89.4	86.0
Good accessibility during evenings/nights	90.0	87.4
Feel uncomfortable about accessibility during weekends/holidays	9.6	14.6
Feel uncomfortable about accessibility during evening/nights	7.5	11.6

approximately 11% of the variance is at the GP level and the remaining 89% at the patient level. Elderly people, people that describe their own health as good or excellent, and people scoring low on the General Health Questionnaire (GHQ)-12 instrument for psychological disorders gave relatively high QoC ratings. However, these variables explain less than 5% of the variance at patient level. Variables at GP level indicate that higher job satisfaction ratings of GPs and the more days GPs are present in the practice facility are associated with higher QoC ratings by patients. Or, in general terms, satisfied GPs have satisfied patients. However, the nature of the study does not allow conclusions about the direction of this relationship.

What to think about it

Dutch patients generally are very satisfied with their GPs. But results show that quality improvement in certain organisational areas (e.g. privacy in the practice facility, waiting times, referral policy, seeing the same GP, accessibility by telephone) is possible and, from the patients' point of view, maybe necessary. Here, GPs with relatively low QoC ratings (the 'learning potentials') may benefit from the way 'best practice' GPs have organised their services. GPs who notice for example that patient ratings for waiting times are relatively low can ask colleagues with relatively high patient ratings on this subject how they managed to (re)organise their practice organisation in order bring down waiting times.

The fact that between 1987 and 2001 many Dutch GPs have reorganised their services with respect to making house calls and their availability outside office hours is reflected in patients' QoC ratings when we compare the results of DNSGP-1 and DNSGP-2. This comparison shows a drop in the way patients evaluate the availability of the GP during the evenings, nights and weekends, as well as the willingness of the GP to do home visits. Here, GPs might have to balance between their own interests ('reasonable working hours and cutting down travelling time and costs') and patients' expectations regarding the availability of GP services.

Finally, the results showed a significant relationship between the patients' psychological wellbeing and the way patients rate their GPs' quality of care. Although this relationship is not very strong it might indicate that, also when QoC ratings are based on 'reports' rather than satisfaction scores, differences in QoC ratings reflect more the respondents' state of mind than differences in the quality of GP care actually received by patients. On the GP level, the fact that GPs' job satisfaction is related to QoC ratings given by patients might open the debate as to whether more satisfied doctors will result in more satisfied patients, or it is just the other way around. Further research in this area might solve such questions about the direction of the relationships between these variables.

References

1 Donabedian A (1988) The quality of care: how can it be assessed? *JAMA*. **260**: 1743–8.

2 Donabedian A (1992) Quality assurance in health care; consumers' role. *Qual Health Care*. **1**: 247–51.

3 Marquis MS, Ross Davies A, Ware JE (1983) Patient satisfaction and change in medical care provider: a longitudinal study. *Med Care*. **21**: 821–9.

4 Wartman SA, Morlock LL, Malitz FE and Palm EA (1983) Patient understanding and satisfaction as predictors of compliance. *Med Care*. **21**: 886–91.

5 Thomas JW (1984) Relating satisfaction with access to utilization of services. *Med Care*. **22**: 553–68.

6 Williams B (1994) Patient satisfaction: a valid concept? *Soc Sci Med*. **38**: 509–16.

7 Strasser S, Aharony L, Greenberger D (1993) The patient satisfaction process: moving toward a comprehensive model. *Med Care Rev*. **50**: 219–48.

8 Fitzpatrick R and White D (1997) Public participation in the evaluation of health care. *Health and Social Care in the Community*. **5**: 3–8.

9 Sitzia J and Wood W (1997) Patient satisfaction: a review of issues and concepts. *Soc Sci Med*. **45**: 1829–43.

10 Rubin HR, Ware JE and Hays RD (1990) The PJHQ questionnaire: exploratory factor analysis and empirical scale construction. *Med Care*. **28**: S22–9.

11 Hays RD, Shaul JA, Williams VS *et al.* (1999) Psychometric properties of the CAHPS 1.0 survey instrument. Consumer Assessment of Health Plans Study. *Med Care*. **37** (3 suppl): 22–31.

12 Coulter A and Cleary PD (2001) Patients' experiences with hospital care in five countries. *Health Aff*. **20**: 244–52.

13 Jenkinson C, Coulter A and Bruster S (2002) The Picker Patient Experience Questionnaire: development and validation using data from in-patient surveys in five countries. *Int J Qual Health Care*. **14**: 353–8.

14 Wilde Larsson B and Larsson G (2002) Development of a shortform of the Quality from the Patient's Perspective (QPP) questionnaire. *J Clin Nurs*. **11**: 681–7.

15 Hall JA and Dornan MC (1988) What patients like about their medical care and how often they are asked: a meta-analysis of the satisfaction literature. *Soc Sci Med*. **27**: 935–9.

16 Wensing M, Grol R and Smits A (1994) Quality judgements by patients on general practice: a literature analysis. *Soc Sci Med*. **38**: 45–53.

17 van Campen C, Sixma H, Friele RD, Kerssens JJ and Peters L (1995) Quality of care and patient satisfaction: a review of measuring instruments. *Med Care Res Rev*. **52**: 109–33.

18 Cleary PD and Edgman-Leviton S (1997) Health care quality. Incorporating consumer perspectives. *JAMA*. **278**: 1608–12.

19 Wensing M, Grol R, van Weel C and Felling A (1998) Quality assessment by using patients' evaluations of care. *Eur J Gen Pract*. **4**: 150–3.

20 Grol R, Wensing M, Mainz J *et al.* (2000) Patients in Europe evaluate general practice care: an international comparison. *Br J Gen Pract*. **50**: 882–7.

21 Sixma HJ, Kerssens JJ, van Campen C and Peters L (1998) Quality of care from the patients' perspective: from theoretical concept to a new measuring instrument. *Health Expect*. **1**: 82–95.

22 Bryk A and Raudenbush S (1992) *Hierarchical Linear Models*. London: Sage, London.

23 Woodhouse G (1993) *A Guide to ML3 for New Users*. Multilevel Models Project, Institute of Education, University of London, London.

24 Snijders T and Bosker J (1994) Modeled variance in two-level models. *Sociol Methods Res*. **22**: 342–62.

Chapter 25

Adherence to pharmacotherapeutic advice in the guidelines of the Dutch College of General Practitioners

Feikje Groenhof, Carlijn Wefers Bettink, Liset van Dijk, Willem Jan van der Veen and Betty Meyboom-de Jong

What is this chapter about?

The guidelines of the Dutch College of General Practitioners were used to assess the adherence to pharmacotherapeutic advice for three diagnoses with a high prevalence: hypertension, depression and cystitis. Medication prescribed in 2001 was analysed for adherence to these guidelines. Adherence varies according to guideline across the diagnoses. General practitioners (GPs) adhered best to the cystitis guideline (70.4%), followed by the hypertension guideline (55.6%), the 2003 depression guideline (50.2%) and worst to the 1994 depression guideline (11.1%). One should be careful in interpreting these results in terms of rationality or quality. There are many reasons why GPs would consciously deviate from the guidelines.

Introduction

The goals of good prescribing, or rational pharmacotherapy, are to maximise effectiveness, minimise risks and costs, and to respect patient preferences.[1] At the 1987 World Health Organization (WHO) conference in Nairobi, the following statement was agreed upon: 'rational use of drugs requires that patients receive medication appropriate to their clinical needs, in doses that meet their own individual requirements, for an adequate period of time and at the lowest costs to the community'.[2] Guidelines facilitate effective, efficient, and cost-aware prescribing. Since 1989, the Dutch College of General Practitioners (Nederlands Huisartsen Genootschap, NHG) has published about 80 guidelines, approximately 50 of which contain pharmacotherapeutic advice. These guidelines are developed in a transparent way and are evidence based as much as possible. They are revised on a regular basis. Monitoring adherence to such guidelines is a logical way to assess prescribing behaviour and, based on this, improve prescribing quality in general practice.[3] Braspenning *et al.* show in Chapter 22 of this book that Dutch GPs follow these guidelines to a large extent. They have developed 139 indicators based upon the NHG guidelines, including diagnostic, prescription and referral indicators. Adherence was 74% on average, but it was lower for the indicators related to prescribing: 62%. There was a large variation in the degree of adherence between the different guidelines and between different advice in guidelines. For example, when it comes to the prescription of antibiotics, GPs adhere better to advice not to prescribe anti-biotics for certain diagnoses than to advice on the choice of a certain antibiotic.

The present study compares GPs' adherence to pharmacotherapeutic advice given in three guidelines of the Dutch College of General Practitioners: hypertension (1999), depression (1994/2003) and cystitis (1999). These three guidelines cover diagnoses that are frequently presented in Dutch general practice. The second Dutch National Survey of General Practice (DNSGP-2) prevalence rate of hypertension was 57.1 per 1000 patients in 2001, for depression 21.2 per 1000 patients and for cystitis 38.5 per 1000 patients.

How was it done?

For a description of the methods of the first and second Dutch National Surveys of General Practice, i.e. DNSGP-1 (1987) and DNSGP-2 (2001), *see* Chapter 2. The following is specific for the study decribed in this chapter.

Selection of general practitioners

Of the DNSGP-2 participants 102 GPs working in 67 practices provided data of sufficient quality. For different reasons a number of GPs were not included in the analyses: the registration period was too short (4 practices), prescriptions could not be linked to individual GPs (20 practices) or less than 40% of the prescriptions were provided with a diagnosis (13 practices). GPs included in these analyses did not differ significantly from the other GPs who participated in the DNSGP-2 (*see* Table 25.1). Only the number of single-handed practices was relatively over-represented in our selection.

Table 25.1 Features of GPs included and not included in this study

	Included (*n* = 102)	Not included (*n* = 93)
GPs in single-handed practice (%)	42	20[a]
GPs in dispensing practice (%)	7	13
Urbanisation level (%)		
non- and small urban	40	44
moderate urban	17	20
(highly) urban	43	37
Female GPs (%)	22	32
Age (mean years)	48	46
Number of peer review group meetings visited	8	7
Use of guidelines, precepts or formularies (mean; 1 = never, 5 = often)	4	4
Use of other information of pharmaceutical industries (1 = never, 5 = often)	1	1
Number of representatives from pharmaceutical companies in the last 4 weeks	2	2
Number of hours of education a year	50	50

[a]$P < 0.01$ (*t*-test).

Adherence to guidelines of the Dutch College of General Practitioners

Prescriptions for three diagnoses with a high prevalence were selected on the basis of the diagnostic code registered with the prescription: hypertension (International Classification of Primary Care (ICPC): K86), depression (ICPC: P76) and cystitis (ICPC: U71). If the prescribed drug matched the advice given in the most recent guideline for that indication, irrespective of restrictions mentioned in the guideline (e.g. comorbidity), we considered the prescription as 'adherent'. For hypertension and cystitis, the guidelines of 1999 were used, for depression the 1994 guideline was used. The depression guideline was revised in 2003. Because of a possible effect of GPs anticipating to this revision, the prescriptions for depression were also checked with the 2003 guideline.

The GPs included in these analyses recorded a total of 1 138 889 prescriptions. Of these prescriptions, 6.3% involved hypertension, 2.0% depression and 1.5% cystitis.

What was found?

Table 25.2 summarises the degree of adherence per guideline. GPs adhered best to the cystitis guideline (70.4%), followed by the hypertension guideline (55.6%) and the 2003 depression guideline (50.2%) and worst to the 1994 depression guideline (11.1%).

Hypertension

The pharmacotherapeutic advice in the hypertension guideline differs for various groups of patients. For all patients the guideline offers first, second and third preferences. For patients without relevant comorbidity, as well as for patients with diabetes mellitus, diuretics are the most preferred choice, followed by beta-blockers and angiotensin-converting enzyme (ACE) inhibitors. Depending on the type of comorbidity other preferences are given. For example, GPs are advised to prescribe beta-blockers when a patient has coronary heart disease; diuretics are second choice for these patients; ACE inhibitors third choice. Beta-blockers are contra-indicated for asthma/chronic obstructive pulmonary disease (COPD), which is why they do not show up in the list of preferred antihypertensives for these patients. While for the largest groups of patients the guideline prefers diuretics, GPs slightly preferred to prescribe beta-

Table 25.2 Percentage of adherence to pharmacotherapeutic advice in the guidelines for hypertension, depression and cystitis

Disease	Publication year	Prescriptions (n)	Adherence DNSGP-2 (%)
Hypertension (K86)	1999	71 295	55.6
Depression (P76)	1994	23 281	11.1
	2003	23 281	50.2
Cystitis (U71)	1999	16 850	70.4

blockers (*see* Table 25.3). Atenolol was the most frequently prescribed beta-blocker (11.7% of all prescriptions for antihypertensives), followed by metoprolol (8.5%). Hydrochlorothiazide was the diuretic most frequently

Table 25.3 Medication considered as adherent according to the guidelines of the NHG and percentage of the prescriptions for the specific indications[a]

Disease	NHG-guideline	ATC code	Medication		Prescriptions (%)
Hypertension (K86)	1999	C07AB03	Atenolol (2)		11.7
		C03AA03	Hydrochlorothiazide (1)		10.8
		C07AB02	Metoprolol (2)		8.5
		C09AA02	Enalapril (3)		8.0
		C08CA01	Amlodipine		4.3
		C08CA05	Nifedipine (3)		3.8
		C03BA04	Chlorothalidone (1)		3.5
		C03EA01	Hydrochlorothiazide with potassium-saving diuretics (1)		3.4
		C09AA01	Captopril (3)		2.2
		C09CA01	Losartan		2.2
		C09AA03	Lisinopril		2.0
		C07CB03	Atenolol with other diuretics (2)		1.7
		C07AB07	Bisoprolol		1.5
		C09BA02	Enalapril with diuretics (3)		1.1
		C09BA01	Captopril with diuretics (3)		0.7
		C07BB02	Metoprolol with thiazide (2)		0.2
		C07FB03	Atenolol with other anti-hypertension medication (2)		0.0
Depression (P76)			1994 guideline	2003 guideline	
		N06AB05	Paroxetine	Paroxetine	32.8
		N06AB03	Fluoxetine	Fluoxetine	6.5
		N06AA09	Amitriptyline	Amitriptyline	6.2
		N06AX16	Venlafaxine	Venlafaxine	5.1
		N05BA04	Oxazepam	Oxazepam	4.8
		N06AB08	Fluvoxamine	Fluvoxamine	4.6
		N06AX11	Mirtazapine	Mirtazapine	4.5
		N06AB04	Citalopram	Citalopram	4.0
		N06AA04	Clomipramine	Clomipramine	2.7
		N05CD07	Temazepam	Temazepam	2.4
		N06AB06	Sertraline	Sertraline	2.4
		N06AA10	Nortriptyline	Nortriptyline	1.2
		N06AA02	Imipramine	Imipramine	0.4
Cystitis (U71)	1999	J01EA01	Trimethoprim		31.1
		J01XE01	Nitrofurantoin		26.1
		J01MA06	Norfloxacin		6.0
		J01EE01	Co-trimoxazole		5.0
		J01CR02	Amoxicillin/clavulanate		4.3
		J01CA04	Amoxicillin		4.0
		J01MA02	Ciprofloxacin		3.1
		G04AC01	Furadantin		3.0

[a]The items in bold indicate that the medication matches the advice in the guidelines.
The figures between brackets indicate whether the medication is a first, second or third preference according to the guidelines for patients without comorbidity.
ATC: Anatomical Therapeutic Chemical classification.

prescribed (10.8%), followed by chlorothalidon (3.5%); for ACE inhibitors, GPs' first choice was enalapril (8.0%). These antihypertensives are all mentioned in the guidelines and the prescription is considered as adherent. The most prescribed non-matching antihypertensive drug was amlodipine, a calcium channel blocker. More than 5% of all prescriptions for hypertension consisted of the relatively new angiotensin II receptor blockers like losartan, candesartan and valsartan. These prescriptions do not match the advice in the guidelines.

Depression

A lack of adherence was found for the 1994 depression guideline (*see* Table 25.3). Only 11.1% of all prescriptions matched the advice in this guideline. In 2003 the guideline was revised. The adherence to this new guideline was much higher than to the 1994 one, although public action took place two years after the data collection. The main difference between the 1994 and 2003 guideline is that tricyclic antidepressants (TCAs) and selective serotonin reuptake inhibitors (SSRIs) were both first-choice products in 2003, while in 1994 TCAs were preferred. Within both groups of medication the 2003 guideline prefers certain specific drugs. For SSRIs these are paroxetine, fluvoxamine and sertraline. The difference in adherence between the 1994 and 2003 guideline is mainly due to the prescription of paroxetine. It was by far the most frequently prescribed drug for depression and accounted for 32.8% of all prescriptions for depression in 2001. Within the group of TCAs, amitryptiline (6.2%) and clomipramine (2.7%) were most frequently prescribed; both TCAs match the advice in the 2003 guideline. The most frequently prescribed non-adherent drugs were fluoxetine and venlafaxine, both responsible for more than 5% of all prescriptions for depression. Also a number of benzodiazepines, like oxazepam, temazepam and diazepam, were prescribed in considerable amounts, respectively 4.8%, 2.4% and 1.4%.

Cystitis

For cystitis the NHG guideline provides different advice for uncomplicated and complicated cystitis. Both trimethoprim and nitrofurantoin are first-choice medication for uncomplicated cystitis. In 2001, trimethoprim accounted for 31.5% of all prescriptions for cystitis; nitrofurantoin for 26.1% (*see* Table 25.3). For complicated cystitis as well as for cystitis in children under the age of 12 years, the guideline advises amoxicillin (combined with clavulanate), or, in cases of hypersensitivity, co-trimoxazole. Together these drugs accounted for 13.3% of all prescriptions for cystitis in 2001. The most frequently prescribed medication which was considered as non-adherent is norfloxacin (6.0%).

What to think about it

In this study, we examined the adherence to three guidelines. More than half of the prescriptions for hypertension were as suggested in the guidelines. Our study, however, does not provide insight into the 'stepwise following' of the guideline. Moreover, it does not distinguish between choices made for patients with and without comorbidity. GPs make different choices, taking the situation of the individual patient into account. A study carried out by van Dijk *et al.* (2004) among 180 Dutch GPs showed that GPs claim to prescribe according to the guidelines for asthma/COPD, coronary heart disease (CHD) and heart failure.[4] However, for diabetes mellitus, most of the GPs stated they were be non-adherent to the guideline. While the first-choice antihypertensive for patients with diabetes mellitus is a diuretic, only 11% of the GPs claim diuretics to be their first choice. Three-quarters (74%) prefer ACE inhibitors, while another 8% have angiotensin II receptor blockers as their first-choice anti-hypertensive for diabetics. These GPs substantiated their choice by stating that ACE inhibitors and angiotensin II receptor blockers better protect the patient's kidneys. The substantial contribution of relatively new classes of drugs, like the not recommended angiotensin II receptor blockers prescribed for hypertension, is also found in the literature. They are prescribed despite the still limited evidence on outcomes.[5]

For depression, little more than 10% of the prescriptions were suggested in the guidelines. A reason for this is that the first depression guideline, published in 1994, was conservative in its pharmacotherapeutic advice and did not include SSRIs that had already been available in 2001 for several years. Considering the 2003 guideline, half of the prescriptions were adherent.

GPs adhere to the depression guidelines for about 10% of the prescriptions.

The reason to look further into the adherence to the depression guideline of 2003 was to discover if the prescription behaviour of the GPs was ahead of the new guideline. This was based on the assumption that the GPs considered the guideline of 1994 as obsolete and therefore changed their prescribing behaviour based on recent literature about new medication. This assumption was confirmed in a study by Volkers *et al.* (2005).[6] From that study it also became clear that GPs prefer SSRIs because they assume these to be more effective or to have fewer adverse effects compared to TCAs. Despite the fact that SSRIs are now also first-choice antidepressants, adherence to the guideline of 2003 is not as high as might have been expected. Two types of frequently prescribed drugs (fluoxetine and venlafaxine), both responsible for more than 5% of all prescriptions for depression, are not recommended in the 2003 guideline. Also the prescription of benzodiazepines, considered as non-adherent, was responsible for at least 10% of all prescriptions for depression.

For cystitis we found the highest degree of adherence: 70%. No distinction was made between uncomplicated and complicated cystitis. Van Dijk *et al.* (2004) found that at practice level, trimethoprim and nitrofurantoin accounted on average for 42.3% of the prescriptions in *first episodes* of cystitis.[7] We found that GPs chose these two drugs in 57.2% of *all prescriptions*. The difference between these two figures can probably be explained by the fact that a patient can have more than one episode of uncomplicated cystitis during a one-year course.

One should be careful to interpret these results in terms of rationality or quality. There are many reasons why GPs would consciously deviate from the guidelines. Recently, for instance, a new approach, called concordance towards suboptimal use of medication has been proposed.[8] Herein, prescribing is seen as a process of shared decision making between the patient and the prescribing doctor. In this interaction process both the patients' and professionals' view and the perception about medication, and the associated harms and benefits are shared and negotiated with the intention of making the patient more compliant. Although concordance might be a satisfying target in the communication between doctor and patient, this new approach might conflict with the adherence to guidelines.

References

1 Barber N (1995) What constitutes good prescribing? *BMJ*. **310**: 923–5.
2 World Health Organization (WHO) (1985) The rational use of drugs and WHO. *Dev Dialogue*. **2**: 1–4.
3 Hutchinson A, McIntosh A, Cox S and Gilbert C (2003) Towards efficient guidelines: how to monitor guideline use in primary care. *Health Technol Assess*. **7 (iii)**: 1–97.
4 van Dijk L, Hermans I, Jansen J and de Bakker D (2004) *Voorschrijven bij Hypertensie in de Huisartspraktijk*. [Prescribing in hypertension in general practice.] NIVEL, Utrecht.
5 Greving JP, Denig P, van der Veen WJ *et al.* (2004) Does comorbidity explain trends in prescribing of newer antihypertensive agents? *J Hypertens*. **22**: 2209–15.
6 Volkers A, de Jong A, de Bakker D and van Dijk L (2005) Doelmatig Voorschrijven van Antidepressiva in de Huisartspraktijk. [Effective prescribing antidepressants in general practice.] NIVEL, Utrecht.
7 van Dijk L, Schiere AM and Braspenning J (2004) Voorschrijven van antibiotica. [Prescribing antibiotics.] In: Braspenning JCC, Schellevis FG and Grol RPTM (eds) *Tweede Nationale Studie naar Ziekten en Verrichtingen in de Huisartspraktijk. Kwaliteit huisartsenzorg belicht*. [Second Dutch National Survey of General Practice. Focus on quality of GP care.] NIVEL/RIVM, Utrecht/Bilthoven, pp. 103–14. *See also* www.NIVEL.nl/ nationalestudie
8 Elwyn G, Edwards A and Britten N (2003) 'Doing prescribing': how might clinicians work differently for better, safer care? *Qual Saf Health Care*. **12** (Suppl 1): i33–i36.

Part 6

International perspective and the future

Chapter 26

Activities of the general practitioner: are they important?

Peter Davis

What is this chapter about?

There is growing international interest in the functioning and performance of health services in the primary care sector. While this in part stems from concerns about the future of the sector in troubled times,[1] it mainly derives from an increasing recognition of the strategic role of primary care in the health systems of the developed world.[2–4] The second Dutch National Survey of General Practice (DNSGP-2) is one of a series of 'monitors' of primary and ambulatory care in a growing number of countries. Traditionally it has been hospital and related services that have drawn the bulk of research and policy attention, with general practice being somewhat neglected. This survey helps to redress the balance.

Introduction

One difficulty with primary care has been that it is still to an extent a 'cottage industry' of small operators without the glamour and financial power of the thriving and medically exciting secondary and tertiary sectors. Primary care has been something of an information 'black box' for decision makers and professional leaders, with only episodic and partial illumination provided by regional and other *ad hoc* data collections.

Primary care is still to an extent a 'cottage industry'.

This picture of relative neglect is now improving. There is much greater interest in understanding the primary healthcare sector. While still in many respects functioning like independent, small businesses, primary care providers are being increasingly acknowledged as of much wider policy significance. With no apparent let-up in the growth of health expenditure, the potential 'gatekeeper' role of general practitioners (GPs) is of great interest.[5] There has also been an increasing assertiveness and strengthening professional identity among providers in this sector.[6]

These developments highlight the importance of DNSGP-2. Firstly, it adds another nationally representative data collection to a growing number available for the United States, the United Kingdom, Australia, and now New Zealand.[7–10] Secondly, it places the spotlight on the crucial role played by GPs and allied health professionals in primary care, a role that is being challenged and tested by a rapidly changing social and professional environment.

General practice in a time of social change

The Dutch model of general practice is similar to that found in a number of other countries such as the UK, Australia and New Zealand, in that it has sought to combine the best aspects of the GP as family doctor with the role of gate-keeper. This pattern of primary care delivery was consolidated and enjoyed its heyday in the period of relative social and economic stability following the Second World War. Yet, many of the conditions that were conducive to this pattern of practice have changed; one set – largely social – has challenged the traditional concept of the family doctor, while another has placed the gate-keeper function at risk. The social conditions for the post-war accommodation were stable nuclear family life, full employment, and relative social homogeneity. This has now altered, with changing patterns of family life (more single parents, more women at work), greater disparities and inequalities, and increasing ethnic diversity. These challenge the stable and established social pattern sustaining the role of the traditional family doctor. Other changes have occurred in the wider health system – greater consumerism, the rise of complementary and alternative medicine, more professionally assertive non-medical colleagues, the scrutiny of the state, greater specialisation, and the overwhelming cultural and financial dominance of the hospital and related services. These challenge the gatekeeper role of the GP.

Combine the best aspects of the GP as family doctor with the role of gatekeeper.

Key challenges to general practice

In most respects the Dutch survey – like others of its kind – is a 'monitor' of primary and ambulatory care, and thus essentially descriptive rather than analytical in emphasis. Yet, a question of crucial policy importance underlies these relatively bland data – what is the future of the 'cottage industry' model of healthcare in an era when the social context is less sympathetic to its aims and functioning, and when corporate and specialist medicine is increasingly dominant in the health system?

General practice today: cross-national comparisons

On the surface, the results on the activities of GPs from the Dutch survey do not bear out these concerns. It appears that the use of general practice services has risen over time and that, overwhelmingly, these services are sufficient to meet most patient needs. But how do the key results compare with findings elsewhere? While it is hard to get directly comparable data across countries, recent national surveys of general practice in Australia and New Zealand give us an opportunity to assess selected characteristics of primary care work.

Table 26.1 provides some key system characteristics for these countries, with data drawn from a recent monograph survey of comparative health policy in selected developed countries.[11] As the data show, these are three gatekeeper systems with a lot in common, but some important differences. On the face of it, these countries evidence distinct financing structures and contrasting societal value systems (as judged by the monograph authors), and yet their patterns of expenditure and demographic ageing are very similar, being close to the Organization for Economic Cooperation and Development (OECD) average. It is noteworthy that New Zealand appears to have greater racial/ethnic diversity (a higher proportion of non-'European' individuals).

There are three core activities of GPs that can be compared across systems – writing a prescription, ordering a test or investigation, and initiating a referral for another service. These are compared in the top panel of Table 26.2. In very approximate terms, about two-thirds of visits to GPs resulted in the writing of a prescription in all three countries, with New Zealand ahead of Australia and the Netherlands.[9,10] This pattern – of New Zealand being rather out on its own – is also evident for the other measures, test orders and referrals. This is where cross-national comparisons run up against differences in data collection. In the case of the Netherlands, the data include telephone consultations as well as home visits. These are excluded in the other two countries. In the case of the Australian data, a low response rate means that perhaps some of the busier practitioners did not take part in the study. In the instance of both these countries, rates of activity may well be lower than New Zealand's on account of these factors. The number of visits a year per patient is within the same range – 5 to 6 – and there is a wide range of similarities in the leading problems addressed by doctors and in the drugs prescribed.

On a generous interpretation of these data, there is a good deal of similarity in the pattern and level of clinical activity across three contrasting GP gatekeeper systems. Yet, without common data collection protocols and procedures, we cannot be sure about the comparability of these results. For example, on each of the clinical activity measures, the Netherlands rests at the lower end of the scale – fewer prescriptions, tests, and referrals – but could these be an arte-

Table 26.1 Characteristics of three 'gatekeeper' systems

	Australia	New Zealand	The Netherlands
Expenditure			
% gross domestic product	8.6	8.1	8.7
% public expenditure	70	77	69
Population			
% aged 65+ years	12.2	11.7	13.6
% Caucasian	92	75	91
System values	Individualist	Egalitarian	Communitarian
Financing healthcare	Mixed public/private	National health system	Social insurance with private elements

Table 26.2 GP activity in three countries

	Australia	New Zealand	The Netherlands
Clinical			
prescriptions (%)	57.5	66.2	57.0
tests (%)	19.7	24.8	13.0
referrals (%)	10.0	15.8	4.0
Number of contacts with general practice per patient per year	5.5[a]	5.3 (estimate)[b]	6.0[c]
Top problems	Respiratory, circulatory in common across all three countries (also musculoskeletal, skin, nervous system)		
Top drugs	Cardiovascular in common across all three countries (also antibiotics, nervous system, respiratory, musculoskeletal, alimentary tract etc)		

[a]Contact during consultation hours.
[b]Contact during consultation hours.
[c]Contact during consultation hours, including telephone contact, home visits and contact with the assistant.

fact of DNSGP-2's methodology? Australia and New Zealand are reliant on conventional practitioner self-completion surveys, while the Netherlands, with its patient enrolment system, has distinct technical advantages in the collection of data and in the estimation of rates. This is something that the two Antipodean countries could fruitfully adopt from the Dutch model.

The Netherlands rests at the lower end of the scale – fewer prescriptions, tests, and referrals.

The changing role of the GP: the New Zealand case

For much of the period since the Second World War, the State in New Zealand has largely suspended any proactive engagement in issues to do with the funding and organisation of primary care.[12] Thus, more recently, the system has been left to evolve some distance from the family doctor-dominated, gatekeeper concept, with the emergence of private accident and medical (A&M) practices, and the important role that hospital emergency departments (EDs) play in ambulatory care, both catering particularly to after-hours care.[13,14]

Are there any insights here about potential challenges to these traditional functions of general practice? In Table 26.3, comparisons are made by demographic group and by diagnostic grouping of presenting problems across urban and rural locations in general practice, and A&M (North Island urban) and ED (largely urban) sites, for patients in the standard working hours of 8 am to 6 pm, Monday to Friday. These data are drawn from a national ambulatory care

Table 26.3 Characteristics of patients and diagnoses by site of care, 8 am to 6 pm, Monday to Friday

	GP urban	GP rural	A&M	ED
No of practices	146	41	12	4
Number of practitioners	197	47	67	–
Number of patients	31 991	8686	590	6484
	logs	logs	visits	visits
Age group (years) (%)				
0–24	31.8	33.3	51.5	34.6
25–64	45.3	44.1	41.0	42.4
65+	22.3	21.8	6.3	23.0
Missing	0.6	0.8	1.2	–
Ethnic group (%)				
NZ European	74.9	75.6	59.7	60.7
Maori	10.1	20.2	11.2	12.4
other	15.0	4.2	29.1	26.9
Number of patients	7315	1957	590	6484
	visits	visits	visits	visits
Number of diagnoses	12 371	3079	707	5914
Diagnosis group (%)				
respiratory	14.5	15.6	20.8	8.6
actions	11.4	11.0	8.5	8.0
cardiovascular/circulatory	9.3	8.7	2.4	12.3
nervous system/sense organs	8.3	7.8	8.1	4.9
injury/poisoning	6.6	9.2	27.3	32.5
symptoms non-specific	3.6	3.0	2.8	8.1
other	46.3	44.7	32.9	25.6

survey, details of which are presented in an appendix to this chapter, together with key definitions.

At this time of day the age distribution of presenting patients is similar across the general practice sites, and hospital EDs. But while about one-third of these patients are aged under 25 years, this same group accounts for half those attending A&M practices. Assessing the ethnic distribution of patients, the two non-GP sites are much more likely to be visited by persons from ethnic affiliations outside the two major ones in New Zealand (European and Maori). On the matter of presenting problem, injury is much more prevalent in the two non-GP sites, along with respiratory problems for A&M, and cardiovascular and non-specific symptoms for EDs. Therefore, even during normal working hours, there are indications of demographic, ethnic and epidemiological differentiation between traditional GP and non-GP sites in the New Zealand setting (although the concentration of A&Ms and EDs in urban North Island sites guarantees a greater ethnic diversity, with proportionately fewer Europeans).

What about after hours? Here we do not have a strictly comparable group in GPs since we do not have information on any cases handled by GPs at this time of the working week, but it can safely be assumed that in most cases they are dependent on deputising and other services. The picture that emerges in Table 26.4 seems to be one accentuating the tendencies evident in Table 26.3. Patients visiting A&Ms are even more youthful – two-thirds are aged under 25 years – and A&Ms and EDs have an even higher proportion of patients who are neither European by heritage or Maori (about one-third). Epidemiologically, this trend continues. Respiratory conditions are even more dominant in A&Ms and injury at EDs, along with injury for the former and cardiovascular and non-specific conditions for the latter.

Conclusion

These results from the New Zealand survey are indicative only, but they do suggest that a system that fails to work actively to shore up the traditional role of the GP will start to erode this function in sociodemographic and epidemio-logical terms, and new sites of care will start to open up to cater for needs that are being underserved. Thus, in New Zealand – at least in the larger urban areas – the young and mobile, more recent immigrant groups, and those with certain acute problems (respiratory, injury) are looking elsewhere for assistance, espe-cially 'after hours'. Similarly, a whole new sector of community-governed practices has emerged to cater for the most socially disadvantaged (ethnic

Table 26.4 Characteristics of patients and diagnoses by site of care, 'after hours' and weekends

	A&M	ED
Number of practices	12	4
Number of practitioners	67	–
Number of patients	840 visits	9171 visits
Age group (years) (%)		
0–24	62.8	43.2
25–64	31.9	41.9
65+	4.4	14.9
missing	0.9	–
Ethnic group (%)		
NZ European	58.0	56.4
Maori	8.0	12.5
other	34.0	31.1
Number of patients	840 visits	9171 visits
Number of diagnoses	963	8319
Diagnosis group (%)		
respiratory	27.9	12.4
injury/poisoning	17.8	31.2
nervous system/sense organs	11.6	4.9
infectious/parasitic	11.0	3.5
symptoms non-specific	3.5	10.4
cardiovascular/circulatory	1.1	9.4
other	27.1	37.2

minority groups, low-income families), although they still only represent about 5% of the sector.[15] These, then, may be harbingers of the shifting social bases for general practice in the rapidly changing circumstances of the urban setting in most western, developed countries.

There is a challenge here to decision makers and professional leaders. If these are trends – even if only incipient – how best to respond if the family doctor concept and the gatekeeper role are to be protected? Or, couched in terms expressed earlier in this chapter, what is the future for a 'cottage industry' of family-oriented health practitioners in social conditions that are less conducive to their work and in an environment dominated by specialist and hospital-focused medicine?[16]

What is the future for a 'cottage industry' of family-oriented health practitioners?

There is evidence that the strength of general practice – as judged by service profiles – is related to its gatekeeping role.[17] Although patients feel ambivalent about some aspects of this gatekeeping function, they appreciate the first-contact and co-ordinating role of primary care doctors, they favour small practices and full-time GPs, and prefer in-person consultation over telephone contact (for after-hours services).[18–20] Therefore, there are indications here for policy makers and professional leaders as to the likely model of primary care practice that will prove to be sustainable over the long term.

Crucial to this work, of course, is the regular availability of accurate, timely and pertinent information of strategic significance to the sector. This is what we have in the DNSGP-2. The survey has certain valuable features. Data are collected on all interactions between the GP and patients (not just face-to-face), and non-medical personnel are included, thus providing a much more rounded picture of primary care than the Australian and New Zealand studies. The survey also provides crucial information on the informal sector of care – people making health and self-care decisions outside the practice setting – and it has a denominator from which to calculate rates. These are great advantages.

Ambulatory and primary care monitors in other countries could well take note of these useful qualities of the data collection system in DNSGP-2. But data collection in this survey may also need to accommodate a range of sites, including hospital EDs and commercial practices, if we are to get a more complete picture of the future of the primary care sector. Only then will we be in the position to ensure that the valuable qualities provided by this sector – continuing, comprehensive, first-contact care in sustained partnership with patients – flourish in the rapidly changing circumstances of the developed welfare democracies.[6]

References

1 Moore G and Showstack J (2003) Primary care medicine in crisis: toward reconstruction and renewal. *Ann Intern Med*. **138**: 244–7.
2 Faulkner A, Mills N, Bainton D *et al.* (2003) A systematic review of the effect of primary care-based service innovations on quality and patterns of referral to specialist secondary care. *Br J Gen Pract*. **53**: 878–84.

3 Salisbury C and Munro J (2003) Walk-in centres in primary care: a review of the international literature. *Br J Gen Pract.* **53**: 53–9.

4 Powell J (2002) Systematic review of outreach clinics in primary care in the UK. *J Health Serv Res Policy.* **7**: 177–83.

5 Dixon J, Holland P and Mays N (1998) Developing primary care: gatekeeping, commissioning and managed care. *BMJ.* **317**: 125–8.

6 Sox HC (2003) The future of primary care. *Ann Intern Med.* **138**: 230–1.

7 Schappert S (1996) *National Ambulatory Medical Care Survey 1994.* National Center for Health Statistics, Hyattsville, MD.

8 McCormick A (1995) *Morbidity Statistics from General Practice: fourth annual study 1991–92.* HMSO, London.

9 Britt H, Miller G, Knox S *et al.* (2002) *General Practice Activity in Australia 2001–02.* General Practice Series, number 10. Australian Institute of Health and Welfare, Canberra.

10 Raymont A, Lay-Yee R, Davis P and Scott A (2004) *Family Doctors: methodology and description of the activity of private GPs.* The National Primary Medical Care Survey (NatMedCa), Report 1. Ministry of Health, Wellington.

11 Blank RH and Burau V (2004) *Comparative Health Policy.* Palgrave, New York.

12 Crampton P (2000) Policies for general practice. In: Davis P and Ashton T (eds) *Health and Public Policy in New Zealand.* Oxford University Press, Auckland. pp. 201–18.

13 Hider PH, Lay-Yee R and Davis P (2005) *The Work of Doctors in Accident and Medical Clinics.* The National Primary Medical Care Survey NatMedCa Report 5. Ministry of Health, Wellington.

14 Raymont A, von Randow M, Patrick D, Lay-Yee R and Davis P (2005) *Ambulatory Care in Hospital Emergency Departments.* The National Primary Medical Care Survey NatmedCa Report 8. Ministry of Health, Wellington.

15 Crampton P, Lay-Yee R and Davis P (2004) *Primary Health Care in Community-Governed Non-profits: the work of doctors and nurses.* The National Primary Medical Care Survey (NatMedCa), Report 2. Ministry of Health, Wellington.

16 Forrest C (2003) Primary care gatekeeping and referrals: effective filter or failed experiment. *BMJ.* **326**: 692–5.

17 Boerma WG, van der Zee J and Fleming DM (1997) Service profiles of general practitioners in Europe. European GP Task Profile Study. *Br J Gen Pract.* **47**: 481–6.

18 Grumbach K, Selby JV, Damberg C *et al.* (1999) Resolving the gatekeeper conundrum: what patients value in primary care and referrals to specialists. *J Am Med Assoc.* **282**: 261–6.

19 Wensing M, Vedsted P, Kersnik J *et al.* (2002) Patient satisfaction with availability of general practice. An international comparison. *Int J Qual Health Care.* **14**: 111–18.

20 Leibowitz R, Day S and Dunt D. (2003) A systematic review of the effect of different models of after-hours primary medical care services on clinical outcomes, medical workload, and patient and GP satisfaction. *Fam Pract.* **20**: 311–17.

Appendix

The National Primary Medical Care Survey was undertaken in 2001–2002 to describe primary healthcare in New Zealand, including the characteristics of providers and their practices, the patients they see, the problems presented, and the management offered.[14] The study covered private general practices (i.e. family doctors), community-governed organisations, Maori providers, accident and medical (A&M) clinics and hospital emergency departments (EDs).

A nationally representative, multistage probability sample of private GPs, stratified by place and practice type, was drawn. Each participating GP kept a log of all patients seen and reported in detail on a 25% sample in each of two week-long periods separated by an interval of six months. Over the same period, all community-governed practices in New Zealand were invited to participate, as were a 50% random sample of all A&M clinics, and four representative hospital EDs. Maori providers were identified during the course of sampling private GPs and community-governed practices. Similar data collection methods were used for all practice types, though A&M practitioners reported on their patients for one week only, with participants spread over the year. Routinely collected data were obtained on all attendances at four EDs for one week each quarter in 2001.

The distributions from the 1996 Census are shown for age, sex and ethnicity for different sections of the New Zealand population. In general, age and sex distributions are similar across Auckland, other cities, and rural areas and small towns. The ethnic distribution varies, however. In Auckland, Europeans are under-represented, and 'other' ethnic groups over-represented, in comparison with the overall New Zealand totals (*see* Table 26.5).

Table 26.5 Population comparison (1996 Census)

	New Zealand	Auckland cities	Hamilton, Wellington, Christchurch, Dunedin cities	Total rural and towns sampled	Total rural and towns not sampled	Total sampled
Total population	3 618 306	927 774	872 463	1 150 425	667 644	2 950 662
Males (%)	49	49	49	50	49	49
Females (%)	51	51	51	50	51	51
Age (years) (%)						
under 5	8	8	7	8	8	8
5–19	23	22	21	23	23	22
20–64	58	60	60	56	56	58
over 64	12	10	12	13	13	11
Ethnic group (%)						
European	72	60	77	76	73	71
Maori	14	12	10	17	20	13
other	14	28	13	7	7	15

In this paper, GPs (n = 244) include those from 167 private, 6 community-governed and 14 Maori provider practices. Data were contributed by 199 private GPs who logged 36 211 visits and provided detailed information on 8258 of them; 24 community-governed GPs with 2088 logs and 463 detailed visits; and 21 Maori provider GPs with 2378 logs and 551 detailed visits. In the case of A&M clinics, data were collected at 12 sites (8 in Auckland) by 67 medical practitioners who logged 6205 visits and provided detailed information on 1430 of them. Data on 15 655 contacts were collated from routine, administrative sources at four public hospital EDs (two in the North Island, two in the South Island; three in cities, one in a provincial town).

The following definitions were used:

- *community-governed organisations* had a community board of governance, and no equity ownership or profit distribution for GPs
- *Maori provider practices* had to be independent, target Maori patients, and have a Maori management and governance structure
- *accident and medical (A&M) clinics* have X-ray equipment on site, are staffed by non-specialist medical practitioners and nurses, and provide extended-hours primary healthcare cover, allowing access without an appointment
- *emergency departments (EDs)* are operated at public hospitals in large towns.

Chapter 27

Health status of the elderly in the future: demography, epidemiology and prevention

Nancy Hoeymans and Anneke van den Berg Jeths

What is this chapter about?

People get older. In fact, more people than ever before get older. An ageing population has all kind of consequences, not the least regarding healthcare requirements. In this chapter, we focus on the health status of future generations of elderly people and the role of prevention in healthcare. We expect that, if disease trends of the past 10 years continue, the number of elderly people with a disease will increase enormously. However, a powerful and effective prevention policy can partly diminish this increase in chronic diseases in the elderly.

How healthy will we be in the future?

No matter how insecure the health status of the future generation of the elderly is, it will certainly be characterised by rising life expectancy and ageing of the group of people from the post-war baby boom. We start by describing the most important demographic developments, and their influence on the occurrence of chronic diseases in the elderly. On top of the demographic developments, epidemiological trends in chronic diseases influence future health status. Observed trends in diseases in the past are used to predict diseases in the future, the so-called 'epidemiological trend projection'. The direction of these trends can be changed through preventive and medical-technological developments. We will estimate the health effects of prevention concerning two risk factors, i.e. smoking and overweight.

The number of elderly people with a chronic disease will increase enormously in the years ahead.

How was it done?

Health of the elderly

The elderly are defined as people aged 65 years and over. Health is focused on chronic diseases: the prevalence of diseases and disorders is defined as the number of individuals who have a particular disease in one year. Prevalence data were derived from the second Dutch National Survey of General Practice (DNSGP-2) combined with various sets of other primary care records. These concerned, amongst others, the Nijmegen Continuous Morbidity Registration and the Registration Network for Primary Care practices in Limburg, maintained by the University of Limburg, Maastricht. Disease-specific registries, for example the national cancer registry, have also been used. For an overview of the sources for each disease, see the Dutch National Compass on Public Health.[1] For the current study, the diseases are grouped into 10 disease clusters according to the clusters used in the Social and Cultural Planning Office (SCP) model (*see* Table 27.1). The SCP used these clusters in its model that estimates the future use of care facilities for the elderly.[2] This information about the health status and determinants of health in the current generation of elderly people, as well as information on the demand for and use of healthcare facilities, such as home care, homes for the elderly and nursing homes, can be found elsewhere.[3]

Demographic and epidemiological projections

Projections of future numbers of patients are made until 2020. The effects of growth of the elderly population are presented for the 10 selected clusters of diseases. In this demographic projection the prevalence rates of diseases (per 1000 persons by sex and five-year age groups) are kept constant. The expected future numbers of elderly people by age and sex are based on the forecasts made by Statistics Netherlands. These future numbers of elderly people are influenced by hypotheses on future mortality, birth and migration patterns. The hypothesis on mortality patterns results in an increasing life expectancy at birth. For men, life expectancy will rise from 75.5 years in 2000 to 78.0 years in 2020. For women, life expectancy will increase from 80.6 years in 2000 to 81.1 years in 2020. The difference in life expectancy between men and women will then decrease from 5.1 to about 3 years.[4]

Table 27.1 Defined disease clusters and selected diseases

Disease cluster	Diseases
Cancer	Oesophagus, stomach, colorectal, lung, skin, breast, prostate, non-Hodgkin lymphomas
Diabetes mellitus	Diabetes mellitus
Mental diseases	Depression, anxiety, schizophrenia
Diseases of the nervous system	Parkinson's disease, epilepsy, multiple sclerosis
Stroke	Stroke
Heart disease	Myocardial infarction, angina pectoris, heart failure
Lung disease	COPD, asthma
Diseases of the musculoskeletal system	Arthrosis of hip and/or knee, rheumatoid arthritis, dorsopathies
Serious injury	Accident with permanent disability
Dementia	Dementia

For the ten disease clusters we have also performed an epidemiological trend projection. This projection is based on the epidemiological trend of individual diseases in the period 1990–2000. For each disease cluster, the most important diseases were selected (*see* Table 27.1). An epidemiological trend is a significant increase or decrease of the prevalence rate of a disease, irrespective of changes in size or distribution by age and sex of the population as projected in the former step. We performed linear regression analyses that were based on the prevalence of diseases in the Nijmegen Continuous Morbidity Registration, the national cancer registry and the national registration for injuries. In these registries diseases are registered yearly in a similar way. From the trends per disease, we have calculated a 'summary' trend for each cluster based on the relative contribution of the disease to the cluster. These trends of 1990–2000 were then projected to 2020 in a straight line.

Prevention of smoking and overweight

The effects of two theoretical reductions in risk factors were calculated, both based on eliminating socio-economic differences in lifestyle. The first effect assumed that the percentage of elderly smokers will be as low in the whole population of elderly people as it is now for the highly educated elderly. The second effect assumed the same for the percentage of elderly people with normal body weight. The information on socio-economic differences came, among other sources, from DNSGP-2. For smoking, the effects on the prevalence of seven related diseases were calculated: lung cancer, cancer of the oesophagus, myocardial infarction, angina pectoris, heart failure, stroke, and chronic obstructive pulmonary disease (COPD). Nine diseases are related to overweight: colorectal cancer, breast cancer, prostate cancer, diabetes mellitus, myocardial infarction, angina pectoris, heart failure, stroke, and osteoarthritis.

These calculations were based on the Chronic Disease Model.[5] In this model, the Dutch population was distributed over sex- and age-specific classes of the various risk factors, for example, smoker, non-smoker, ex-smoker, and diseases. The model contained age- and sex-specific relative risks for each combination of risk factor and related disease. These relative risks came from literature reviews. The Chronic Disease Model calculated the effects of lower rates of smoking and overweight on the prevalence of the related diseases, taking postponement of diseases into account.

What was found?

Demographic developments

The total number of elderly people is expected to rise from almost 2.2 million in 2000 to more than 3.2 million in 2020 (49% increase). This is due to an increase in life expectancy, but mainly because of the ageing of people from the post-war baby boom.

The increase is much greater in men (68%) than in women (35%). The reason is that life expectancy of men will increase more than that of women.

Nevertheless, in absolute terms, the Netherlands will still have more elderly women than men.

The number of elderly people in 2020 will be two-thirds higher for men and one-third for women.

Because of this rise in the total number of elderly people, we also expect a rise in the number of elderly people with a chronic disease (*see* Table 27.2). This rise varied from 39% (dementia) to 52% (diseases of the nervous system).

Epidemiological projections: how ill will we be?

Many diseases showed an increasing epidemiological trend in 10 years (1990–2000) after demographic adjustments. Adjusted for age and sex, there was a significant rise in the number of patients with diabetes mellitus, stroke, heart disease, lung disease, diseases of the musculoskeletal system and injuries. Diseases of the nervous system decreased. No significant changes were observed for total cancer incidence. For mental diseases and dementia, reliable trends in prevalence were lacking.

The strong increase in diabetes mellitus was partly due to the unfavourable trend in overweight. Furthermore, the recognition of the disease in primary care has improved. The observed increase in prevalence of stroke and heart disease was the result of an increase in stroke and myocardial infarction in women and heart failure in men. These increases were partly caused by an increasing trend in smoking behaviour in women, and improvements in the quality of healthcare, resulting in higher survival rates of myocardial infarctions

Table 27.2 Four different projections for the number of patients (×1000) in 2020 compared to 2000 (between brackets, the percentage increase)

	2000	2020 Demographic projection	Epidemi-ological projection[a]	Prevention: smoking[a]	Prevention: overweight[a]
Cancer	91	137 (51)	137 (51)[b]	134 (47)	136 (49)
Diabetes mellitus	211	312 (48)	386 (83)	–	272 (29)
Mental diseases	200	288 (44)	288 (44)[c]	–	–
Diseases of the nervous system	45	69 (52)	51 (13)	–	–
Stroke	127	188 (47)	217 (71)	182 (43)	185 (46)
Heart disease	301	447 (49)	497 (65)	439 (46)	431 (43)
Lung disease	268	397 (48)	515 (92)	381 (42)	
Diseases of the musculoskeletal system	911	1311 (44)	1331 (46)	–	1281 (41)
Serious injury	62	88 (42)	107 (73)	–	–
Dementia	203	281 (39)	281 (39)[c]	–	–

[a]Epidemiological trend and prevention projections include demographic changes.
[b]No significant epidemiological trend.
[c]Epidemiological trend unknown.

and stroke. The increase in the prevalence of lung diseases was the result of rising asthma prevalence, which increased because of higher rates of allergies and better recognition in primary care. The increase in the cluster of diseases of the musculoskeletal system was the product of two trends: osteo-arthritis increased, and dorsopathies decreased. It is not easy to tell why these trends occur. There is a negative influence of the unfavourable trend in overweight and a positive influence of decreasing rates of people with occupational hazards. No significant changes in total cancer incidence are observed in the period 1983–1998, resulting from diverging trends in specific cancers. The incidence of lung cancer, for example, increased in women and decreased in men. The trend for mental diseases is unknown. In primary care, the prevalence increased, but it is unclear to what extent this is caused by better recognition of symptoms by both patients and physicians. Other data sources show no trend. The decrease in the prevalence of diseases of the nervous system is caused by a decrease in Parkinson's disease. This decrease is difficult to explain. Possibly it is related to the death of the first generation of patients treated with dopatherapy. This therapy led to postponement of death. No changes were observed in the incidence of Parkinson's disease. Finally, the prevalence of dementia did not change significantly in 10 years, as recorded in primary care registrations. However, this trend is not very reliable, because dementia is not always registered in primary care registrations.

The number of patients with diabetes and lung diseases will be doubled in 2020.

These observed epidemiological trends in disease clusters are projected to 2020. Table 27.2 shows the number of patients based on the epidemiological trend, including the demographic changes. Diabetes and lung diseases show the largest increase: 83% and 92% respectively.

What about prevention? The case of smoking and overweight

If the smoking rates decreased and were as low for the total population of elderly people as they are today for the more highly educated elderly, the prevalence of a large number of diseases would decrease (*see* Table 27.2). In 2020, compared to the demographic projection, there would be 3000 fewer patients with cancer (mainly lung cancer, but also cancer of the oesophagus), 8000 fewer with heart disease (myocardial infarction and angina pectoris), 6000 fewer with stroke and 16 000 fewer with lung disease (COPD and asthma).

If socio-economic differences in overweight disappeared, the prevalence of diabetes would decrease by as much as 40 000 patients in 2020 compared to the demographic projection (*see* Table 27.2). This means that prevention can flatten the expected demographic and epidemiological increase in diabetes (*see* Figure 27.1). Furthermore, in 2020, we would have 30 000 fewer patients with diseases of the musculoskeletal system, 16 000 fewer with heart disease, 3000 fewer with stroke, and the prevalence of cancer (breast cancer and colorectal cancer) would decrease by 1000 patients.

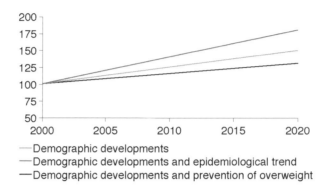

Figure 27.1 Three different projections for the future number of diabetes patients aged 65 years and over. Trends are shown starting from a baseline of 100 in 2000.

Conclusion

The number of elderly people will increase in the future. And, if disease trends of the past 10 years continue, the number of elderly with a disease will increase even more. However, a powerful and effective prevention policy can partly diminish this increase in chronic diseases in the elderly.

What to think about it

The validity and reliability of these results are largely based on the appropriateness of the methods used. The demographic projection seems reliable. Birth rates play no role, since all elderly people of 2020 are already born in 2000; mortality trends are reasonably reliable, and migration is not an important factor in the demography of the elderly population. The reliability of the epidemiological projection depends on the reliability of the estimations of the past trends *and* on the appropriateness of projecting these trends into the future. Even if a past trend is reliable, temporary effects can make it unlikely that this trend will continue for the coming 20 years. Diabetes, for example, has increased rapidly, (partly) because of a better detection of cases. It is unlikely that this increase will continue at the same rate.

The future elderly are more highly educated and for that reason might have a healthier lifestyle.

The assumed reductions in the prevalence of risk factors are hypothetical and theoretical situations. We chose these rates of smoking and overweight, because they are already attained in the highest socio-economic groups, and are thus theoretically also attainable in other groups. We do not think that socio-economic differences will disappear entirely. However, it is not certain whether these rates will drop as much as we have assumed in our projections. In the past decade, smoking rates have been more or less stable, and the percentage of overweight elderly people has increased. On the other hand, because of the increasing educational levels of tomorrow's elderly, it is to be expected that the rates of smoking and overweight will decrease. This is, of course, based on the assumption that smoking and overweight will remain stable within educational levels.

In this chapter, we have only quantified two possible reductions in risk factors. However, many more preventive activities exist, for example the prevention of hip fractures, primary prevention through medication, and vaccination. Primary prevention through medication is already common practice for different risk factors, for example blood pressure and blood cholesterol, although more health gains are still possible. A possible new development is the combination of different medications to tackle different risk factors simultaneously. An example is the so-called 'polypill', which will reduce four cardiovascular risk factors at the same time: low-density lipoprotein cholesterol, blood pressure, serum homocysteine, and platelet function.[6] The formulation of this pill is a statin, three blood pressure-lowering drugs, folic acid, and aspirin. The researchers have estimated that this combination reduces events of ischaemic heart disease by 88% and stroke by 80%. One-third of people taking this pill from the age of 55 years would benefit, gaining on average about 11 years of life free from ischaemic heart disease or stroke. We did not quantify this prevention strategy in our analyses, because the effects and safety still have to be confirmed in other follow-up studies.

The introduction of the 'polypill' might make a huge difference to life expectancy.

These effects of prevention, but also healthcare developments, point to a further postponement of mortality. The hypothesis that the life expectancy will rise to 78.1 years for men and 81.1 years for women in 2020 could possibly be too 'conservative'. The possibilities of prevention and healthcare are still increasing, causing a further increase in healthy life expectancy, and, probably, a further delay of death.

Concluding, prevention is not only important at young and middle age, but is still important at old age.[7] To improve the health status of the current as well as future generations of elderly people, promoting a healthy lifestyle remains essential. Investing in existing prevention strategies, like the campaigns against overweight, and reinforcing prevention within healthcare is important. General practice can play an important role in this task.[8]

References

1 www.nationaalkompas.nl (in Dutch) (accessed 20 September 2005).

2 Timmermans J and Woittiez I (2004) Verpleging en verzorging verklaard. (Nursing and care explained). Hagg: *Sociaal en Cultureel Planbureau*. Den Haag.

3 van den Berg Jeths A, Timmermans JM, Hoeymans N and Woittiez IB (2004) *Ouderen nu en in de Toekomst. Gezondheid, verpleging en verzorging 2000–2020*. [Elderly now and in the future. Health and care 2000–2020] Bohn Stafleu Van Loghum, Houten.

4 de Jong A (2003) Bevolkingsprognose 2002–2050: veronderstellingen. [Population prognosis 2002–2050] In: *Bevolkingstrends* [Population trends]. **51**(1): 27–33.

5 van Genugten M, Hoogeveen R and de Hollander A (2001) Incorporating risk factor epidemiology in mortality projections. In: Tabeau E, van den Berg Jeths A and Heathcote C (2001) *Forecasting Mortality in Developed Countries. Insights from a statistical, demographic and epidemiological perspective.* Kluwer Academic Publishers, Dordrecht/Boston/London, pp.189–204.

6 Wald NJ and Law MR (2003) A strategy to reduce cardiovascular disease by more than 80%. *BMJ.* **326**: 1419–24.

7 van Oers JAM (ed) (2003) *Health on Course? The 2002 Dutch Public Health Status and forecasts report.* Bohn Stafleu Van Loghum, Houten.

8 Jones R, Schellevis FG and Westert GP (2004) The changing face of primary care: the second Dutch National Survey. *Fam Pract.* **21**: 597–8.

Chapter 28

The need for general practitioners in the Netherlands until 2020: an exploration of demographic and epidemiological changes in general practice

Johan Polder, Ronald Gijsen, Nancy Hoeymans, René Poos and Henriëtte Treurniet

What is this chapter about?

Healthcare needs of people living at home will increase in the next decades, due to an ageing population and expected epidemiological changes. In this paper, we present demographic and epidemiological projections for general practice in the near future. We estimate by what percentage the number of general practitioners (GPs) must increase in the period 2005–2020 to meet the increasing demand for primary care. We have used data from the second Dutch National Survey of General Practice (DNSGP-2 Netherlands Institute for Health Services Research (NIVEL)) and the 2002 Dutch Public Health Status and Forecasts Report (National Institute for Public Health and the Environment (RIVM)), in combination with population forecasts of Statistics Netherlands. We conclude that the number of GPs must increase by 4.1–6.3% in 2005–2010, while in the period until 2020 an increase of 13.0–20.1% is needed.

These demographic and epidemiological developments together with other changes in demand and supply will confront the Dutch government as well as the whole primary care sector with important questions about the sustainability of general practice in the future. In further research, in addition to this paper, we will explore policy options of enlarging the number of positions in the education of GPs, task delegation and task shifting, triage systems and new models of co-operation, such as walk-in centres and integrated primary care institutions. In our final report, published early in 2005, we sketch an integrated picture of all primary care disciplines.[1]

The need for care and for doctors

In the Netherlands, care from GPs increasingly attracts a lot of attention. This development is not out of the blue. Since the 1970s, primary care has been a spearhead of Dutch health policy. A strong and coherent primary care sector with the GP as gatekeeper for medical specialists and advanced health provision was seen as a foundation for a successful and cost-effective healthcare system. Measures were taken to give primary care more coherence and to facilitate the development of the different disciplines. In later years, the attention shifted towards education and professionalisation, for instance by the development and introduction of guidelines.

In spite of all the attention and measures, rather than increasing, the bottlenecks in primary care decreased. The intended coherence among the different disciplines was at best partially realised. The dissatisfaction about workload, work stress and remuneration grew stronger and stronger. Understaffing appeared a serious and persistent problem, especially in general practice because more and more physicians preferred a part-time job. There is a general feeling that capacity problems cause trouble with the access, continuity and quality of primary care, at least in certain areas.

In the recent past, many experiments started trying to manage these bottlenecks. Triage systems were developed and implemented, by physicians themselves as well as by some leading health insurance companies. A report on task shifting in healthcare by the Council for Public Health and Health Care fuelled the debate about task delegation and new organisational structures in primary care.[2] In 2004, the government proposed to drop the requirement that patients who visit a physical therapist need a referral from the GP. For occupational physicians the government created possibilities to refer employees directly to medical specialists, without the obligation to consult a GP, as before.

Meanwhile, the Dutch government, realising that primary care is facing increasing demands and expectations, started a trajectory to develop a new political view on primary care.[3] The Ministry of Health commissioned RIVM and NIVEL to set up a study on the most promising organisational changes to match diverging trends in demand and supply of primary care. DNSGP-2 plays an important role in this study.[4]

In this paper we focus on a part of this study, namely the need for physicians in primary care. Our objective is twofold: (1) to describe healthcare consumption in general practice from the perspective of the health status of the Dutch population and trends in incidence or prevalence of major diseases; and (2) to anticipate the number of GPs needed in 2010 and 2020 to take care of increasing health demands resulting from expected demographic and epidemiological developments.

How was it done?

The description of health status in the Netherlands is based on the 2002 Dutch Public Health Status and Forecasts Report of the RIVM,[5] while DNSGP-2 provided the data for the description of healthcare use.[4] The former study and its underlying 1990–2000 data from recent health surveys and registries of general practice were also used to calculate about 50 major diseases trends in prevalence or incidence using linear regression techniques.

We have made a demographic projection of the number of GPs needed in 2010 and 2020. In such a projection, the effects of changes in the number of inhabitants and the age structure of the population are calculated. Ageing is the most important demographic phenomenon for primary care in the next decades, since the post-war baby-boom cohorts will reach the age of increasing morbidity and health demands. For this projection, we have used the 2002 population forecasts from Statistics Netherlands,[6] in combination with the results from DNSGP-2.

Demographic projections are based on the 'business as usual' assumption that healthcare consumption per inhabitant in each age–sex category remains constant. It is obvious, however, that healthcare needs will change due to epidemiological developments. Therefore, we have also made epidemiological projections based on the above-mentioned trends, assuming that the provided care per patient in each disease–age–sex category will remain constant. The trend figures were age standardised and clustered in major disease categories (*see* Table 28.1). For this study, we assumed that all statistically significant trends will continue in the next decades with doubling as a fixed maximum. For the non-selected diseases we made a distinction between two variants: in the A variant, incidence and prevalence are assumed to remain constant; in variant B we hypothesised that incidence and prevalence follow the average pattern of the selected diseases in the same cluster.

What was found?

Actual health status

The Dutch population lives, on average, in good health.[5] Since 1980, male life expectancy has increased by 3.1 years while female life expectancy has grown by 1.4 years. In 2000, the Dutch could expect an average life span from birth of 75.5 and 80.6 years respectively for men and women. The years that have been added over the last decade are generally spent in good health. Statistics Netherlands predicts that life expectancy will increase even more over the next 20 years. Around the year 2000, both men and women experienced roughly the same number of healthy years: 61 years are spent in self-perceived good health, more than 70 without disabilities, and 68 in good mental health. Consequently, the number of subsequent unhealthy years is considerably higher for women than for men, about 5 years. Considering that neither the incidence nor the duration of chronic disorders has decreased, certain healthcare provisions, such as medical devices and pharmaceuticals, seem to have effectively improved the social participation of the chronically ill.[7]

Information about the diseases and disorders that underlie the unhealthy years comes from different sources, varying from questionnaires and epidemiological population surveys to morbidity registers. Among the self-reported diseases malaise complaints such as fatigue, tiredness and headache were most frequently mentioned, followed by upper respiratory infections (*see* Table 28.1). Hypertension, migraine and mental problems were also very common, with a self-reported prevalence in 2001 varying from 9.7% to 20.9%.

Morbidity figures from general practice show a quite different picture. Infectious diseases and hypertension were in 2001 the most commonly registered diagnoses in general practice, followed by mental and social problems (*see*

Table 28.1 Occurrence of major diseases in the population[a] and in general practice (% of the population by disease cluster and specific diseases per year)

Disease cluster/specific disease	Prevalence or incidence (%)	
	Self-reported	Visiting GP
Infectious diseases (incidence)		
upper respiratory infections	41.6[b]	9.3
otitis	2.1[b]	4.0
Chronic somatic diseases (prevalence)		
migraine	15.0	1.1
hypertension	9.7	6.4
Musculoskeletal diseases (prevalence)		
peripheral arthrosis	8.8	1.3
Injuries (incidence)		
contusion, bruising	2.3	0.6
Other somatic complaints (prevalence)		
tired	42.4[c]	2.5
headache	32.8[c]	1.5
Mental and social problems (prevalence)		
sleeping disorders	20.9[c]	2.4
depression	10.3[d]	2.6

[a]Diseases that are most frequently reported in health surveys among the general population.
[b]Self-reported infectious disease in the past 2 months, population of 12 years and older.
[c]Self-reported health problems in the past 2 weeks, population of 4 years and older.
[d]Self-reported depressive symptoms for at least 2 weeks in the past year, population of 12 years and older.
Source: Van Oers (2002); Westert (2005).[4,5]

Table 28.1). The prevalence in general practice of nearly all diseases is much lower than self-reported in health surveys. This is known as the 'iceberg phenomenon', meaning that in healthcare only a small proportion of total morbidity is visible. The less severe the disease is, the less the patient is inclined to visit a physician. For a lot of diseases people do not need a physician or other types of care at all.

Epidemiological trends

The future health status and healthcare needs also depend on epidemiological developments. Looking back over the last decade it is quite clear that the dynamics in population health cannot be solely explained by demographic change. Table 28.2 shows age-standardised trends in prevalence or incidence of some major diseases between 1990 and 2000.[5] The incidence of some infectious diseases has declined substantially. The incidence of some major cancers has also decreased. For instance, the incidence and mortality of stomach cancer have been declining for several decades. This is probably connected with the

Table 28.2 Major trends in incidence or prevalence of some diseases in 1990–2000 (age- and sex-standardised change)

Disease cluster/specific disease	Incidence (I)/prevalence (P)	Change in %		
		Men	Women	Total
Infectious diseases				
infectious intestinal disease	I	−50	ns	
Meningitis				−42
AIDS	I			−63
upper respiratory infections	I	−42	−32	
cystitis	I	ns	37	
Chronic somatic diseases				
stomach cancer	I	−32	−33	
colorectal cancer	I	14	ns	
lung cancer	I	−24	54	
melanoma	I	22	50	
prostate cancer	I	60	–	
diabetes mellitus	P	71	ns	
Parkinson's disease	P	ns	−60	
glaucoma	P	91	169	
coronary heart disease	P	ns	73	
heart failure	P	35	ns	
stroke	P	ns	39	
asthma	P	140	177	
COPD	P	ns	41	
congenital anomalies of the heart and circulatory system	P			−44
Musculoskeletal diseases				
rheumatoid arthritis	P	70	ns	
dorsopathies	P	−18	ns	
osteoporosis	P	ns	118	
Injuries				
sport injuries	I			−16
road and traffic accidents	I	ns	13	
home and leisure accidents	I			17
violence	I			56
Other somatic problems				
inflammatory bowel diseases	P	ns	−87	
cataract	P	96	96	
Mental/social problems				
depression	P	142	283	
anxiety disorders	P	ns	++	

ns: not significant; ++: very strong increase.
Source: van Oers (2002).[5]

replacement of pickling as a means of preserving food in favour of refrigeration in the second half of the 20th century, in view of the fact that the previously high salt intake would have increased the chance of stomach cancer. Moreover, *Helicobacter pylori*, a bacterium that is involved in the development of stomach cancer, is becoming less common.

Among men the incidence and mortality of lung cancer are decreasing rapidly, as a result of the fact that men are smoking less. This decline in mortality started in the early 1980s. For women the opposite is true: because increasing numbers of women smoke, the incidence of lung cancer is sharply increasing. For other cancers such as melanoma, colorectal cancer and prostate cancer incidence has also increased.

The sharp increase in diabetes mellitus is at least partly attributable to an increased alertness to symptoms on the part of GPs and patients themselves. The increase of obesity, however, must also be mentioned here. There has been a decrease in the number of hospital admissions for diabetes mellitus, however. Apparently, complications associated with diabetes mellitus occur less often or are treated in primary healthcare and outpatient clinics.

Partly because of decreasing mortality, the prevalence of most diseases of the circulatory system has increased. Among the other chronic somatic diseases the prevalence of asthma and, to a smaller extent, chronic obstructive pulmonary disease (COPD) has increased, while there was a visible decline in the number of children being born with a congenital abnormality of the cardiovascular system. Among the musculoskeletal diseases, opposite trends were shown for rheumatoid arthritis and osteoporosis, which showed increasing prevalence among men and women respectively, and dorsopathies that have decreased among men.

Certain diseases appear to show a trend, while in reality the increase or decrease must be attributed to changes in diagnostics and demand for care. Anxiety disorders and depression, which are common and sometimes major disorders, have been recorded more frequently by GPs in recent years. It is unlikely that any 'real' increase (trend) is involved here. Other factors, the relevance of which is beyond doubt, are the improved ability of GPs to recognise the disorders, the enhanced therapeutic possibilities and the introduction of standards. Furthermore, there are indications that people with minor mental problems are increasingly inclined to visit professional caregivers.

Actual healthcare use

On average, people visit the GP 4.6 times per year, referrals and prescriptions excluded. The frequency increases with age, from an average of 3.1 visits among children to 8.7 visits for people of age 75 years and older.

The reasons for visiting the GPs were most frequently associated with chronic somatic diseases, followed by somatic complaints and infectious diseases (*see* Table 28.3). Musculoskeletal diseases rank fourth. An important phenomenon here is that not all people with complaints seek professional help. For example, the number of GP visits relating to mental and social problems is low compared to the number of complaints in the population. Another, opposite, explanation is the use of professional care in mental health institutions by some of the patients. Similarly, the availability of emergency care units and midwives can explain the relatively low contact frequency for injuries and childbirth in general practice. Finally, the time that GPs spend on screening and prevention is also very limited.

Table 28.3 Workload of GPs by disease category (share of disease clusters in total number of contacts in %)

Disease cluster	2001
Infectious diseases	16.1
Chronic somatic diseases	19.2
Musculoskeletal diseases	12.8
Injuries	3.6
Other somatic complaints	17.3
Other somatic diseases	10.4
Mental and social problems	7.3
Fertility, pregnancy and childbirth	3.3
Screening and prevention	2.1
Unknown	8.0
Total	100.0

Source: Westert *et al.* (2005).[4]

Need for GPs: demographic projection

In the next decades, ageing will cause the most important demographic change. The proportion of people aged 65 years and older will increase from 13.6% in 2002 to 14.8% in 2010 and about 20% in 2020. Given the age pattern in healthcare consumption, the demand for primary care will increase, additional to the effects of population growth. In a simple demographic projection, the required number of GPs for care will increase by 3.4% from 2005 to 2010, and by 10.6% in the period 2005–2020 (*see* Table 28.4), all other things remaining unchanged. Because chronic somatic diseases are most prevalent among elderly people, ageing will cause the largest increase within this cluster, and, similarly, in the clusters of other somatic diseases, musculoskeletal diseases and screening and prevention. The decreasing needs in the cluster of fertility, pregnancy and childbirth result from the expected decline in birth rates.

Need for GPs: epidemiological projections

In our epidemiological projection we assumed that the significant linear trends in the past will continue in the future. We have distinguished two variants: in the A variant incidence and prevalence are assumed to remain constant; in variant B we hypothesised that incidence and prevalence follow the average pattern of the selected diseases in the same cluster. According to variant A, the total number of GPs has to increase by 0.7% in the period 2005–2010 and 2.1% in 2005–2020, assuming that all other things remain constant (*see* Table 28.4). In variant B the growth rate is anticipated at 2.9% and 8.6%, respectively. The need for mental and social problems will show the highest increase, followed by care for chronic and other somatic diseases. The demand for care due to infectious diseases and musculoskeletal diseases will decline.

Table 28.4 Projected need for GPs in 2010 and 2020 (increase in number of GPs in % compared to 2005 by demographic change and epidemiological trends in two variants)

Disease cluster	2010 Demo	Epi A	Epi B	Total A	Total B	2020 Demo	Epi A	Epi B	Total A	Total B
Infectious diseases	1.5	−1.6	−3.6	−0.2	−2.1	5.1	−4.9	−10.7	0.0	−6.1
Chronic somatic diseases	6.1	3.4	7.0	9.7	13.5	19.2	10.2	20.9	31.4	44.1
Musculoskeletal diseases	3.5	−1.2	−3.0	2.3	0.4	9.6	−3.6	−9.0	5.7	−0.3
Injuries	2.0			2.0	2.0	5.6			5.6	5.6
Other somatic complaints	3.0			3.0	3.0	9.2			9.2	9.2
Other somatic diseases	4.1	0.3	11.1	4.4	15.7	12.1	0.9	33.4	13.1	49.5
Mental and social problems	3.0	5.7	17.3	8.9	20.8	8.7	17.2	51.9	27.4	65.2
Fertility, pregnancy and childbirth	−1.8			−1.8	−1.8	−0.7			−0.7	−0.7
Screening and prevention	4.1			4.1	4.1	14.1			14.1	14.1
Unknown	3.1			3.1	3.1	10.8			10.8	10.8
Total	3.4	0.7	2.9	4.1	6.3	10.6	2.1	8.6	13.0	20.1

Demo: demographic projection; Epi: epidemiological projection.
Variants:
A = trends were only calculated for diseases selected in the Dutch Public Health Forecasts Report
B = average trends of selected diseases within each cluster were also applied to diseases within that cluster about which no trend information was available.

Demographic and epidemiological projections combined

Combined with demographic change, total need for GP care will increase by 4.1–6.3% in the period 2005–2010, and by 13.0–20.1% in the period 2005–2020. Given the workload of GPs (*see* Table 28.3), the need for care of chronic and other somatic diseases will show the highest increase in absolute terms.

What to think about it

According to our projections the number of GPs must increase in the next 15 years by 10.6% for demographic changes and by 13.0–20.1% for the combination of demography and epidemiology. Because ageing mainly results from the post-war baby-boom, which implies that all these people are already living now, the demographic projection is more certain than the epidemiological projections, which show a wide range.

All projections, however, are based on some major assumptions. First, we assumed that trends from the past will continue in the future. For some diseases this hypothesis will be valid, but for others the trends might change, for instance as a result of changing (un)healthy behaviour in the population. Second, we have seen that some trends were unclear due to external factors such as changes in remuneration system and detection rates. Infectious diseases and mental disorders must be mentioned here. Third, we had no information about trends in help-seeking behaviour. There are indications, however, that for some diseases people are more or less inclined to visit GPs more often than in the past.[4] Diabetes could be a good example of a disease with a rather high detection rate which confuses the real trend in prevalence. Fourth, we assumed 'business as usual'. It is likely, however, that the provision of healthcare will also change. Nurse practitioners, for instance, can take over part of the care for chronically ill patients from the GPs. The importance of this task delegation will increase if the number of physicians does not match the projected need.

General practice has to deal with increasing demands from the chronically ill and patients with somatic diseases. Also, the need for primary psychiatric care will increase. If the number of GPs increases less than the estimated need, organisational changes like task delegation can be required to match supply and demand.

All these demographic, epidemiological and other developments confront the Dutch government, as well as the whole primary care sector, with important questions about future sustainability of general practice. Many policy options need to be explored to tackle future problems in care delivery, e.g. increasing the number of places in the education of GPs, task delegation and task shifting, triage systems and new models of co-operation, such as walk-in centres and integrated primary care institutions.

In the next chapter, the future development of the supply side will be described and contrasted with the expected need for care predicted in this chapter.

References

1 de Bakker DH, Polder JJ, Sluijs EM et al. (2005) *Op één lijn. Toekomstverkenning eerstelijnszorg 2020.* [Public health forecast for primary care in the Netherlands in 2020.] RIVM, Bilthoven/NIVEL, Utrecht.

2 Raad voor de Volksgezondheid en Zorg (RVZ) (2003) *Taakherschikking in de Gezondheidszorg.* [Council for Public Health Care: Task re-arrangement in health care.] RVZ, Zoetermeer.

3 Ministerie van Volksgezondheid, Welzijn en Sport (VWS) (2003) *De toekomstbestendige Eerstelijnszorg (brief met kenmerk: CZ/EZ-2431353).* [Ministry of Health: Future sustainability of primary health care (letter with reference number: CZ/EZ-2431353).] VWS, Den Haag.

4 Westert GP, Schellevis FG, de Bakker DH *et al.* (2005) Monitoring health inequalities through General Practice: the Second Dutch National Survey of General Practice. *Eur J Public Health.* **15**: 59–65.

5 van Oers JAM (ed) (2002) *Health on Course? The 2002 Dutch Public Health Status and Forecasts Report.* Report No: 270551002. RIVM, Bohn Stafleu Van Loghum, Bilthoven, Houten.

6 de Jong A (2003) Bevolkingsprognose 2002–2050: anderhalf miljoen inwoners erbij. [Population prognosis 2002–2005: one and a half million extra inhabitants.] *CBS Bevolkingstrends.* **51**: 21–6.

7 van den Berg Jeths A, Timmermans JM, Hoeymans N and Woittiez IB (2004) *Ouderen nu en in de Toekomst – Gezondheid, verpleging en verzorging 2000–2020.* [Elderly people now and in future – Health, nursing and caring 2000–2020.] RIVM, SCP, Bohn Stafleu Van Loghum, Bilthoven, Houten.

Chapter 29

The supply of general practitioners in the Netherlands

Lud van der Velden and Lammert Hingstman

What is this chapter about?

In the previous chapter, Polder *et al.* give a description of the developments in the need for general practitioner (GP) care in the Netherlands. To complement this need-analysis, we will give a description of the supply developments that can be expected. In order to make a supply prognosis, we will also look into the developments in the supply of the past decade. Therefore, we will answer the following research questions:

- how has the supply of GPs developed in the last decade and how will this supply develop up to the year 2020?
- to what extent will there be a shortage or a surplus of GPs in 2010 and 2020, if the demand for GP care develops according to the demographic and epidemiological projections made in the previous chapter?

Manpower policy for GPs in the Netherlands

The Netherlands has a relatively low number of GPs. According to the Organization for Economic Cooperation and Development (OECD) Health Data, the population to GP ratio in the Netherlands is about 2000:1. This ratio can also be found in Ireland and Portugal. In most other European countries, the ratio is lower: 1667 in Great Britain, 1111 in Italy, 909 in Germany and 625 in France. One of the reasons of the relatively low number of GPs in the Netherlands is that the manpower planning policy for GPs was always directed at limiting the total number of GPs in order to limit the costs of GP care.

The population to GP ratio in the Netherlands is about 2000:1.

Healthcare manpower policy in the Netherlands is characterised by a highly fragmented structure. Many organisations play a part in it and a complicating factor is that the organisations involved in planning are not the same as those involved in financing the educational system.[1] However, a more centralised planning organisation for the training capacity of the medical professions was established in 1999 on the initiative of the Ministry of Health. This so-called Capacity Body is an advisory committee on the training capacity for all officially recognised medical and dental specialities. The Capacity Body consists of representatives of professional organisations, training institutes and health insurance companies.[2–4]

How was it done?

The supply analysis and prognosis are partly based on empirical data and partly on estimates from the Capacity Body. The supply of GP care is measured through the total number of full-time equivalents (fte) GPs. Data on the number of active GPs and the number of fte GPs are drawn from the register of professionally active GPs from NIVEL.[5] Every year, data are published on the total number of GPs, their characteristics and the geographical dispersion of GPs in the Netherlands. Based on the sex- and age-specific outflow rates of the past, a prognosis for the development of the number of male and female GPs is made. Multiplied by the mean number of ftes per man and woman, this also gives a prognosis for the total number of fte GPs.

What was found?

Developments in the supply of GPs are mainly the result of inflow and outflow. These will be dealt with in the next two sections. In the third section the total supply of GPs (head count and fte count) will be described. Finally, the supply development will be compared to the need development.

Inflow

The inflow of new GPs is mainly the result of the inflow in GP training. The inflow in GP training has risen from less than 300 per year in the early 1990s, to about 350 per year at the end of the 1990s (*see* Figure 29.1). In 2000 the Capacity Body advised to enlarge the intake. From then on the intake has risen to 500 in the year 2003. The proportion of women in GP training has risen from 41% in 1990 to 68% in 2003.

The number of women in GP training has risen from 41% in 1990 to 68% in 2003.

For the future, we assumed the input in GP training to remain constant at 500 per year, with 68% women. Although the inflow could rise a little bit further, the training capacity of the training institutes is already at its maximum. The percentage of women will probably not rise any more, because the percentage of women studying medicine is not increasing any more.

The training period for GPs was two years until 1993, and three years from 1994 onwards. An intake of 500 in GP training will not lead to 500 GPs three year later, since not all trainees will succeed. Moreover, not all who succeed will actually start working in general practice, and not all who start working will continue working as a GP for their whole career. In the prognosis for the future supply, we have not only taken into account the dropout during training (approximately 5% for both men and women) and the dropout immediately

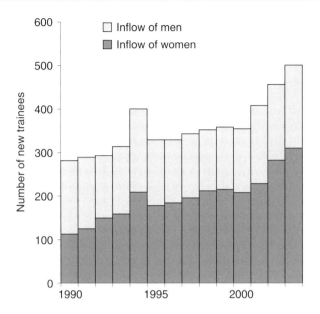

Figure 29.1 Developments in the inflow in GP training. Source: NIVEL.[5]

after training (also 5% for both men and women), but also a 1% outflow rate per year after certification for men and a 2% outflow rate per year for women. These percentages are assessed on the basis of inflow and outflow figures of the past decade for newly trained GPs.

Beside an inflow of new GPs from the Dutch GP training, there is also an inflow from abroad. The main inflow from abroad is from Belgium. These are Dutch students that could not participate in the Dutch GP training but who could participate in the Belgium GP training and then returned to the Netherlands. In total, there were about 50 GPs per year that came from abroad. With the extra number of trainees in the Netherlands, we can already see that the inflow from abroad is decreasing. Nowadays, 35 GPs per year are coming from abroad. This is also the number that we have accounted for in the future.

Outflow

We have also investigated the outflow of already active GPs in more detail. The number of GPs leaving practice varied in 1990 to 2004 between 200 and 300 per year (*see* Figure 29.2).

As mentioned previously, there are different outflow rates for men and women. Of all male GPs aged 50 years, about 20% have already left practice (*see* Figure 29.3). For women this is 33%. So, the outflow of GPs is certainly not restricted to outflow for pensioning. In fact, almost no GP continues working until the official pensioning age of 65 years. Almost 60% of all men and 80% of all women have already ceased working as a GP at the age of 60 years. Most GPs who stop working as a GP at an early age, start working as a physician in another specialty (e.g. nursing home care). Most GPs who stop working around the age of 60 years, retire from work.

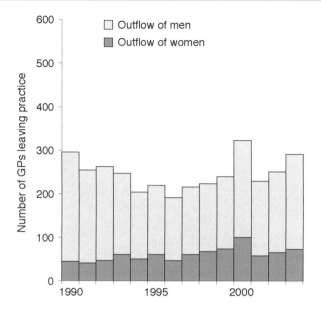

Figure 29.2 Developments in the outflow of GPs. Source: NIVEL.[5]

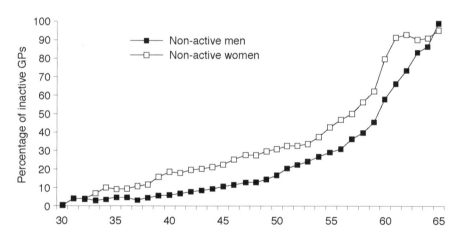

Figure 29.3 Percentage of GPs not actively working as GP, by age and sex. Source: NIVEL.[5]

We made a prognosis of the outflow by relating the age and sex composition of the current GP population with the age- and gender-specific outflow rates. In this way, we calculated the future outflow, which will rise from some 300 to more than 450 per year. Although the outflow rates for women are proportionally higher than for men, the men in the outflow will outnumber the women, in absolute numbers.

Size of the active GP population: 'stock'

The number of GPs has risen from 7147 in the year 1990 to 8495 in the year 2003 (*see* Figure 29.4). At the beginning of the year 2005, there will probably

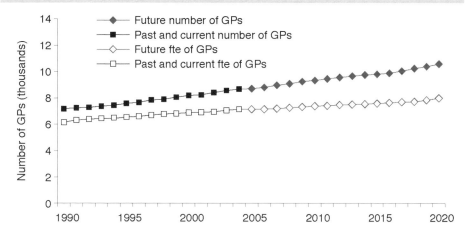

Figure 29.4 Developments in the supply of GP care: head count and fte count. Source: NIVEL.[5]

be 8687 GPs. This amounts to a 22% increase in 15 years' time. Maintaining the current inflow and outflow, the number of GPs will grow further to 9287 in the year 2010 and 10 465 in the year 2020. For the period 2005–2010, this will be a 7% increase in 5 years. For 2005–2020 it is a 20% increase in 15 years.

While the number of GPs increased by 22%, the total number of fte GPs increased by only 13% in 1990–2005. The difference between the development in the head count and fte count can also be seen for the future. Although the number of GPs will grow by 20% in the next 15 years, the number of fte GPs will grow by 12%.

The number of GPs will grow further to 9287 in the year 2010 and 10 465 in the year 2020.

The difference in growth rate for the head count and fte count is due to the fact that the number of women will rise more sharply than the number of men. The percentage of women in the GP population will rise from 30% nowadays to 56% in the year 2020 (*see* Figure 29.5). In 1990, the number of women was 15%. From a male-dominated group, the GPs will turn into an evenly mixed group within the next 10 years. This will have an effect on the number of part-time GPs. For 2015 we assessed each man for 0.91 fte and each woman for 0.63 fte. This is equal to the current situation.[5]

Supply and demand

According to the demographic and epidemiological projections from Polder *et al.* (*see* Chapter 28), the need for GP care will rise by 4–6% in the period 2005–2010. The supply analysis shows that the amount of GP care that will be available will rise by 4%. Therefore, in 2010, we will get about the same equilibrium as in 2005 or a 2% shortage. For 2020, Polder *et al.* expect a 13– 20% higher need compared to 2005, and the supply will be 12% higher. This can be translated into a 1–8% shortage.

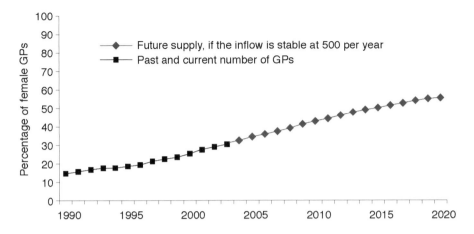

Figure 29.5 Developments in the percentage of female GPs. Source: NIVEL.[5]

What to think about it

For the developments in the demand, Polder *et al.* made a projection on the basis of demographic and epidemiological developments (*see* Chapter 28). Their need analysis did not include any unfulfilled demand. The Capacity Body, however, predicts that there is a 5% unfulfilled demand. The Capacity Body also assumes that other factors apart form demographic and epidemiological developments will influence the future demand for GP care. For instance, it is hypothesised that social and cultural developments will lead to a higher demand for care in the future and, furthermore, that some of the care that nowadays is delivered by medical specialists, should be met by GPs in future. In the analyses that we have made for the Capacity Body, this resulted in a higher shortage for the coming years compared to the analysis we made in this article.

The second question that one could raise is: if the analysis is correct, what could we do to prevent a shortage? Prevention of the occurrence of shortages could involve both reducing the use of care and extending the supply of care. Measures were already being proposed regarding reducing care use, i.e. by introducing a contribution of the patient to the GP via the so-called no-claim refunds. Such measures are meant to make patients more aware of their use of care and limit unnecessary use of GP care.

Apart from reducing care use, solutions for the shortages in capacity could be found in feasible measures to extend the supply of GP care. The simplest solution would be to raise the intake in GP training institutes. However, the problem is that training institutes have already reached their maximum intake. Traineeships for GPs in training are hard to find. Reducing the outflow of GPs by introducing a special policy on senior GPs is another frequently mentioned measure. For example, GPs of certain age could be exempted from nightshifts or weekend shifts. This would make it more interesting for older GPs to continue working. On the other hand, research has shown that a special policy on senior GPs has only limited effects and the costs are high.[6] This is due to the fact that exemption from shifts for older GPs creates the need for many substitute GPs.

Organising the practice more efficiently could be another option to extend GP care supply. Data from the second Dutch National Survey of General Practice (DNSGP-2) show that, over the last 10 years, GPs have managed to do more in less time.[7] Organisational characteristics of these GP practices are: practice visits are replaced by contacts by phone, fewer home visits, visits on appointment solely, evening night and weekend shifts are organised differently via central GP co-operatives and, lastly, delegation of tasks, in particular to practice assistants. GPs have already delegated many tasks to the assistants in the past few years. The total amount of assistance turns out to affect the work-load of GPs positively. Also, the option to delegate tasks to assistants has not been used to the full, as research has shown. GPs delegate their tasks not only to assistants but also to assistants at higher education level, like nurse practitioners. The nurse practitioners, however, apparently only lighten the burden of the GPs in a limited way: they rather improve the quality of care in general.

Practice management can be made more efficient, which could lead to more capacity within the practice by measures such as outsourcing the supporting facilities (administration, ICT, purchase, management) and by ICT and automation improvements. The opportunities offered by the electronic prescription system and electronic medical records are worth mentioning in this context.

In conclusion we can say that to solve the present shortage of GPs a further increase of the intake in GP training is difficult because of the limitation of the training institutes. Thus, to find a solution, measures are necessary to reduce the use of care on the one hand, and organisational changes in GP practice are needed to treat more patients in less time on the other hand.

References

1 van der Velden LFJ and Hingstman Groenewegen PP (1999) Verkenning van vraag en aanbodontwikkelingen binnen medische en paramedische zorg: knelpunten en oplossingen. [Identification of developments in offer and demand in medical and paramedical care: bottlenecks and solutions.] In: *RVZ. Achtergrondstudies bij het Zorgaanbod in de Toekomst.* [RVZ. Background studies concerning future offer in care.] Den Haag/Zoetermeer, Den Haag.

2 Capaciteitsorgaan (2001) *Capaciteitsplan 2001 voor de Vervolgopleidingen van de Medisch Specialisten.* [Capacity Body. Capacity Plan 2001 for follow-up training of medical specialists.] Capaciteitsorgaan, Utrecht.

3 van der Velden LFJ and Hingstman L (2001) *Vraag en Aanbod Huisartsen: Bronnenoverzicht en raming 2000–2010.* [Sources outline and estimates 2000–2010.] NIVEL, Utrecht.

4 Leliefeld HJ and Holland PCHM (2002) Toekomstig evenwicht, de cijfers van het Capaciteitsorgaan. [Future equilibrium, figures of the Capacity Body.] *Medisch Contact.* **57:** 660–2.

5 NIVEL (1980–2004). *NIVEL Registratie van Huisartsen.* [NIVEL GP registration.] NIVEL, Utrecht.

6 de Jong J, van den Berg M, Brouwer W and Heiligers PH (2004) *Effecten van Seniorenbeleid voor Huisartsen.* [Effects of policy on senior GPs.] NIVEL, Utrecht.

7 van den Berg MJ, Kolthof ED, de Bakker DH and van der Zee J (2004) *De Werkbelasting van de huisarts.* (Tweede Nationale Studie naar Ziekten en Verrichtingen in de Huisartspraktijk). [GPs'workload. (Second Dutch National Survey of General Practice).] NIVEL, Utrecht. *See also* www.NIVEL.nl/nationalestudie

Chapter 30

Collecting information in general practice: 'just by pressing a single button'?

Robert Verheij and Jouke van der Zee

What is this chapter about?

What did we have to do to get the data for the second Dutch National Survey of General Practice (DNSGP-2)? Will all this be necessary for a possible third survey as well? Can policy information be derived from raw electronic medical records, just by pressing a single button? These questions will be addressed below, resulting in recipes for acquiring and using data from general practices for research purposes. We start with a brief history.

A brief history of Dutch national surveys

DNSGP-2 has its roots in the Netherlands Information Network of General Practice (LINH), which, in turn, has its roots in the first DNSGP (*see* Figure 30.1). Before the first DNSGP (1987/1988) little was known about what was going on in general practice, with the exception of data on how many people were referred to secondary care. Given the fact that, as we know now, more than 95% of the health problems presented in general practice are dealt with by the general practitioner (GP) himself, this lack of information was considered an undesirable situation.

DNSGP-1

The first DNSGP was inspired by the National Morbidity Surveys in England and Wales.[1,2] For DNSGP-1 data on referrals, contact diagnoses, episodes of illness and socio-economic characteristics were collected. A population census was conducted among the total practice populations, extensive health interview surveys were carried out among a sample of patients, GP questionnaires were sent and even video observations were made. Except for the video observations, data were collected using paper and pencil.[3]

For a number of years, the first DNSGP provided enough information for policy and research. It served as a basis for 18 PhD theses, many scientific publications, and numerous policy documents.

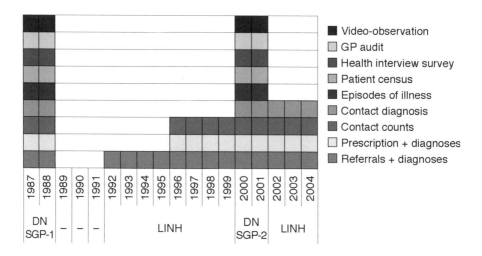

Figure 30.1 The history of LINH and the Dutch National Surveys on General Practice (DNSGP).

The birth of LINH

PhD students can continue studying old data for quite a long time. Policy makers, on the other hand, are always in need of the most recent data. Already in the early 1990s, the Dutch Ministry of Health felt a need to monitor referrals from general practice to specialist medical care. By that time, personal computers had entered general practice and many GPs had started recording patient data in their computers. It went without saying that these data could be used for monitoring purposes: the Netherlands Information Network of General Practice (LINH) was born (*see* Box 30.1).[4] At first, only referral data were collected, including the indications for the referral. By the mid-1990s the rising costs of drugs made monitoring of prescriptions necessary. Later on, data on prescriptions, as well as on numbers of consultations in LINH were collected as well (*see* Figure 30.1). It is important to note that these data about delivered care are routinely recorded, primarily for use by the GP practice itself.

DNSGP-2

In the meantime, NIVEL and National Institute for Public Health and the Environment (RIVM) had started lobbying for a second national survey to be financed by the Dutch Ministry of Health. The plan was to use the data that were already collected in LINH as a basis. This basis would have to be extended substantially to collect the same dataset as in the first national survey: video observations, GP audits, health interview surveys, patient census and information on episodes of illness. The big difference between the first and the second survey was the fact that everything was recorded electronically.

> **Box 30.1 Features of Netherlands Information Network of General Practice (LINH)**
>
> ---
>
> - Joint project of NIVEL, the Centre for Quality of Care Research (WOK), the National Association of GPs (LHV) and the Dutch College of GPs (NHG)
> - Data collection since 1992
> - 80–100 practices (varies by year)
> - 350 000 patients
> - Deals with 5 different GP software packages (situation in 2004)
> - Comprehensive recording of morbidity, referrals and prescriptions
> - Diagnoses coded with International Classification of Primary Care (ICPC)
> - Individual patient linkage
> - Extraction of data every 6 months
>
> Source Verheij *et al.* (2005).[4]

LINH after the DNSGP-2

Not only did the second national survey benefit from LINH, but it was also the other way around. The DNSGP-2 created the opportunity to start collecting morbidity data (contact diagnoses) on a routine basis. For LINH this meant the transition from a network recording interventions with the associated morbidity into a network recording morbidity with the associated interventions. Since 2001, all diagnoses in all patient contacts, referrals and prescriptions are recorded on a routine basis.

In sum, LINH nowadays collects data on morbidity, prescription and referrals, each of these with the associated diagnosis code, and all these data can be linked to individual patients and thereby to each other, opening the possibility to study comorbidity, comedication, and time series at the individual level. It is, in short, a permanent mini-national survey, based on data that are routinely recorded in general practice.

What is required to collect useful data in general practice? The ingredients and the cooking utensils

The history outlined above makes clear that there is a distinction between the routinely collected data on contacts, prescriptions and referrals on the one hand, and the data that are collected only once in a while, e.g. health interview surveys, census data, on the other hand. Because LINH collects data routinely, we focus on the prerequisites for routine data collection.

Preventing sloppy and incomplete recording

A number of factors may cause sloppy and incomplete recording. The GP or the assistant may be too busy to record properly. In particular, telephone encounters, home visits and repeat prescriptions may suffer from this. Frequent computer failure may be another factor inhibiting reliable recording routines. GPs and assistants are stimulated and motivated in different ways. Training is provided on a regular basis. GPs receive an annual feedback report on the morbidity presented in their practice, the number of contacts, referrals and prescriptions. And last but not least, practices are paid 1500 euro (2004) per full-time GP equivalent (fte).

Necessity of good coding systems

Analysing free text is very impractical where large datasets are involved. Therefore, a classification system and accompanying thesaurus is indispensable for morbidity recording. GPs of LINH and of both DNSGPs use the International Classification of Primary Care (ICPC). In the Netherlands, the ICPC is the standard for coding morbidity in general practice. It is included in all electronic patient record (EPR)-based morbidity recording systems. It has been developed especially for general practice and leaves room to record properly in situations where a real diagnosis can not yet be made: symptom/complaints coding as opposed to diagnoses. A disadvantage is the limited linkage possibilities with Dutch International Classification of Disease (ICD)-coded hospital databases.

Episodes of illness

A third problem of using routinely collected computer data, especially for public health purposes, is the necessity of grouping patient contacts into episodes of illness. Episodes are important for the calculation of disease incidences and prevalences. This is a major problem as most GP software is still contact based, not episode based.

In the DNSGP-2, this problem was tackled by deploying medical students as 'episode constructors', who grouped patient contacts into episodes of illness. This was necessary in spite of the fact that GPs (or assistants) were asked to electronically indicate whether the problem was new or existing.

Software-associated obstacles

Software-associated obstacles make it difficult to obtain data that are representative. There are seven different software systems for 4600 general practices in the Netherlands. None of these seven really has the economic strength to make large investments. Also, their flexibility in adding complementary tools to their systems is very limited.

Unfortunately, a number of outcome parameters vary systematically between the software systems. Choosing only one of these systems would negatively affect the network's representativeness. Therefore, it was necessary for the DNSGP-2 (and LINH) to include as many of the seven software packages as possible. The DNSGP-2 managed to include the five largest. All additional software that was developed for the DNSGP-2 had to be tested for each of the five GP software systems.

Identifying a proper denominator

The problem of identifying a good denominator represents a fifth possible limitation to using routinely recorded data from general practice. Indeed, we need to have at least some idea of the size and composition of the practice population to relate prescriptions, referrals and other outcomes to. In the Netherlands, however, this is only a minor problem, since there are (more or less) fixed patient lists.

Non-routine data

LINH collects routinely recorded data. Obtaining the non-routinely collected dataset of the DNSGP-2 was not as easy as it might seem. Questions arise about what data to collect, how to collect them and on how many people. For example: how do you measure people's socio-economic position; do you want that information from all people or would a sample be enough? And once these questions have been answered and translated in measurement instruments, the data actually have to be collected!

What else is needed?

The problems and their solutions outlined above give an impression of the prerequisites for collecting useful data in the GP practices themselves. In terms of recipes, these were just the ingredients and the utensils. This, of course, is not the whole story: we need cooks as well. In order to get reliable data in a research database, data have to be transported from the practices to a central database, and their quality has to be checked continuously.

During the DNSGP-2 period, extraction software was sent to the practices every three months; in LINH this is every six months. In an accompanying letter, practices are asked to retrieve the data from their systems and send it to the LINH organisation by email or on floppy disks by ordinary mail. The quality of the data is subsequently checked on a number of key variables and stored in a central database.

Logistic assistants and ICT experts monitor this whole process closely. The logistic assistants are the intermediates between the practices and the database. They keep in close contact with the GPs and stimulate them to continue recording meticulously. They send the extraction software to the practices, receive the data and perform a first quality check. To improve the quality of the data, regular feedback on data quality is sent to the participating practices.

The ICT experts are responsible for keeping the extraction software up to date. All software has to be compatible with each of the five GP software systems. But it is perhaps even more important to make sure that it *keeps* working. Extraction software, for example, has to be tested for every update of each of the GP software systems.

Putting usefulness into practice: what are the data used for?

Once the data are in the central database they will have to be used. This requires an experienced team of researchers who are aware of the pitfalls that are inevitably associated with the use of these data.

The results of the DNSGP-2 have been published in a number of reports describing the key results (for an excerpt, *see* this book). The number of additional studies has grown to more than 100 in 2004. DNSGP-2 data are often used for secondary analyses. Also, for a limited number of projects, the study population of the DNSGP-2 was used as sampling frame for follow-up studies, e.g. on the time course of dermatological infections in children, and of musculoskeletal symptoms of the upper and lower extremities.[5, 6]

Furthermore, the routinely recorded data that are collected in the DNSGP-2's successor LINH are used to publish annual reports on morbidity, contacts, prescriptions and referrals (*see* www.linh.nl, also in English[4]). This information is used in many policy documents. This is facilitated by the fact that the outcomes are presented graphically as well as in a tabular form. LINH data are used for a large and growing number of studies using either the LINH methodology, or the LINH data themselves (*see* Box 30.2).

Box 30.2 Examples of research projects with data from the Netherlands Information Network of General Practice (LINH)

- *Monitoring health effects of a firework disaster.* On 13 May 2000, the city of Enschede was struck by a massive explosion in a firework depot. It made 400 households homeless. LINH data show that more than 2 years later, the health effects are still noticeable.
- *Off-label prescribing.* Not all drugs are prescribed exclusively for the health problems they are intended for. LINH data show the extent to which off-label prescribing actually takes place in general practice.
- *Monitoring influenza vaccination campaign.* During the influenza season, Dutch citizens are invited by their GP for influenza vaccination. Coverage and effectiveness of this campaign are evaluated yearly using LINH data. About 75% of the target population is covered by the vaccination scheme.
- *Evaluation of electronic prescribing system (EVS).* During the late 1990s, EVS was introduced in the Netherlands. LINH provided reference data for the evaluation. The results of the study show that the introduction of EVS enhanced the quality of prescribing behaviour, but did not result in cost reduction.

Looking into the future

Particularly in recent years, the role and position of GP care within the healthcare system is changing. On the one hand, this makes it even more necessary to monitor the activities of the GP. On the other hand, some of the recent developments affect the representativeness of the data that are collected in general practice.

An example of this are the 'call centres' that have been introduced in some regions. These call centres take over part of the gatekeeping role of the GP. More specifically, these call centres act as a first filter, deciding which patients with which health problems should consult the doctor, and which not. Furthermore, co-operativess for out-of-hours services are now operational in many areas. Practice nurses, nurse practitioners, and physician assistants are introduced in some practices; occupational health services have been allowed to refer to secondary care since 1 January 2004; and physiotherapy will soon be accessible without referral. These phenomena have one thing in common: tasks that traditionally belong to the GP are increasingly taken over by other professionals. This will cause part of the DNSGP-2 data to become rapidly outdated. It is therefore very important for the DNSGP's successor LINH, to adapt to these changes.

Another challenge is to further develop the possibilities that are already there. One of these is the possibility to start monitoring public health. As was indicated above, after the DNSGP-2, LINH was transformed from a system recording interventions to a system recording morbidity. This creates the possibility to start monitoring public health developments on a yearly basis as well as the surveillance of infectious diseases on a weekly basis.

The third national survey: a matter of pressing a button?

The above has shown that many problems associated with collecting and using routinely recorded data have to be overcome for a national survey. Increased use of computers in general practice will probably increase the possibilities of routinely recorded data, but it is unlikely that it will become much easier to get sensible results from these data.

Other problems and possibilities are associated with obtaining the enormous set of non-routinely recorded data through video registrations, population censuses, and health interview surveys. It is not wise to include all this in the routinely collected dataset. It would, first of all, increase the workload of general practices beyond imagination. Second, it would seriously limit the possibilities of adapting the information collected to the political and scientific interests and needs of that time.

In other words, creating a system as comprehensive as the DNSGP-2, with which it is possible to generate policy information by pressing a single button, is not only impossible, it is also unwise.

References

1 Office for Population Censuses and Surveys (1974) *Morbidity Statistics from General Practice. Second National Study 1970–71.* Her Majesty's Stationery Office, London.

2 van der Zee J (1982) *De Vraag naar de Diensten van de Huisarts* [dissertation]. [The demand for GP services.] NHI, Utrecht.

3 van der Velden J (1999) *General Practice at Work. Its contribution to epidemiology and health policy* [dissertation]. Erasmus Universiteit, Rotterdam.

4 Verheij RA, Jabaaij L, Abrahamse H *et al.* (2005) *Landelijk Informatienetwerk Huisartsenzorg. Feiten en cijfers over huisartsenzorg in Nederland.* [Netherlands Information Network of General Practice. Facts and figures on GP care in the Netherlands.] LINH, Utrecht. Available from www.linh.nl (accessed 21 September 2005).

5 Koning S, Mohammedamin RSA, Wouden JC *et al.* Impetigo: incidence and treatment in general practice in 1987 and 2001. Results from two national surveys. *Br J Dermatol* (accepted for publication).

6 Bot SD, van der Waal JM, Terwee CB *et al.* (2005) Incidence and prevalence of complaints of the neck and upper extremity in general practice. *Ann Rheum Dis.* **64**: 118–23.

Chapter 31

The future of data collection in general practice in Belgium

Viviane van Casteren

What is this chapter about?

This chapter illustrates that, despite some obstacles related to the organisation of healthcare, valuable initiatives in collecting data in general practice exist in Belgium. Electronic patient record (EPR)-based data collection, however, has only just started and still has a long way to go before we can speak of a nation-wide network with a considerable number of GPs routinely gathering reliable EPR-based information on health problems and associated interventions. Recent findings and developments outlined in this paper might offer prospects in this direction.

Background

Policy makers and researchers all over the world are looking for ways to gather information on morbidity data for public health monitoring and commissioning. General practitioners (GPs) possess a wealth of information on the health of their patients, and general practice computer databases are increasingly appreciated as a potential rich source of data.[1] But how can these data be extracted? The Dutch National Survey on General Practice (DNSGP) is a marvellous example of what you can do with these data. The researchers faced a number of problems, but most of these could be solved. Although Belgium borders the Netherlands, the situation in Belgium is totally different. A nation-wide network of practices participating in a comprehensive EPR-based recording of not only morbidity, but also associated interventions, does not exist in Belgium at the moment. This paper highlights the experiences with the prospects of morbidity recording as well as other types of data collection in general practice in Belgium.

GPs possess a wealth of information on the health of their patients, and general practice computer databases are increasingly appreciated as a potential rich source of data.

Challenges in Belgium

EPR-based data collection and especially morbidity recording in general practice in Belgium is confronted with some basic obstacles. Some are related to the organisation of healthcare, others to the situation regarding electronic patient records (EPR):

- direct access to specialists
- no fixed patient lists per GP (denominator problem)
- the problem of data capture during home visits
- a wide variety of EPR-based software (over 20 packages)
- a moderate coverage of EPR use in general practice (about 60–65%).

These aspects complicate data sampling. New findings and developments, however, might help to overcome these obstacles in the end.

Direct access to specialists: GPs' place in the Belgian healthcare system

Belgian GPs have no gatekeeper function: medical specialists are freely accessible. Nevertheless, the Health Interview Survey (HIS) in 2001 showed that GPs have a key role in the healthcare system.[2,3] Ninety-four per cent of the Belgian population said they have a fixed GP, 80% have at least one encounter per year, with a mean number of 6.5 encounters per patient per year. The survey also revealed that there are no important barriers for the use of the GP. These figures illustrate that it is worthwhile collecting health information on the general population through the GP.

No fixed patients lists per GP: the global medical record in general practice and the Intermutualistic Agency (IMA)

A fixed patient list per GP facilitates the assessment of the denominator for calculating incidence and prevalence data. In Belgium, traditionally GPs did not have fixed patient lists. But times are changing. Since May 2002, the federal public health authorities encourage the whole population to designate one particular GP as the one responsible for their medical record, which is called the global medical record (GMR).[4] The GMR emphasises the role of the GP as the one who keeps a record of all health-related information of one patient. This does not mean that a patient can only consult that GP, but it means that the information should be recorded by the GP responsible for the GMR. An incentive is foreseen for both the patient and the GP. The patient financially contributes less to the consultation and the GP receives a financial stimulus each time he starts a new GMR. In spring 2004, the federal public health authorities launched a national campaign on the GMR, 'The global medical record conserves your medical past for a healthier present'. This campaign was oriented towards the 7 out of 10 million Belgian inhabitants without a GMR. GPs' organisations stress the important surplus value of the GMR. The GMR will facilitate the organisation of activities targeted to specific groups of patients, a correct transfer of information in case of referral, change of GP, or collaboration with other disciplines. Furthermore, it also enables data collections and improves the knowledge of the GPs' population.

Awaiting a better coverage of the GMR in the Belgian population, the yearly contact group denominator (number of patients seen at least once a year in a practice), corrected for the non-attenders, can be considered the best estimate of the practice population in countries where patient lists are not available.[5] The recent development of the Intermutualistic Agency (IMA) offers an opportunity to get information on this kind of denominator. This agency centralises reimbursement data from all medical acts, which were previously scattered over the various mutualities the patients are affiliated to. This agency can calculate a yearly contact group denominator per GP. By applying a correction factor (by age group, sex and district) for the non-attenders, provided by the same agency, a population denominator by age and sex becomes available. This possibility of providing denominator data, based on administrative information (reimbursement data), has to be further explored and validated and has to be compared with the yearly contact group denominator derived from the EPR (*see* 'A certification procedure for EPR software').

The problem of data capture during home visits

In Belgium, about 40% of the encounters are during home visits.[6] In the sentinel network involved in morbidity recording, most of the GPs take the paper registration forms with them on home visits, which should guarantee complete recording. It is known, however, that far fewer home visit data are recorded in the EPR than consultation data.[7] Light devices are being developed in order to bridge that gap (e.g. personal digital assistant or PDA, tablet PC) but these are still unsatisfactory in their use. Recently, the impact of removing home visits from the database was researched, and this will be further explored in the ResoPrim project outlined below.[8]

A wide variety of EPR-based software (over 20 packages): a certification procedure for EPR software for GPs

In 2002, the federal public health authorities launched a certification procedure for EPR software in general practice, followed by a second round in 2003. The software packages have to meet a list of quality criteria.[9,10] Nineteen EPR software packages are presently certified. GPs working with certified software receive an annual incentive. This certification procedure is meant to reduce the number of EPR software packages on the market and to improve their quality. This development can also play a favourable role in EPR-based data collections. Contrary to paper patient records, the EPR can also facilitate the calculation of the yearly contact group denominator. The 19 certified software packages presently cover about 90% of the EPR software on the Belgian market.

A moderate coverage of EPR use in general practice: 60–65%

In 2003, 6100 out of 12 000 GPs contacted the federal public health authorities to ask for the incentive for using a certified EPR-software, which is only 50% of all Belgian GPs! Presumably not all GPs using certified EPR software filled in the forms to receive the incentive. As mentioned above, the certified EPR software covers about 90% of the EPR software on the market, therefore, the global coverage of EPR software use by GPs in Belgium can be estimated at about 60–65% and is still far below the figure in the Netherlands. It can be expected that the certification procedure for EPR software together with its incentive for the GP will increase the coverage of EPR use in the years to come.

In the following we will show how problems are handled to sample reliable data on health and healthcare in the Belgian context. Only nationwide and large regional networks of data collection that have resulted in scientific publications are described.

Registration networks in Belgium

The sentinel network of GPs

This network, existing since 1979, is co-ordinated by the Scientific Institute of Public Health (IPH) and financed through the Flemish- and French-speaking Community in Belgium. Its main characteristics, problems and solutions are outlined in Box 31.1. Every annual registration programme counts about eight different health problems (infectious as well as non-infectious themes).[11–14] The network has contributed to many European initiatives together with several other sentinel networks in Europe.

The Intego network

This network has existed since 1994, is co-ordinated by the Department of General Practice at the Catholic University of Leuven and is financed through the Flemish-speaking Community of Belgium. Its main characteristics, problems and solutions are outlined in Box 31.2.[16] This network recently established collaborations with some regional morbidity-recording networks in the Netherlands.

Other EPR-based recording experiences in general practice, co-ordinated by the IPH

Between 1999 and 2002, the IPH co-ordinated three *ad hoc* studies with EPR-based and paper-based data collections.[8,17–20] All three are situated in the domain of quality of care (for hypertension, diabetes and osteoarthritis). The studies were done in close collaboration with the scientific associations of GPs (WVVH and SSMG) and with an academic research centre. The main characteristics, problems and solutions are outlined in Box 31.3. For the electronic part in each study, data collection was semi-automatic and semi-anonymous. At patient level, a unique code was generated by the GP's software. Only the GP was able to link this code to a patient when additional information was required. At the level of the GP, the GP's scientific associations ensured the anonymity. The latter provided each GP with a unique identification number. Semi-automatic data collection means that, after an automatic data extraction from the EPR, the GP could complete/correct the data before sending them.[21]

Box 31.1 The sentinel network of GPs

Coverage?
- Nationwide network

Number of practices?
- 150 practices with 180 GPs

Purpose?
- To study for a selection of health problems:
  - incidence
  - main epidemiological characteristics
  - management of health problem

What kind of data?
- Age
- Sex
- Other information according to the theme

Method of data collection?
- Paper-based recording

Main problems encountered?
- Estimation of denominator population
- Unknown characteristics (e.g. age and sex) of denominator population

Solutions?
- Denominator is estimated on the basis of yearly number of encounters in participating practices divided by mean annual number of encounters in general practice per inhabitant (denominator population is estimated at 150 000 inhabitants, 1.5% of the national population)[15]
- Age and sex distribution of this denominator population is assumed to be similar to the Belgian population as the participating GPs are representative of the Belgian GPs according to age and sex, and as they are homogeneously spread over the country

---

Comparing the results from the paper-based with the EPR-based recording showed that in the latter much more data were lacking and the drop-out rate of GPs was considerably higher. The findings in these three studies led to a new project 'ResoPrim' which will study thoroughly the necessary conditions for EPR-based data collections in Belgium in the fields of epidemiology, quality of care assessment and socio-economy.

The ResoPrim project: an experimental network in primary care

Recently, a research project was started, ResoPrim, an experimental electronic network with GPs. This project can contribute to the progress in EPR-based data collections in general practice. It is financed by the federal science policy authorities, in the framework of the multi-annual programme for the development of the information society.

The project aims at developing an electronic reference network providing a stable test framework for the collection, analysis, feedback and dissemination of data from general practice. Data will be collected on an individual basis, start-

Box 31.2 The Intego network

Coverage?
• Flanders, northern part of Belgium
Number of practices?
• 47 practices with 55 GPs
Purpose?
• To study:
  – incidence
  – prevalence
  – diagnostic and therapeutic approaches in general practice
What kind of data?
• Year of birth
• Sex
• All diagnoses
• All prescriptions
• All laboratory results
• Weight and height
• Bood pressure
Method of data collection?
• EPR-based
Main problems encountered?
• Only one software involved, hampering representativeness
• Estimation of denominator population
Solutions?
• Other EPR-software to be approached in the future
• The denominator population calculation is based on the yearly contact group (number of patients seen at least once a year) by age and sex, extracted from the EPR of participating GPs (about 60 000 patients)
• This yearly contact group is corrected for non-attenders based on information from the IMA (*see* above); the total denominator population is estimated at about 80 000 inhabitants

ing from the electronic patient records; the data will be anonymised (or pseudonymised) and validated. Every patient will have a unique patient code which remains the same in the course of the project. Through feedback and benchmarking, GPs will benefit from these data. The various scientific research institutes will be able to exploit the data, under the practitioners' control. It will afterwards be possible to disseminate some of these data, after aggregation. These aggregated data will be available to health actors, decision makers, research centres, etc. The project is divided into two phases.

The first phase (2003–2005) will define the framework required for developing a network for useful and realistic purposes: how to organise it, possibilities and limitations of exploitation of the collected data. A specific data collection with a small network of 30 GPs will be organised for answering specific research questions, e.g. 'What is the potential impact of data capture at home on the content of the database?'; 'Does the personal digital assistant (PDA) improve the number of

Box 31.3 *Ad hoc* data collections in general practice, co-ordinated by IPH

Coverage?
- Nationwide networks

Purpose?
- To study:
  - quality of care for osteoarthritis before national campaign on appropriate drug use
  - quality of care for hypertensive and diabetes patients
  - quality of care for osteoarthritis after national campaign on appropriate drug use

Method of data collection?
- For the three studies, GPs could chose between paper form or EPR-based recording (with extraction software)

Number of practices?
1 385 (paper: 233; EPR (5 EPR-software):152)
2 308 (paper: 193; EPR (8 EPR-software): 115)
3 213 (paper: 140; EPR (5 EPR-software): 73)

What kind of data?
- Mainly information on the management (prescriptions, referrals, follow-up) of the studied health problems

Characteristics of EPR-based recording?
- Semi-automatic
- Semi-anonymous
- Asymmetric encryption (PGP technique)
- Weekly data transfer by email or secure medical messaging applications
- Trusted service provider (scientific associations of GPs)
- Common XML-exchange format
- ICPC coding for diagnoses
- ATC coding for drugs

Main problems encountered in EPR-based data collections?
- Considerable dropout of GPs (up to 40%), mainly because of:
  - problems with extraction module (installation and use)
  - problems with encryption procedure
  - problems with sending of files
- Considerable % of missing data (up to 90%) mainly because:
  - data not present in EPR
  - data not captured by module (not coded, not at the right place in EPR, not in the right format)

Solutions?
- Due to *ad hoc* financing, there was no time to thoroughly study the problems and to find solutions, but the findings led to a new project 'ResoPrim' which will study thoroughly the necessary conditions for EPR-based data collections in Belgium

---

Box 31.4 ResoPrim project, first phase

Coverage?
- Experimental nationwide network

Purpose?
- To study:
  - the conditions for EPR-based data collections in field of epidemiology, quality of care and socio-economy
  - the organisation of the network
  - the validity of collected data
  - the added value for participating GPs

Method of data collection?
- EPR-based recording (3 EPR-software)
- Qualitative research for questions on training needs, benefits and drawbacks expected and experienced by GPs

Number of practices?
- 30 (because of budgetary restraints)

What kind of data?
- different data sets will be collected, some retrospectively and automatically:
  - basic patient information
  - diagnosis, referrals, prescriptions
- Other ones, prospectively automatically and semi-automatically:
  - basic patient information
  - diagnosis, referrals, prescriptions
  - cardiovascular risk factors for hypertensive patients

Characteristics of EPR-based recording?
- Semi-automatic and automatic
- Semi-anonymous
- Weekly data transfer by secure medical messaging applications
- Trusted service provider (scientific associations of GPs)
- Common XML-exchange format
- ICPC and ICD coding for diagnoses
- CNK (national code for drugs) coding for drugs
- PDA (personal digital assistant) use for data capturing during home visits

Problems and solutions?
- The purpose is to make an inventory of problems at various levels and to formulate solutions for the future

home encounters registered?'; 'Is it possible to produce a yearly contact group per practice, by age group, sex and eventually by socio-economic status?'; 'Is it possible to relate diagnosis and drug prescriptions/referrals?'; 'What are the educational needs of GPs participating in the project?' (*see* Box 31.4).

In the second phase (2005–2007), a pilot network (about 100 GPs) will be set up, and the test framework will be validated through specific research activities; the results will be disseminated and recommendations will be issued for sustaining the development of other networks. At the end of the second phase, the identification of new objectives will ensure the survival of the ResoPrim pilot network in the long run.

In order to carry out this project, a partnership has been set up between the Scientific Institute of Public Health (IPH), the scientific GPs' associations in Flanders and Wallonia, respectively SSMG and WVVH and the Université Catholique de Louvain (UCL).

What to think about it

Data collection and especially morbidity recording in general practice has already a long history in Belgium. The two most important problems encountered especially in morbidity recording are the denominator and capturing data during home visits. There are new prospects however, for the denominator problem, through the use of administrative data coming from the IMA. Moreover, the EPR also can, if appropriately used, provide a better denominator estimation. However, if Belgium, like other countries, wants to switch to comprehensive automated morbidity recording and associated interventions in general practice by a considerable number of GPs, much greater effort and financial perspectives are needed. All the requirements for valid automated data collection made by Verheij in the previous chapter are also relevant for Belgium e.g. payment of GPs, training, feedback, coding systems, episode-oriented recording, solutions for software-associated obstacles. In our efforts to tackle these problems, we are running behind. At this moment, researchers, GPs' associations and GPs in the field expect a lot from the ResoPrim project and hope that this project will boost EPR-based data collections in Belgium.

References

1 Pringle M, Ward P and Chilvers C (1995) Assessment of the completeness and accuracy of computer medical records in four practices committed to recording data on computer. *Br J Gen Pract*. **45**: 537–41.
2 Demarest S (2001) Health Interview Survey. *Arch Public Health*. **5–6**: 219–21.
3 van der Heyden J, Demarest S, Tafforeau J and van Oyen H (2003) Socio-economic differences in the utilisation of the health services in Belgium. *Health Policy*. **65**: 153–65.
4 Koninklijk Besluit: Tot wijziging van artikel 37bis van de wet betreffende de verplichte verzekering voor geneeskundige verzorging en uitkeringen, gecoördineerd op 14 juli 1994. *Belgisch Staatsblad*. (24 May 2002). [Royal Decree: on amendment to Article 47bis of the law on compulsory insurance regarding medical care and benefits, coordinated at 14 July 1994.]

5 Schlaud M, Brenner MH, Hoopmann M and Schwartz FW (1998) Approaches to the denominator in practice-based epidemiology: a critical overview. *J Epidemiol Community Health*. **52** (Suppl 1): 13–19.

6 de Maeseneer J, de Prins L and Heyerick JP (1999) Home visits in Belgium: a multivariate analysis. *Eur J Gen Pract*. **5**: 11–14.

7 Hamilton WT, Round AP, Sharp D and Peters TJ (2003) The quality of record keeping in primary care: a comparison of computerized, paper and hybrid systems. *Br J Gen Pract*. **53**: 929–33.

8 Vandenberghe H, van Casteren V, Jonckheer P, Lafontaine MF and de Clercq E (2004) Quality of care assessment using GPs electronic patient records: do we need data from home visits? In: Roger-France FH, de Clercq E, de Moor G and van der Lei J (eds) *Health Continuum and Data Exchange in Belgium and in the Netherlands*. IOS Press, Amsterdam, pp. 35–42.

9 Be-Health Telematics [homepage on the Internet]. *Brussel: Federale Overheidsdienst Volksgezondheid. Cel Informatica, Telematica en Communicatie binnen de sector van de Gezondheidszorg* [cited 2004 Dec 16]. Available from www.health.fgov.be/telematics/ (accessed 21 September 2005).

10 Koninklijk Besluit: tot bepaling van de voorwaarden en de modaliteiten overeenkomstig dewelke de verplichte verzekering voor geneeskundige verzorging en uitkeringen een financiële tegemoetkoming verleent aan artsen voor het gebruik van telematica en het electronisch beheer van medische dossiers. [Royal Decree: establishing the conditions and terms of granting financial allowance by the compulsory insurance of medical care and benefits to GPs for using telematica and electronic management of medical files.] *Belgisch Staatsblad* (21 February 2003).

11 van Casteren V and Leurquin P (1992) Eurosentinel: development of an international sentinel network of general practitioners. *Meth Inform Med*. **31**: 147–52.

12 Devroey D, van Casteren V, Sasse A and Wallyn S (2003) Non-consented HIV testing by Belgian general practitioners. *AIDS*. **17**: 641–2.

13 Devroey D, van Casteren V and Buntinx F (2003) Registration of stroke through the Belgian sentinel network and factors influencing stroke mortality. *Cerebrovasc Dis*. **16**: 272–9.

14 Scientific Institute of Public Health [homepage on the Internet]. Brussels [updated 2004 Sep 20, cited 2004 Dec 16]. *Sentinel GPs*. Available from: www.iph.fgov.be/epidemio/epien/index10.htm (accessed 21 September 2005).

15 Lobet MP, Stroobant A, Mertens R, van Casteren V *et al*. (1987) Tool of validation of the network of sentinel general practitioners in the Belgian health care system. *Int J Epidemiol*. **16**: 612–18.

16 Bartholomeeusen S, Buntinx F and Heyrman J (2002) Ziekten in de huisartspraktijk: methode en eerste resultaten van het Intego-netwerk. [Diseases in GP practice: method and first results of the Intego-network.] *Tijdschr Geneesk*. **58**: 863–71.

17 Vandenberghe H, Bastiaens H, Orban T *et al*. (2004) *De Aanpak door Huisartsen van Degeneratief Gewrichtslijden bij Patiënten van 60 jaar en Ouder – Tweede Fase*. [GP intervention in degenerative joint pain in patients of 60 years and older – second phase.] Brussel: Wetenschappelijk Instituut Volksgezondheid, Afdeling Epidemiologie, Brussels. Rapport Nr: D/2004/2505/5. Contract: NSAID Kwaliteit. Gefinancierd door het RIZIV.

18 Vandenberghe H, Bastiaens H, Jonckheer P *et al*. (2003) *Kwaliteitsbevordering in de Huisartsgeneeskunde op Basis van Registratie van Praktijkgegevens: diabetes type 2 en hypertensie*. [Quality improvement in GP medicine based on registration of practice data: diabetes type 2 and hypertension.] Eindrapport. Wetenschappelijk Instituut Volksgezondheid, Afdeling Epidemiologie, Brussels. Rapport Nr: D/2003/2505/18. Contract Nr: N01 – 158Y, N01 – 158Z Gefinancierd door de Federale Overheidsdienst Volksgezondheid, Veiligheid van de Voedselketen en Leefmilieu.

19 Vandenberghe H, Jonckheer P, Bastiaens H *et al.* (2001) *De Aanpak door Huisartsen van Degeneratief Gewrichtslijden bij Patiënten van 60 jaar en Ouder – Eerste Fase.* [GP intervention in degenerative joint pain in patients of 60 years and older – first phase.] Brussel: Wetenschappelijk Instituut Volksgezondheid, Afdeling Epidemiologie, Brussels. Rapport Nr: D/2002/2505/07. Contract Nr: 605/QG/N00–85C. Gefinancierd door het RIZIV.

20 Vandenberghe H, Van Casteren V, Jonckheer P *et al.* (2005) Collecting information on the quality of prescribing in primary care using semi-automatic data extraction from GPs' electronic medical records. *Int J Med Inform.* **74**: 367–76.

21 de Clercq E, Vandenberghe H, Jonckheer P *et al.* (2002) Assessment of a three-year experience with a Belgian primary care data network. In: Roger France F, Hasman A, de Clercq E and de Moor G (eds) *E-health in Belgium and the Netherlands.* IOS Press, Amsterdam, pp. 163–9.

Index